A Colour Atlas of
TRAUMA PATHOLOGY

Hubert Fischer
Professor, Department of Pathology
University of Ulm, Germany

C.J. Kirkpatrick
Professor, Institute of Pathology
The Technical University
Aachen, Germany

with additional material from
Dr M.E. Aronson
Consultant Forensic Pathologist
Philadelphia, Pennsylvania, USA

Wolfe Publishing Ltd

Copyright © Hubert Fischer, C.J. Kirkpatrick, 1991
Published by Wolfe Publishing Ltd, 1991
Printed by BPCC Hazell Books Ltd, Aylesbury, England
ISBN 0 7234 1566 8

A CIP catalogue record for this book is available from the British Library.

This book is one of the titles in the series of Wolfe Medical Atlases, a
series that brings together the world's largest systematic published
collection of diagnostic colour photographs.

For a full list of Atlases in the series, plus forthcoming titles and details
of our surgical, dental and veterinary Atlases, please write to Wolfe
Publishing Ltd, 2–16 Torrington Place, London WC1E 7LT, England.

Contents

Foreword

This compendium of some of the gross and microscopic features of trauma in humans represents a cross section of experiences encountered by the pathologist. But it is also useful to those who treat patients. With brief but thoughtful discussions the authors have carefully presented the material to assist both pathologists and therapists in understanding the significance and implications of the injury or trauma with which they are confronted.

With this book as a guide, pathologists may more accurately diagnose what *has* occurred to the patient who is now deceased, but more important, the treating physicians may be able to further forestall that moment when the patient becomes the exclusive responsibility of the pathologist. When that occurs, as it inevitably must, the pathologist will find here the clues which will permit more sophisticated advice to be passed on to police or other interested parties.

Medical students can also learn from these pages those general processes by which the human body responds to trauma and injury, as well as the characteristic appearances of some forms of trauma. A special section dealing with the changes that occur after death is especially useful for avoiding some of the pitfalls of over-interpretation. A section dealing with histologic dating of wounds will be of paramount importance in some aspects of litigation.

The book is not intended as a 'match the picture' type of catalogue, nor should any book be so used. A system of organisation of the pathology of trauma is presented, with illustrations, that can be used as a framework upon which can be hung the experiences of daily practice, resulting in a background which can be used to judge problem cases. The selection of illustrations reflects the wide and deep experience of the authors' practices, while the organisation reflects the clarity and perspicacity of their thinking.

The authors are to be congratulated on their efforts in the compilation of this atlas.

M.E. ARONSON

Preface

In this atlas we present in pictorial form an overview of the macroscopy and histology of common and important traumatic alterations in the human organism. Knowledge of morphology is an essential foundation of diagnostic and therapeutic activity. Thus, the atlas is of interest to clinical colleagues dealing with various aspects of traumatology. In addition, it is a reference aid to both the clinical and forensic pathologists at both junior and senior levels. The inclusion of basic aspects of tramatic pathology also makes it of use to the medical student.

We have tried as much as possible to present, in particular, histological changes in a form that is encountered in routine practice and not to put the primary emphasis on the aesthetic appearance of the pictures. Thus, there are some illustrations which do not possess optimal quality, but which are 'true to nature', in that the material was available in this state for diagnosis. The latter is a well known phenomenon to the forensic pathologist, who often has to examine material under unfavourable conditions, for example, from corpses that have been lying for considerable periods of time.

The text is intended as an adjunct to the pictorial presentation and not as a literature overview. Thus, only a sample of the very extensive international literature has been included.

Note that for the histological illustrations the magnifications given in the captions are those seen under the microscope.

Finally, we wish to acknowledge the very considerable help from our colleagues who have provided material. A special word of thanks is due in this respect to Dr. M.E. Aronson.

H. FISCHER, M.D., Ph.D.
C.J. KIRKPATRICK, M.D., Ph.D.

Acknowledgements

Apart from those listed below, all the illustrations in this book are from the authors' collections.

From the Institute of Forensic Medicine of the Ludwig-Maximilians University, Munich (director, Prof. Dr. med. W. Spann):
1, 2, 3, 6, 33, 34, 39, 40, 41, 64, 65, 72, 79, 90, 94, 95, 107, 108, 109, 113, 114, 121, 123, 124, 138, 160, 176, 193, 194, 197, 205, 206, 247, 248, 249, 269, 270, 271, 272, 273, 274, 281, 282, 283, 294, 400, 403, 405, 406, 410, 411, 413, 414, 422.

From the Institute of Forensic Medicine of the University of Ulm (director, Prof. Dr. med. G. Reinhardt; photographer, G. Reiter):
4, 5, 7, 13, 74, 78, 96, 97, 98, 99, 100, 101, 102, 104, 105, 115, 117, 118, 119, 120, 122, 137, 139, 175, 183, 184, 187, 188, 261, 262, 376, 377, 378, 382, 399, 401, 402, 412, 420, 421.

From Prof. Dr. med. Spier, formerly of the Accident Hospital, Murnau, Bavaria:
12, 13.

From Medical Director Dr. Med. K. Willner, Bavarian State Criminal Dept., Munich:
487.

1 Introduction—variation in traumatic change

Trauma has always been part of human existence and, particularly in industrialised countries, has increased in significance. In spite of safety legislation and attempts to raise public awareness of the problem, accident rates remain high. Although modern medicine is able to deal with many of the dangerous complications, trauma still represents a more or less serious risk to health, reducing work efficiency and costing money.

The various types of incident that may lead to trauma, in particular to severe trauma, are, in order of importance:

- Accidents in the home.
- Accidents at work.
- Road traffic accidents.
- Sports injuries.
- Homicide and suicide.

Within these groups one finds injuries caused by blunt objects, by sharp objects and, occasionally, by firearms. Thermal injuries and the effects of electricity are also commonly seen. Rarer forms of trauma may present differential diagnostic problems for the morphologist.

2 Sharp instrument injuries

Sharp instrument injuries are usually caused by a knife, glass fragments or sharp metal edges. The lesions are frequently superficial.

The incision shows a break in the continuity of skin and subcutaneous tissue with smooth, gaping wound edges. It is usually accompanied by profuse haemorrhage, particularly if arteries are involved. Moreover, superficial nerves and tendons are also vulnerable and may be severed.

Chop wounds are caused by heavy, sharp-edged instruments, such as an axe, cleaver or hatchet. These injuries tend to be gaping and may involve bone in the depth of the wound.

A stab wound is usually caused by a knife, dagger, awl or file. Although the severed tissues are for the most part well marked and the wound margins smooth, in certain cases they may be irregularly torn—for example, after stabbing with a nail. It is particularly important to note that the superficial wounds may appear insignificant and conceal severe internal injuries to vital organs, often with massive haemorrhage. This has very important practical consequences. Thus, the removal of knives (or other instruments used for stabbing) from the victim must be performed under operative conditions to avoid often fatal haemorrhage.

Impalement is a further form of stabbing. It may occur on the playground or in road traffic accidents. In such injuries, both the pleural and the peritoneal cavities may be involved.

The slit-wound is often a combination of incision and stabbing. Thus, the initial stab-wound is extended by a simultaneous or subsequent cutting action and results in superficial and deep wounds which are much larger than the dimension of the instrument used.

Areas of haemorrhage tend to be confined to the proximity of the wounding instrument. In the case of a knife wound, this would be the incision channel. The plane of separation of the tissue is smooth, and tissue damage outside the incision is minimal. Differentiation between antemortem and supravital changes is difficult, and often impossible. The exudation of fibrin and leucocytes is evidence of an ante-mortem injury, but these characteristics do not show until 6 to 8 hours after the trauma.

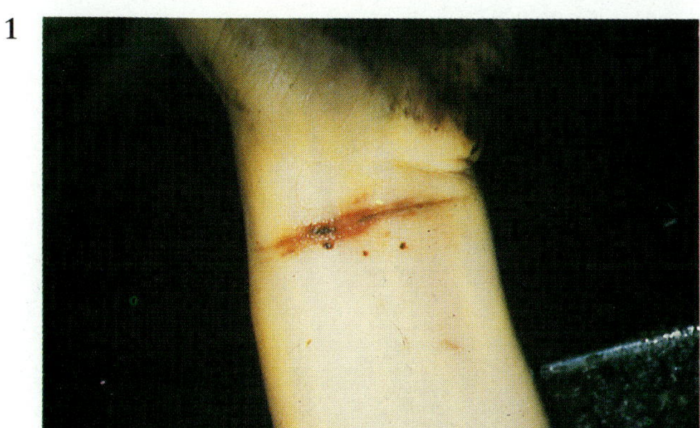

1 Knife wound to the volar surface of the distal forearm proximal to the wrist. A case of suicide. Usually, with this type of wound, only the tendons are severed. A very deep incision is required to puncture the blood vessels. Thus, incisions which haemorrhage rapidly through a cut in the medial artery are longitudinal to the tendons.

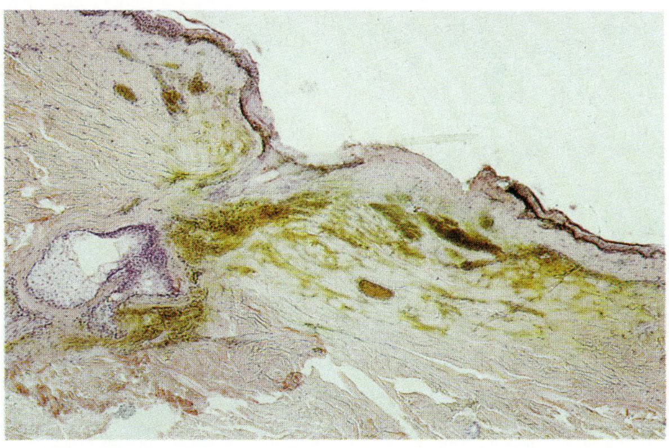

2 Skin: knife wound, showing a superficial epidermal defect and haemorrhage in the dermis and around a sebaceous gland. The right-angled edge at one margin (right) of the wound could correspond to the back of the knife. Almost immediate death after stabbing. Some post-mortem desiccation has occurred. (*H&E ×16*)

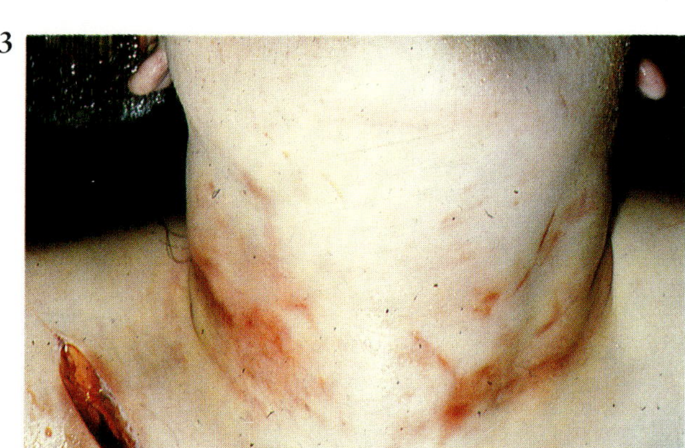

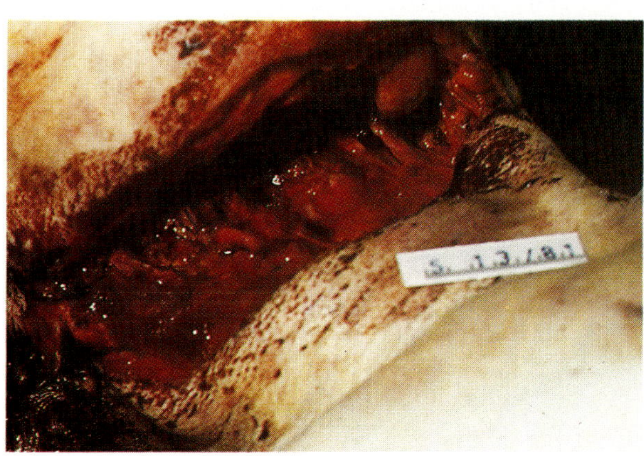

3 Stab wound of the shoulder, without severe haemorrhage. The pre-mortem trauma is seen on the victim's right. The upper end of the incision is characteristic of those caused by the sharpened side of a blade. Additionally, there are strangulation marks on the neck and a small portion of autopsy incision can be seen on the victim's left.

4 Deep incision of the neck.

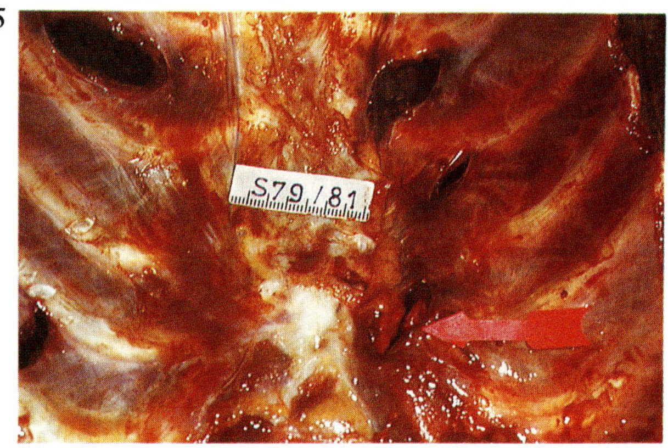

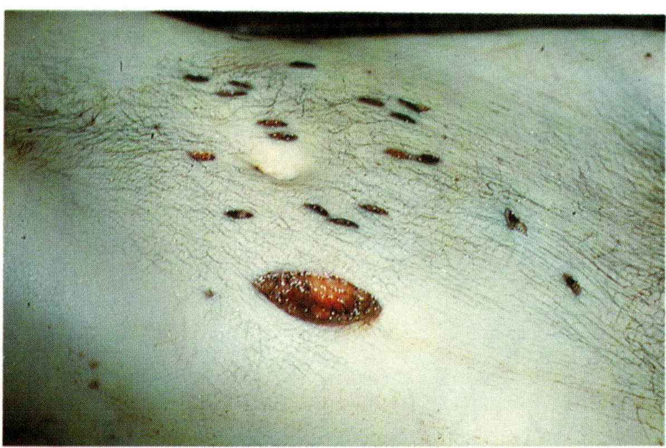

5 Five stab wounds to the anterior thorax. Most are intercostally situated; one stab wound (red arrow) transected the costal cartilage in the parasternal region. The punctures lie deeper (body of the sternum with transition to the xiphoid process), between the third and fourth ribs on both sides, between the fourth and fifth ribs, and between the fifth and sixth ribs, with severance of the cartilage of the fifth rib.

6 Multiple stab wounds, made with a narrow-bladed implement. The lowest wound is deep and extended on the skin surface, due to the relative motion of body and implement. Note that the end closest to the naval is pointed, while the other end is blunt, which indicates that the implement was most likely a knife with only one edge sharpened.

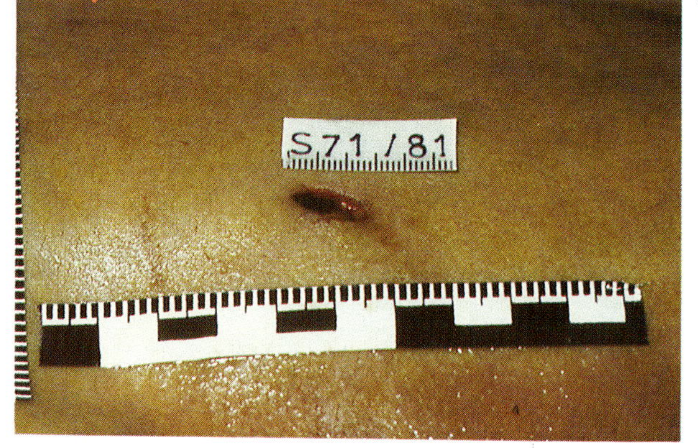

7 File stab wound. A thrust of some force can cause even a blunt instrument (in this case a file) to penetrate the body, even if clothed.

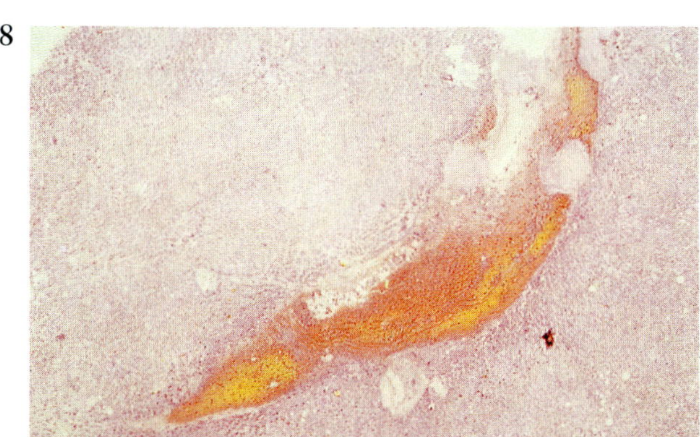

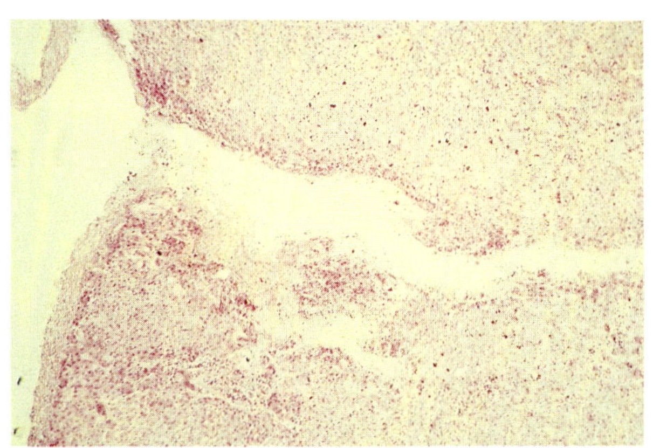

8 and 9   Liver: stab wound with a knife, showing fibrin and blood in the wound channel. Post-traumatic survival time: 4 hours. Note the sharp edge of the wound channel in **8** and compare with the irregular rupture site resulting from blunt injury of the liver shown in **9**. (*H&E ×20*)

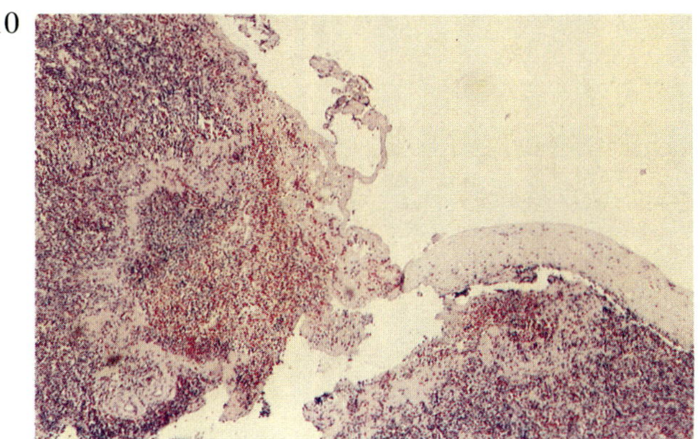

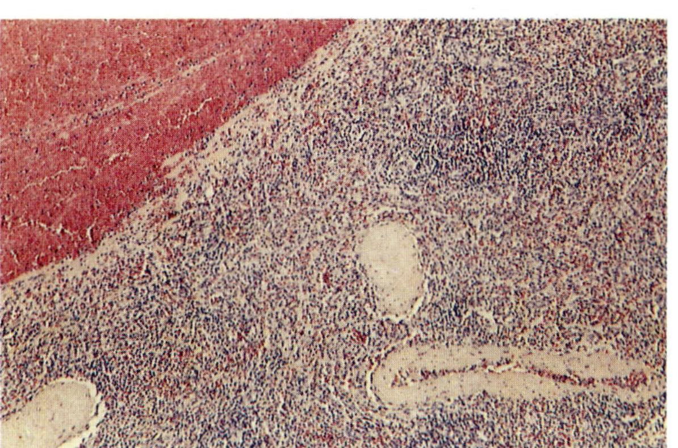

10   Spleen: knife wound in a 26-year-old male (spleen removed operatively). Splitting of the splenic capsule. At the entrance of the wound channel are fibrin and erythrocytes as well as disrupted areas of parenchyma. Irregular edges of the wound channel. (*H&E ×10*)

11   Spleen: knife wound. Same case as in **10**. Deeper portion of the wound channel with smooth edges and filling with blood. (*H&E ×25*)

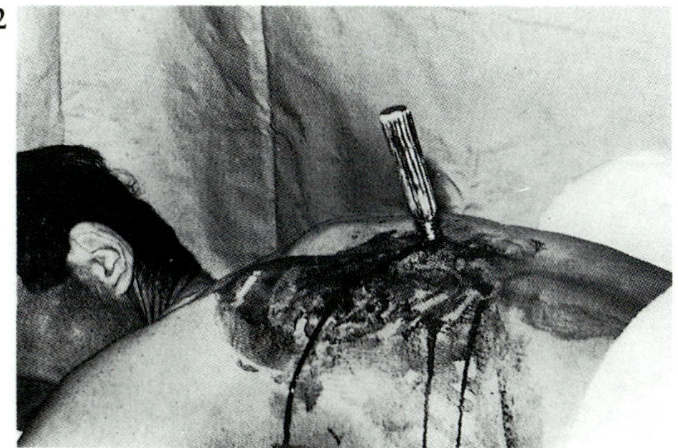

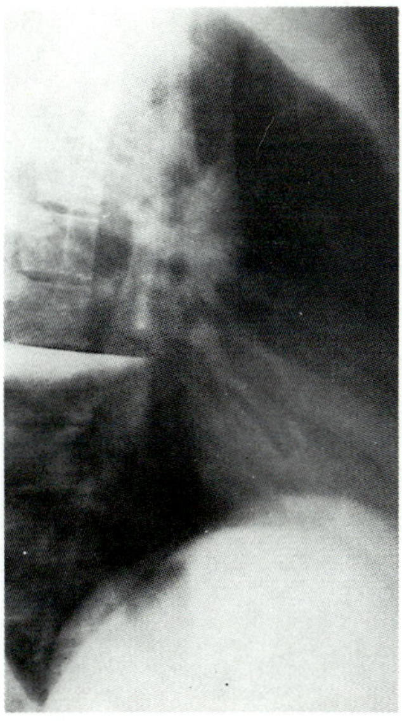

12   A knife wound to the back (paravertebral region). The victim survived.

13   Same case as in **12**. A lateral X-ray of the victim in **12**, showing the traumatised region. The blade of the knife is directly against the aorta and was carefully removed during thoracotomy. The patient survived without neurological complications.

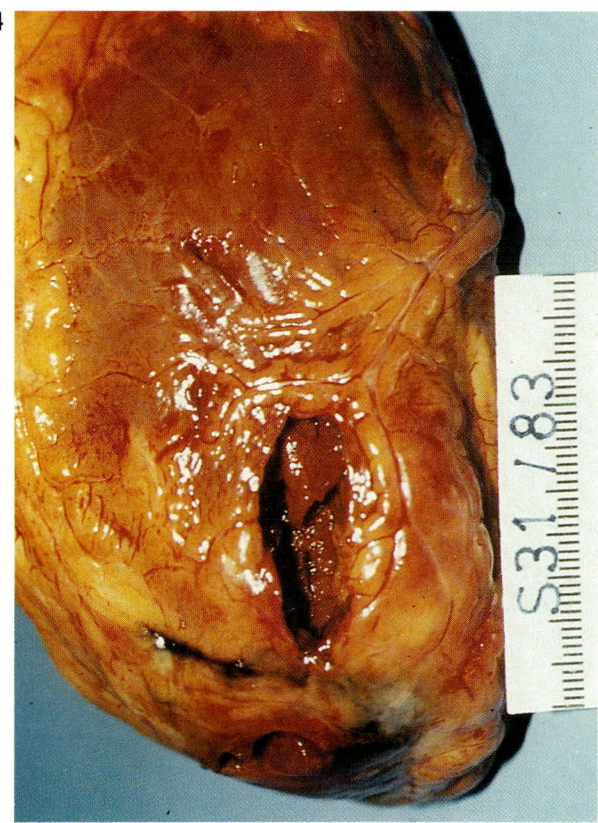

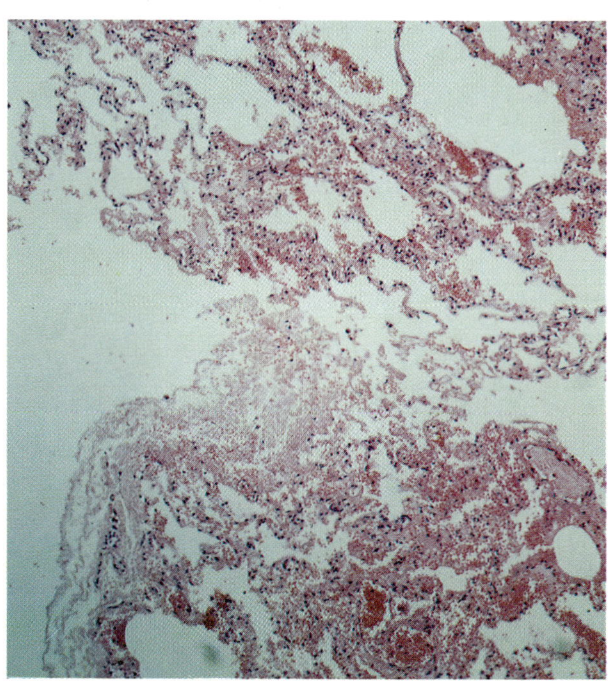

15   Stab wound to the lung, with separation of the pleura and the lung parenchyma. Fibrin and blood are also visible. Almost immediate death. (*H&E ×20*)

14   Stab wound to the heart. Massive and speedy loss of blood following a major haemothorax. The apex of the heart has been punctured.

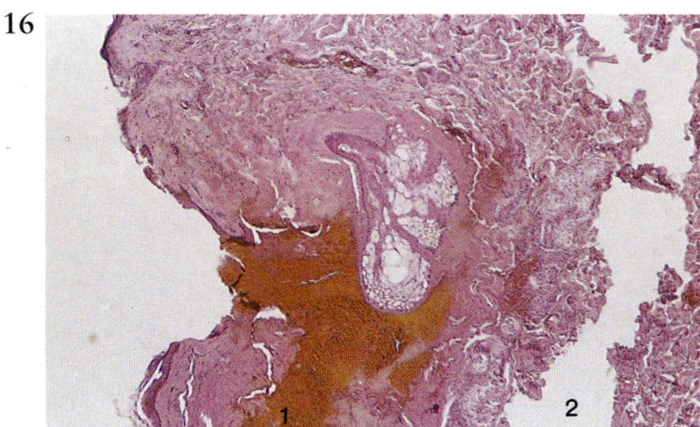

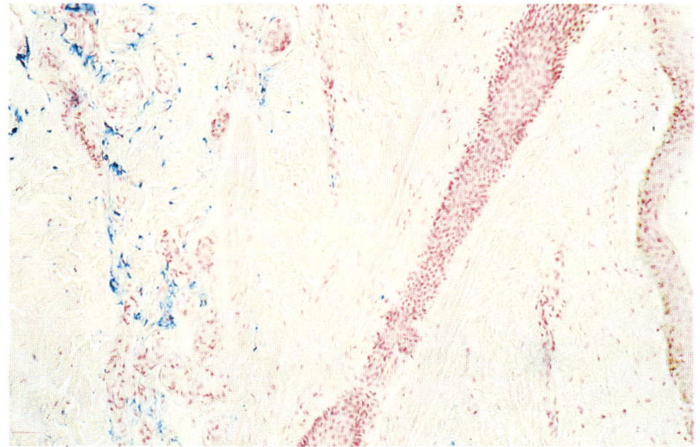

16   Skin from the anterior thorax after catheterisation of a subclavian vein in a patient who died almost immediately after knife wounds to the thoracic aorta. Note the dermal haemorrhage around the puncture wound (1). There is an artefactual tear of the subcutaneous tissue (2). (*H&E ×20*)

17   Subcutaneous tissue. Considerable fibrosis at long-term injection sites in a drug addict, showing the results of repeated haemorrhage into the subcutaneous tissue. (*Prussian blue ×40*)

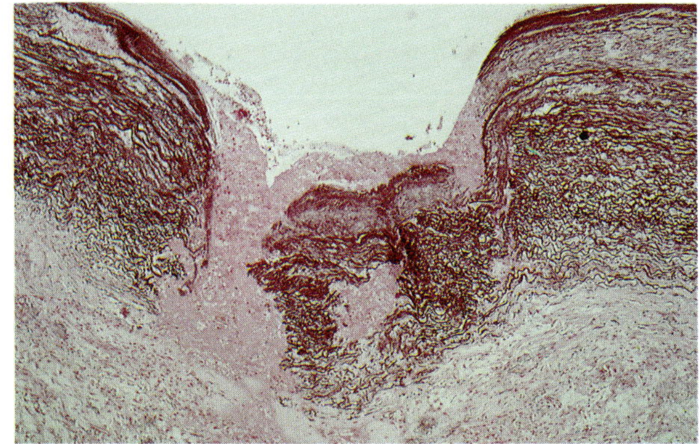

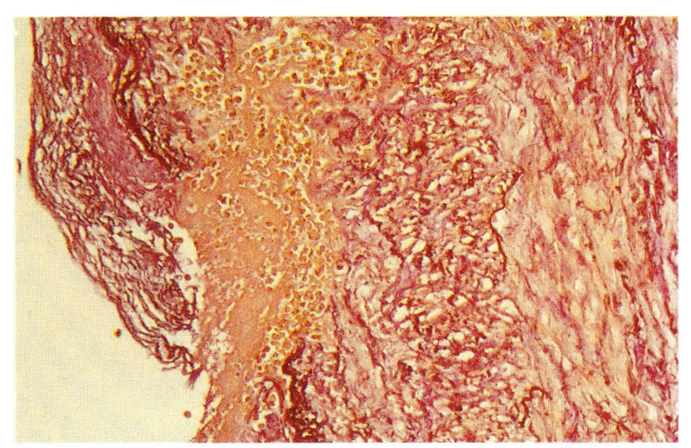

18 **External carotid artery** showing a puncture site caused by cannulation for carotid angiography 24 hours before death. Note the separation of all components of the arterial wall with disruption of the elastic fibres. Fibrin and blood can be seen in the incision channel. Subsequent death was not related to this diagnostic procedure. (*Elastic stain: resorcin–fuchsin ×20*)

19 **External carotid artery.** Site of puncture for carotid angiography. Separation of the intima and the internal elastic lamina. Tearing of the media adjacent to the intima and filling of the tissue defect with fibrin and erythrocytes. The perforation was caused by incorrect insertion. (*Resorcin–fuchsin and van Gieson ×25*)

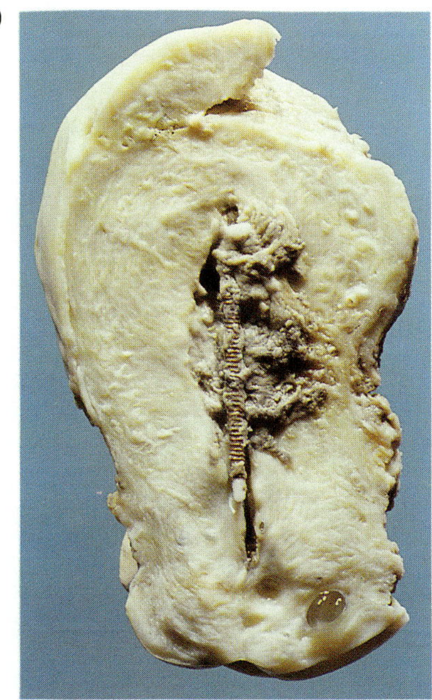

20 **Perforation of the uterus** caused by insertion of an intra-uterine device. (*Formalin-fixed tissue*)

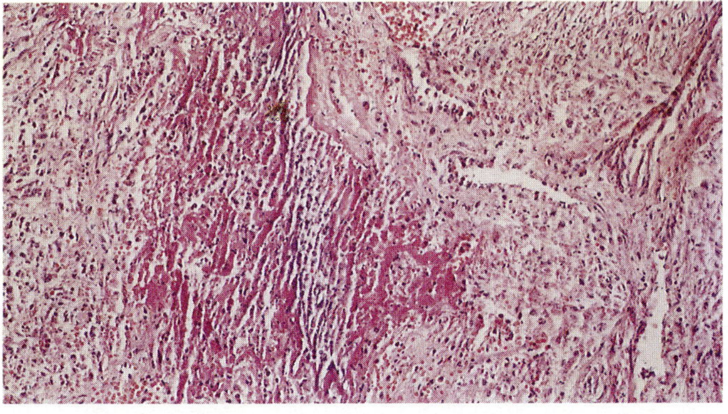

21 **Perforation of the uterus** by insertion of an intra-uterine device in a 28 year-old woman (with subsequent hysterectomy one day later). Central necrosis in the myometrium with a cellular reaction. Single glands can be seen at the right of the picture. Haemorrhage and tissue destruction are clearly visible. (*H&E ×25*)

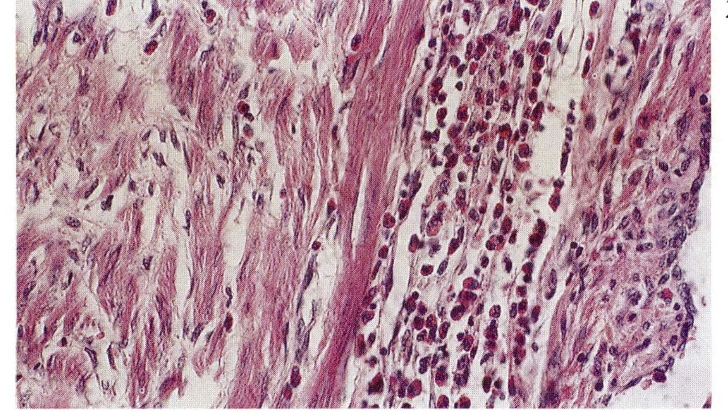

22 **Uterus**: same case as in **21**. Numerous segmented granulocytes (right) are visible in the channel formed by the perforation in the myometrium. (*H&E ×63*)

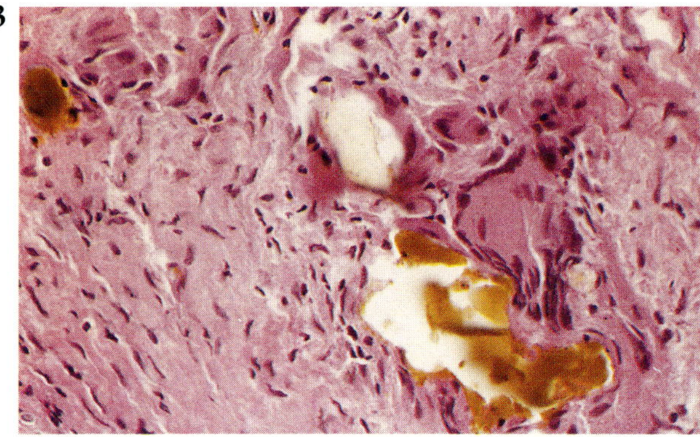

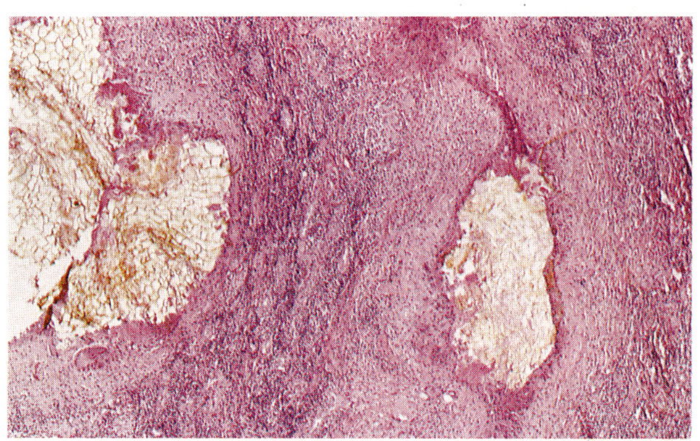

23 Subcutaneous tissue. Penetration of the skin by wood splinters (yellow–brown), showing a typical foreign body reaction with fibrous tissue formation and the presence of multinucleated giant cells around the wood particles. The lesion was recorded many months after injury. (*H&E ×100*)

24 Subcutaneous tissue. Low-power view showing wood particles with a surrounding chronic inflammatory cell infiltration. (*H&E ×16*)

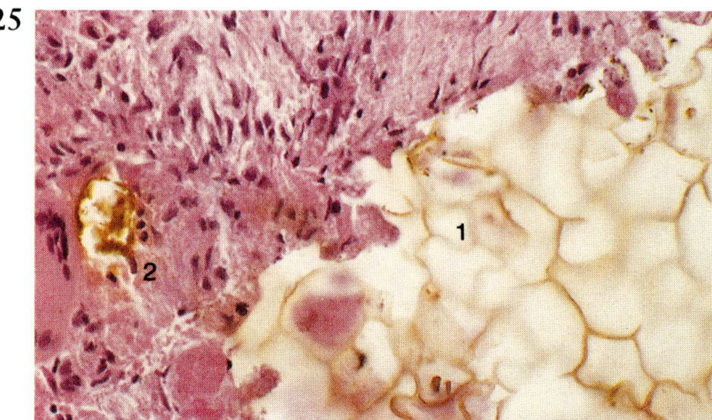

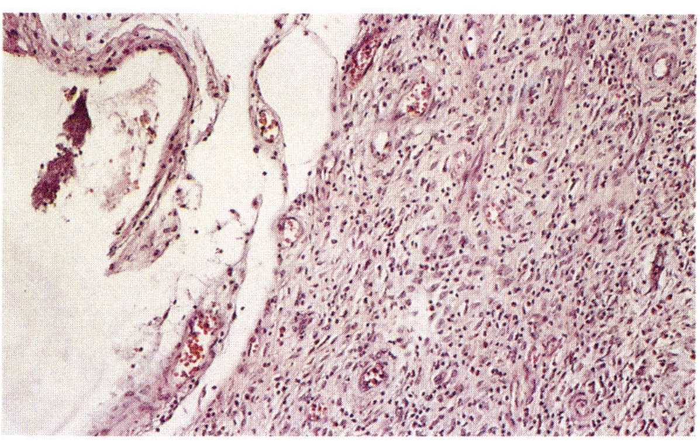

25 Subcutaneous tissue. Higher-power view of **24**, showing the cell wall structure of the wood splinter (1), as well as a foreign body giant cell (2). Only the wood in the plane of the section of the human tissue is in focus. (*H&E ×100*)

26 Tissue from the olecranon bursa: wood splinter trauma. Note the cavity where the wood fragments lay (left) and the marked formation of a very cellular granulation tissue (right). Wood splinters can also be seen. (*H&E ×16*)

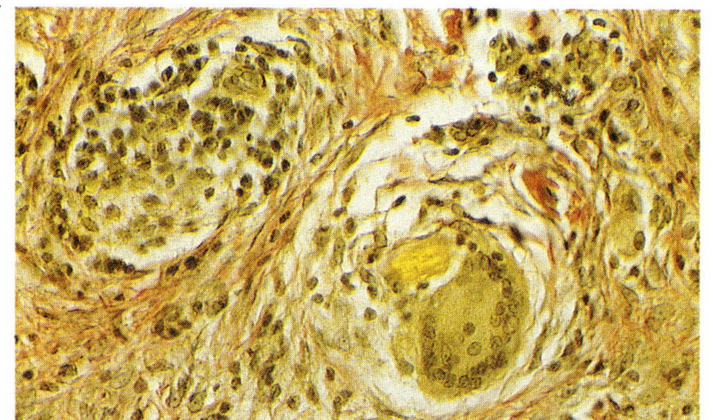

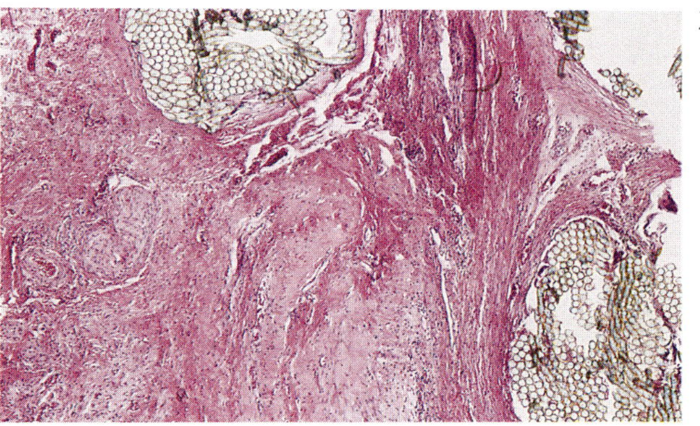

27 Subcutaneous tissue. Foreign body reaction with formation of collagenous connective tissue (red). Note the presence of a multinucleated giant cell adjacent to the foreign material (yellow). (*van Gieson ×100*)

28 Subcutaneous tissue. Surgical suture material (green threads) with a marked granulomatous reaction in the surrounding tissue and formation of considerable quantities of connective tissue. (*H&E ×25*)

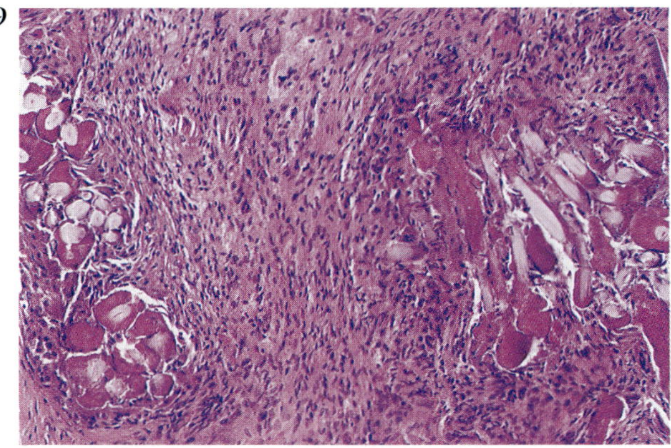

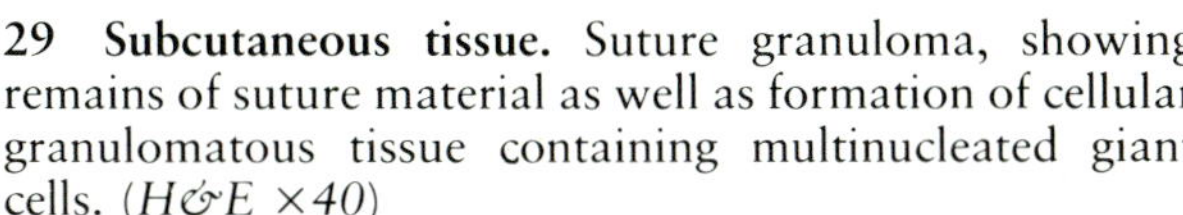

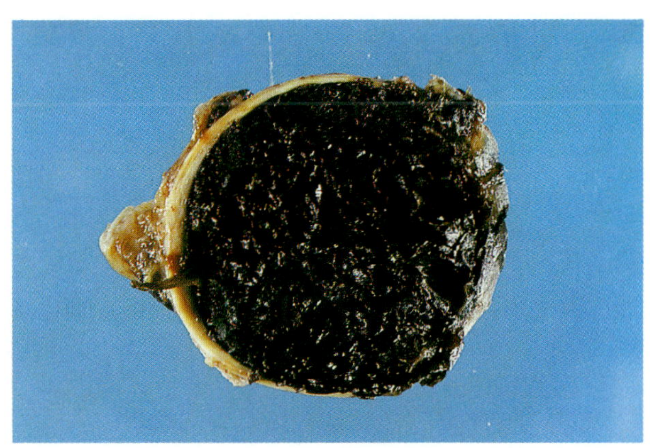

29 Subcutaneous tissue. Suture granuloma, showing remains of suture material as well as formation of cellular granulomatous tissue containing multinucleated giant cells. (*H&E ×40*)

30 Penetrating splinter injury to the eye with massive haemorrhage in the vitreous body. Longitudinal section. (*Formalin-fixed tissue*).

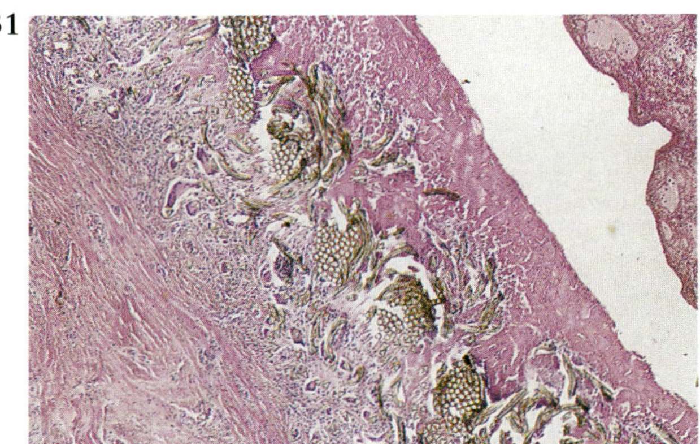

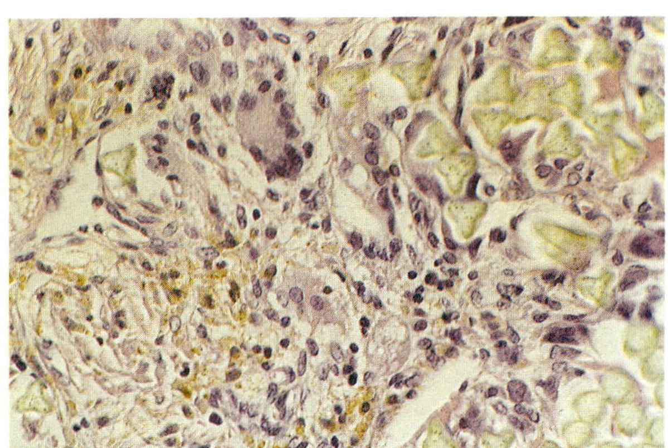

31 Dacron prosthesis of the popliteal artery. Material from a 66 year-old male, demonstrating a foreign body giant-cell reaction to the prosthesis (green threads). Note the formation of a neointima and a thrombus in the vessel lumen (right). (*H&E ×63*)

32 Dacron prosthesis of an iliac artery showing fibres of the prosthesis (light green, right) and foreign body giant cells, as well as considerable amounts of haemosiderin pigment (yellow, lower left) formed as a result of intra-operative haemorrhage. (*H&E ×100*)

3 Gunshot wounds

The extent of tissue destruction in gunshot wounds is determined by the size of the bullet, its speed and angle of entry. Its shape is also significant. Necrotic changes can be observed around the bullet channel with the formation of numerous clefts and tears in the surrounding tissue. These necrotic changes are visible quite shortly after the trauma and are revealed by a reduced or absent nuclear staining reaction.

The boundaries of the bullet channel are not clearly defined, but in the channel or ar its edges, there are always areas of haemorrhage. The bullet channel may also contain tissue fragments. The extent of these changes depends on the kinetic energy of the bullet (low or high velocity).

It is common to find tissue fragments, powder, metal particles and dirt around the entrance wound. According to Menzies *et al.* (1981) entrance wounds caused even by silenced firearms show the usual characteristics of progressive epithelial thermal and mechanical changes as the defect is approached, thermal changes in the dermal collagen, and varying amounts of powder residue in the wound tract and on the surface of the epithelium.

Particles of clothing or bone splinters can occasionally be found in the bullet channel. The connective tissue at the periphery of the bullet channel often shows a basophilia.

High velocity missiles cause characteristic changes. On entering the tissue a temporary pulsating cavity develops, in the walls of which areas of necrosis arise. The resulting bullet channel contains blood and tissue fragments.

Two zones can be distinguished in the periphery of the bullet channel:

- A 'contusion zone' containing amorphous necrotic tissue (for example, muscle cells) along with a cellular infiltration consisting of neutrophilic granulocytes. In the capillaries and venules, hyperaemia, neutrophil margination and thrombosis may be seen.
- A 'concussion zone', in which the degeneration of cells is much less marked. A sharp demarcation between the contusion and concussion zones is not always visible, but they are occasionally separated by a thin zone of neutrophils and/or erythrocytes.

The histopathological changes in both zones become more severe with increasing survival time, and are particularly marked if an infection develops.

Table 1. The comparison of calibres.

Inches	*Milllimetres*
0.22, 0.222 or 0.223	5.56
0.243 or 0.244	6
0.25	6.35
0.264	6.5
0.284	7
0.30 or 0.308	7.62
0.32	7.65
0.323	8
0.357 (0.38)	9
0.45	11 or 11.43
0.50	12.7

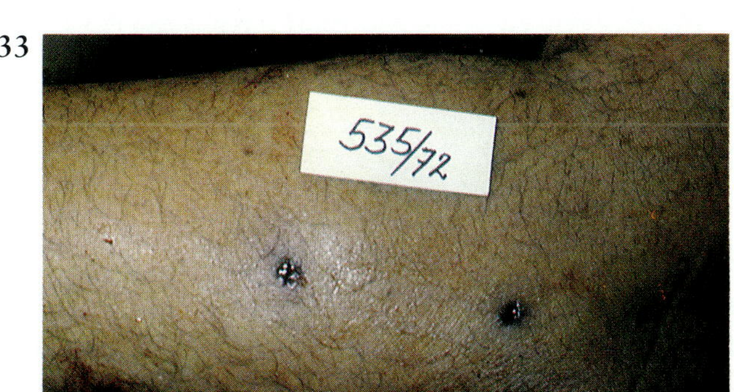

33 **Two entry wounds in the left forearm,** caused by a pistol.

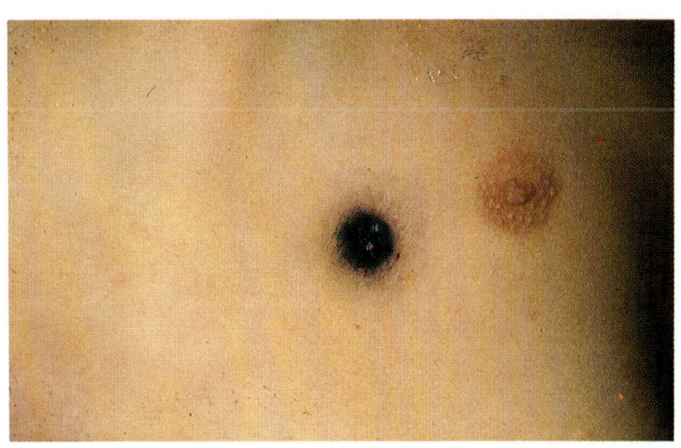

34 **Anterior thorax with an entrance wound over the precordium,** caused by a large-bore pistol.

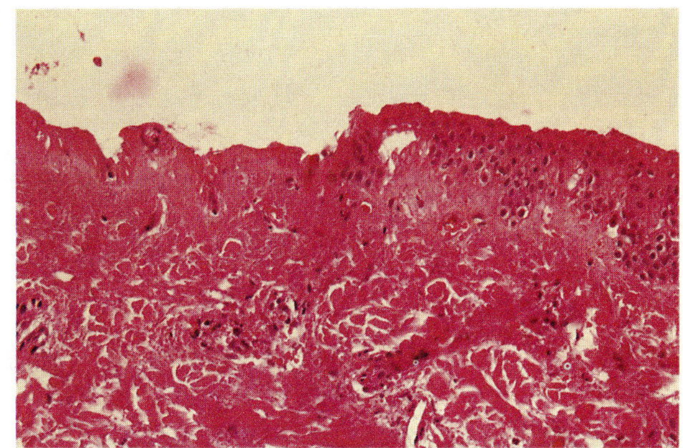

35 **Skin (edge of entrance wound in the forehead of a 15 year-old boy; spherical bullet from a 7.65 mm (0.32 inch) pistol).** Note the transition from well preserved epidermis to the epidermal defect (left) caused by the oblique entry of the projectile. (*H&E ×40*)

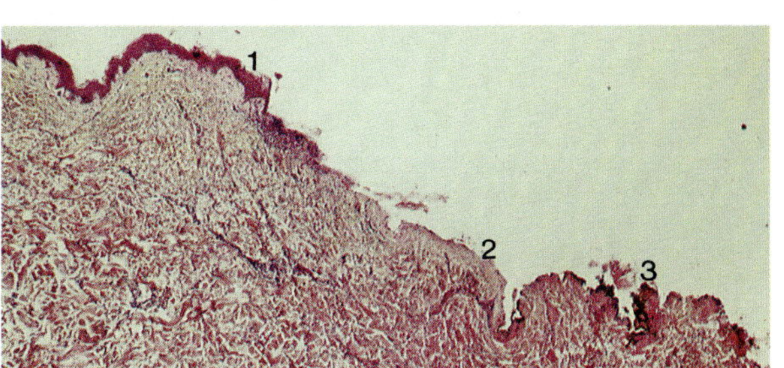

36 **Skin (entrance wound, 7.65 mm (0.32 inch) pistol).** Note the normal epidermis (1), loss of epidermis (2) caused by a bullet entering the skin obliquely, and powder particles (3) embedded in the surface of the entrance wound. (*H&E ×10*)

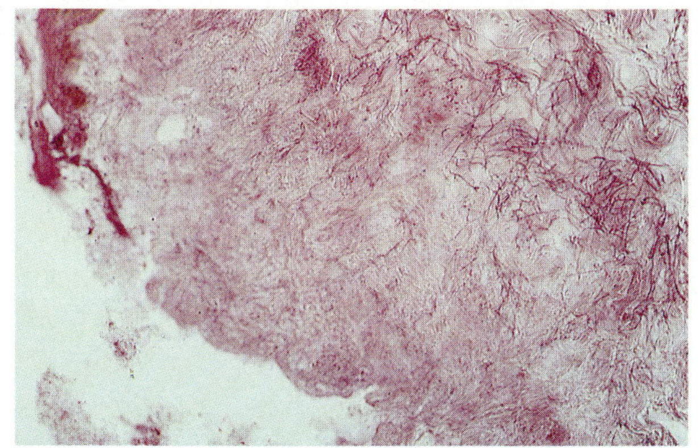

37 **Skin (thorax, entrance wound, 7.65 mm (0.32 inch) pistol).** 30 year-old male. Epidermal destruction, extensive disruption and tearing of elastic fibres. Tissue destruction is considerably clearer than any possible thermal effects. (*Elastic stain: resorcin–fuchsin ×160*)

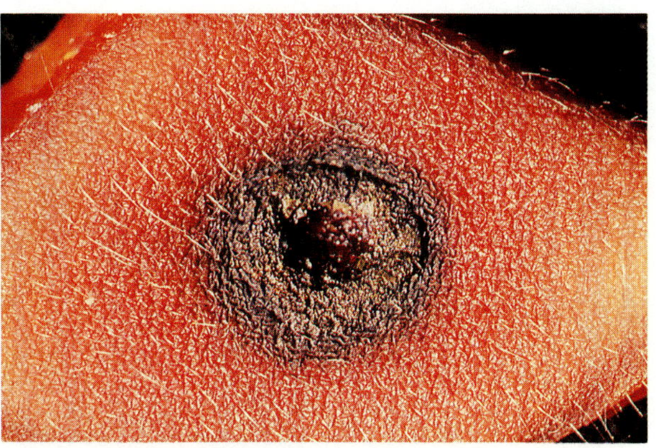

38 **Entrance wound to the thorax,** made at point-blank range (note powder infiltration).

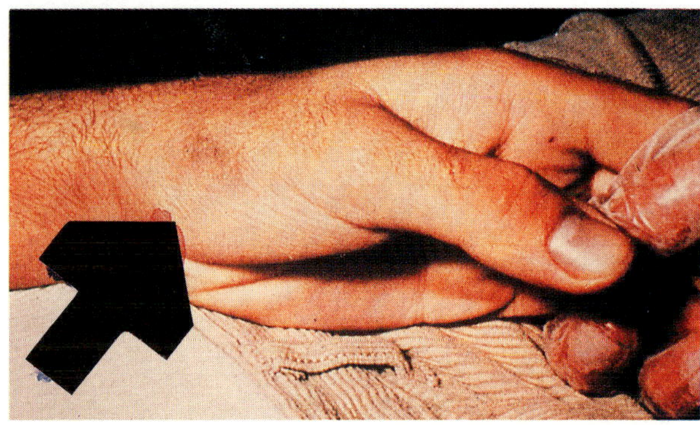

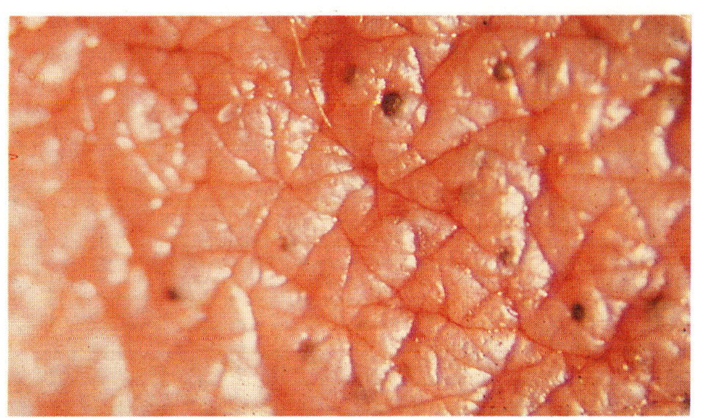

39 and 40 Particles of powder: 39 Gross examination of the hand may not reveal powder particles; **40** Examination of the area arrowed in 39 under slight magnification, by hand-held lens, easily reveals the particles.

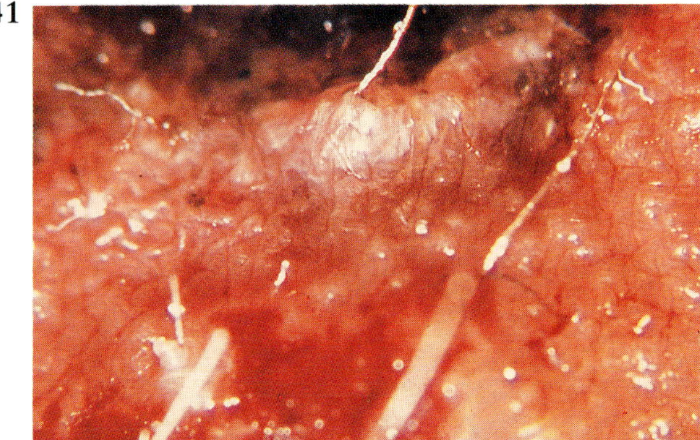

41 Skin: region around the entry wound. Dark colouration caused by particles of powder. The high magnification shows the transition from normal tissue to that darkened by powder deposits.

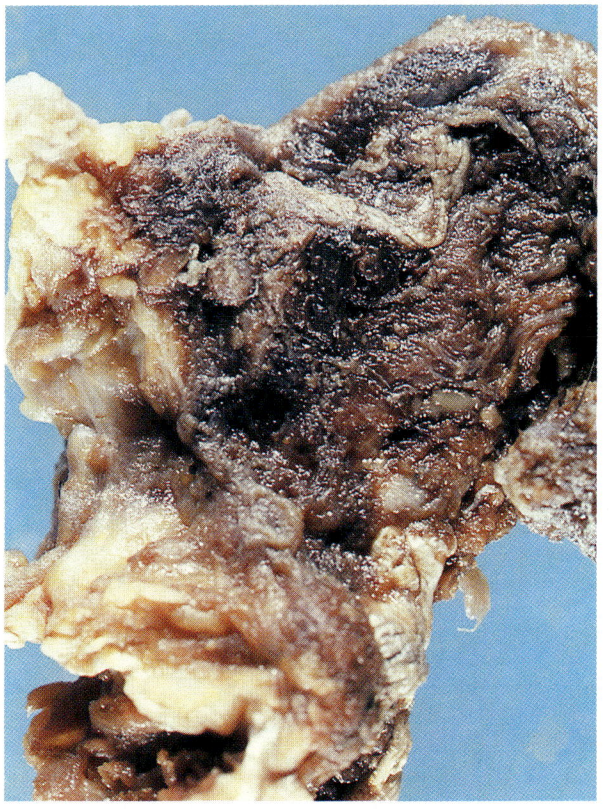

42 Massive accumulation of black powder in subcutaneous tissue. The destroyed tissue is a brownish colour. Entry wound to the temple. (*Formalin-fixed tissue*)

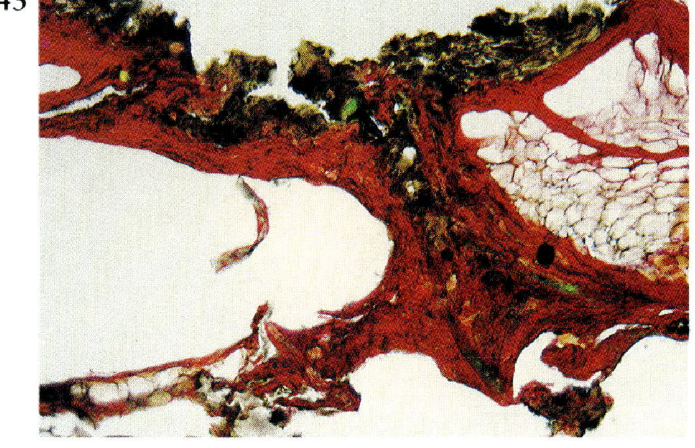

43 Skin (entrance wound, small calibre pistol). Epidermal destruction with formation of large tissue vacuoles (mechanical lesions). Note also the tissue desiccation and the presence of powder particles and dirt. A thicker section was used to preserve the delicate structure of the tissue during sectioning. (*van Gieson ×100*)

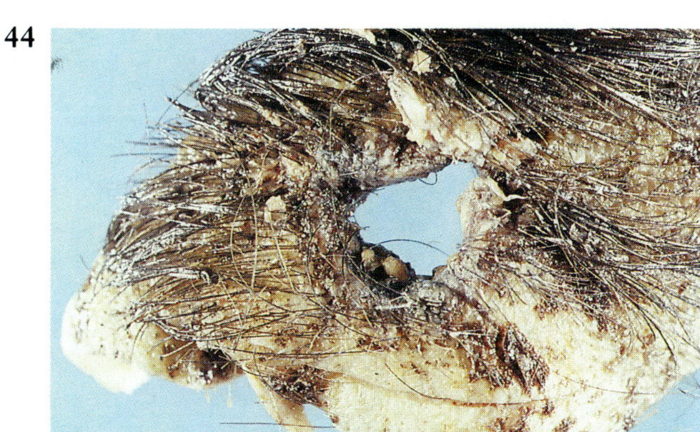

44 Skin: hairline from temple region, entry wound caused by a 9 mm pistol. Gas under high pressure follows the bullet out of the gun muzzle and into the subcutaneous tissue, where it expands and causes the tears in the skin that radiate from the initial bullet perforation. (*Formalin-fixed tissue*)

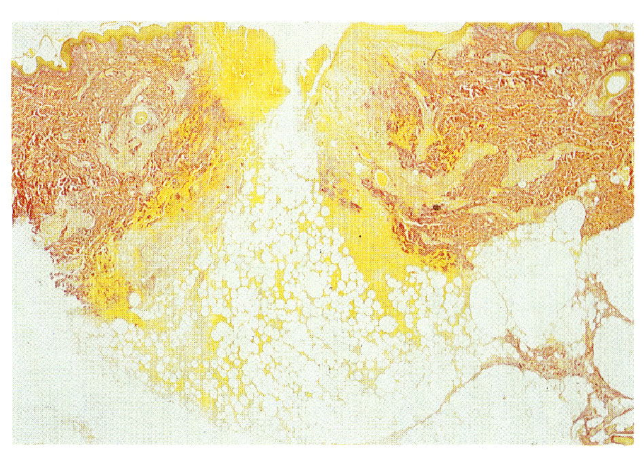

45 Skin (entrance wound, 7.65 mm (0.32 inch) pistol). Post-traumatic survival: 10 days. Massive haemorrhage (yellow) in the bullet tract. (*van Gieson ×10*)

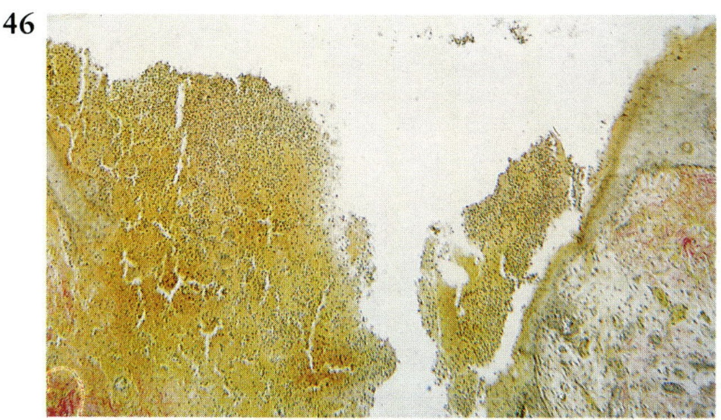

46 Skin (entrance wound, 7.65 mm (0.32 inch) pistol). Part of the entrance wound is shown, with pus formation (left) and granulation tissue (right). There are reparative as well as necrotic changes. (*van Gieson ×100*)

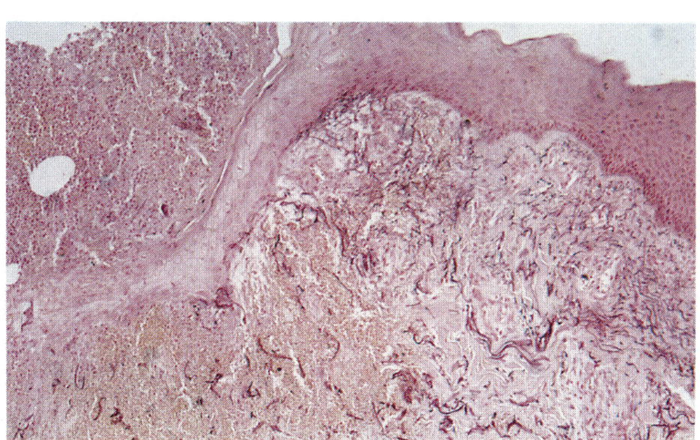

47 Same as **46**, showing the disruption of elastic fibres. (*Elastic stain: resorcin–fuchsin ×100*)

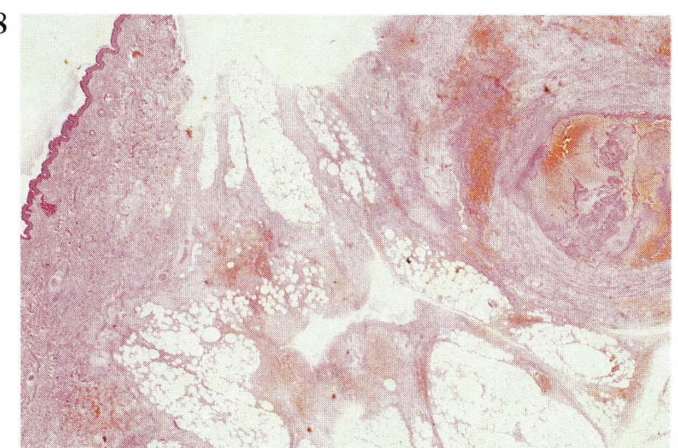

48 Subcutaneous tissue (entrance wound 7.65 mm (0.32 inch) pistol). Note the thrombosis (right) in an artery adjacent to the wound channel. The victim lived for 10 days following the gunshot wound. (*H&E ×10*)

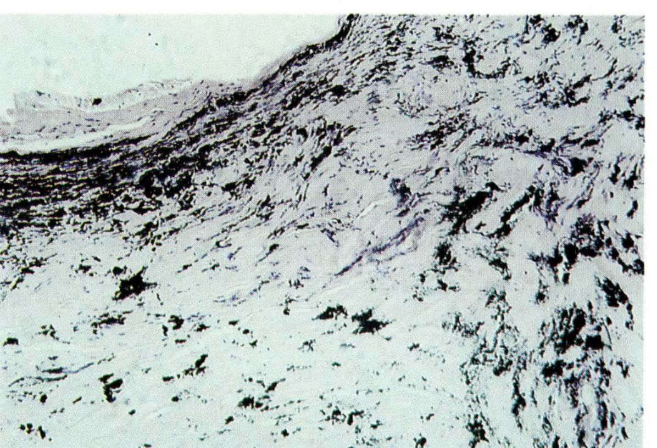

49 Skin: old injury to the skin following a gunshot wound at point-blank range. Note the massive infiltration of the subcutaneous tissue with powder particles (black). (*H&E ×100*)

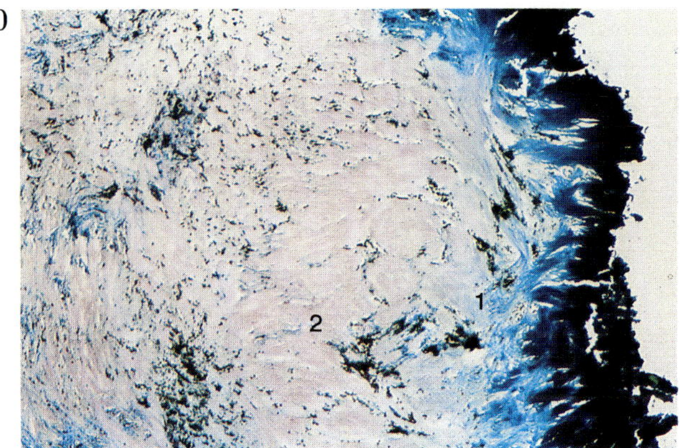

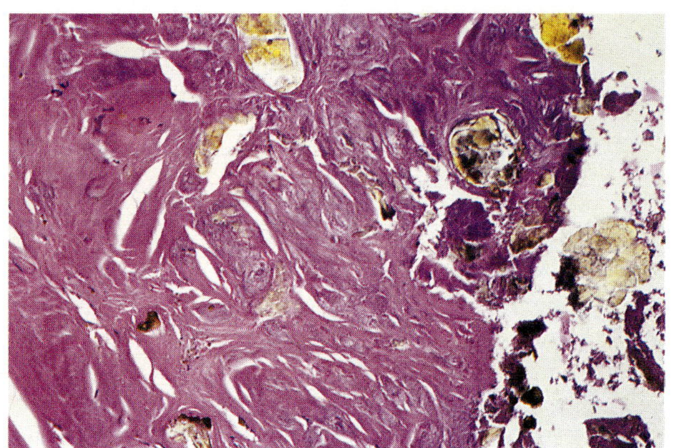

50   Subcutaneous tissue (hand): Injury received 40 years previously from shrapnel. Important features are the iron from metal splinters (especially on the right (1)) and haemosiderin (2), evidence of previous haemorrhage. (*Prussian blue ×100*)

51   Subcutaneous tissue from the material in 50 showing dirt particles in the scar tissue. (*H&E ×100*)

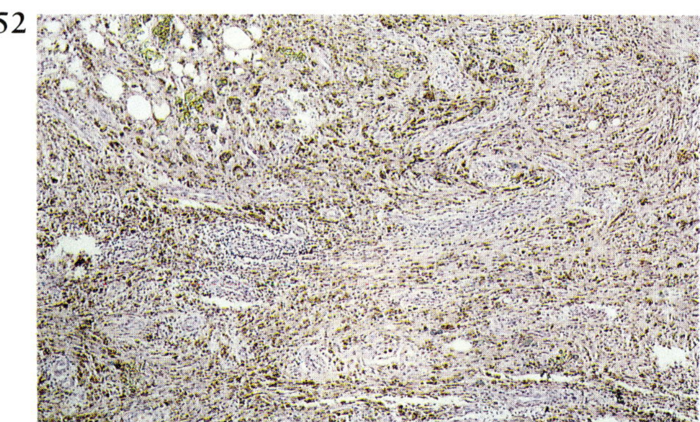

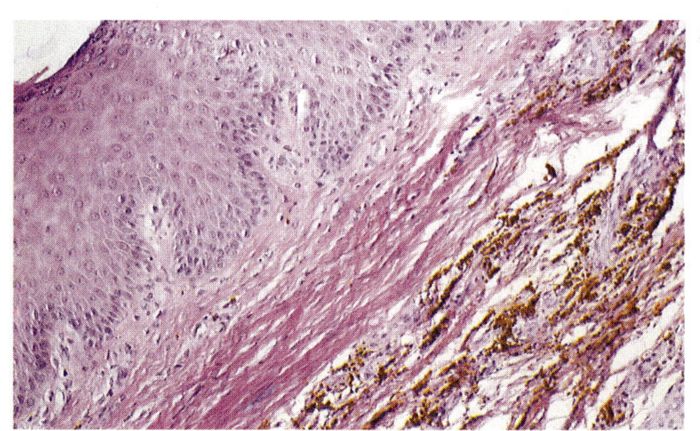

52   Subcutaneous tissue (shin) from a case of tibial fracture following a gunshot wound (rifle, 7.62 mm, 0.30 inch), 9 weeks previously. The picture shows formation of large quantities of cellular connective tissue and haemosiderin (brown). In the upper left are particles of foreign material (green). (*H&E ×80*)

53   Skin and subcutaneous tissue (shin) from a case of tibial fracture 40 years previously. Large amounts of haemosiderin are seen, evidence of previous haemorrhage. Mild acanthosis of the skin. (*H&E ×100*)

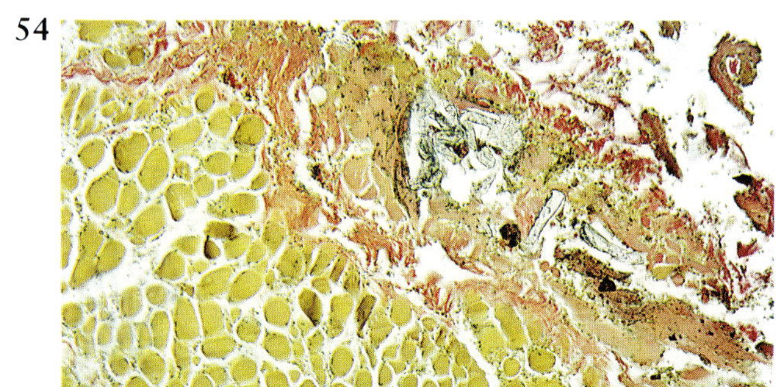

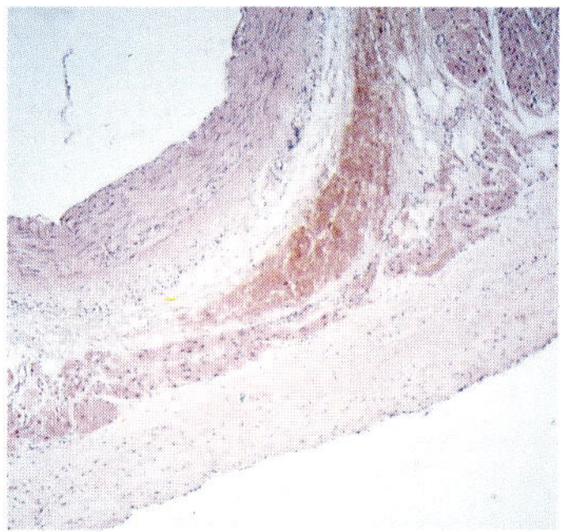

55   Heart. Gunshot wound due to a 7.65 mm (0.32 inch) pistol. Haemorrhage around the right coronary artery (upper left) as a result of blast injury. Almost instantaneous death. (*H&E ×64*)

54   Muscle. Gunshot wound from a 7.65 mm (0.32 inch) pistol. Note the textile fibres (possibly from clothing) present to the right of the muscle fibres. (*van Gieson ×100*)

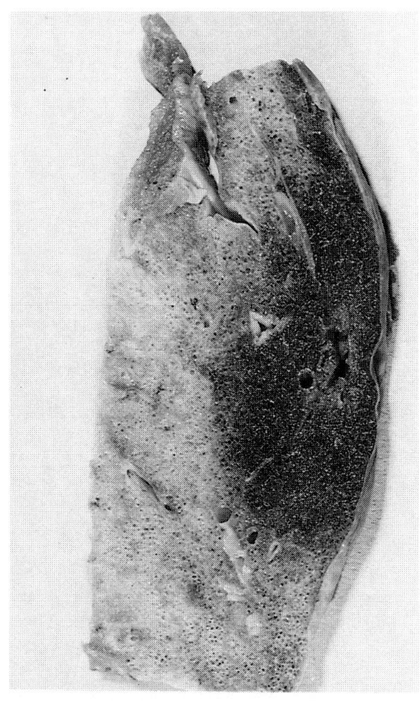

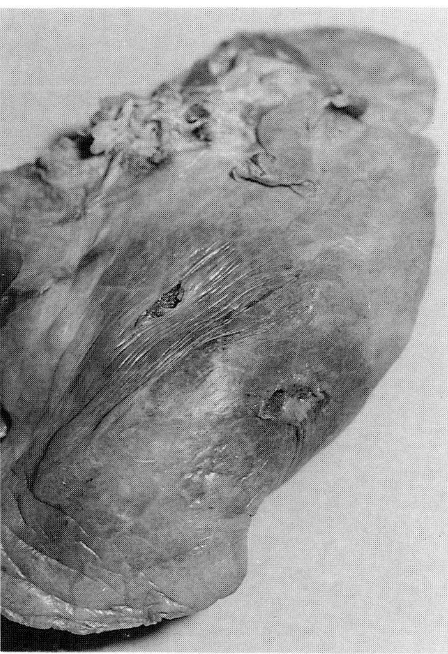

56 **Lung** injury caused by a traversing bullet (pistol 7.65 mm). Massive intrapulmonary bleeding around the subpleural bullet channel.

57 **Lung**. Injuries to the upper lobe of the left lung caused by a bullet from a 7.65 mm pistol. Entry wound left, exit wound right. (*Formalin-fixed tissue*)

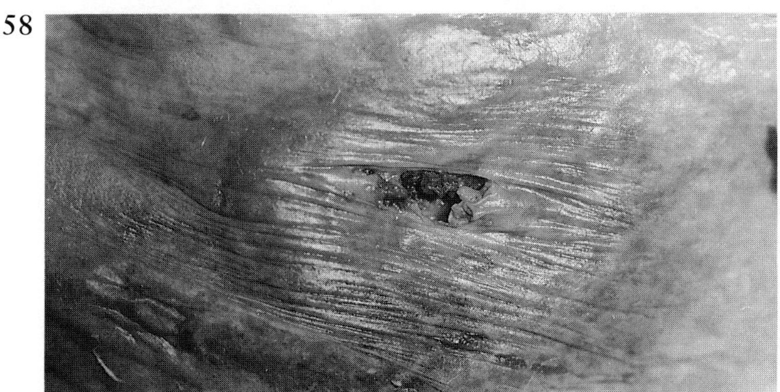

58 Same as 57. Close-up of the entry wound, which has an irregular shape. There is no rib fracture. The passage of the bullet through clothing, skin, subcutaneous tissue and muscle caused a change in trajectory and angle of entry.

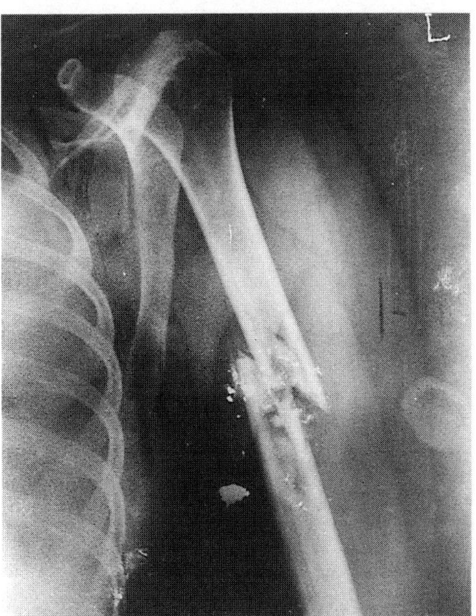

60 **Fracture of the left humerus** caused by a 6.35 mm bullet, which disintegrated on impact.

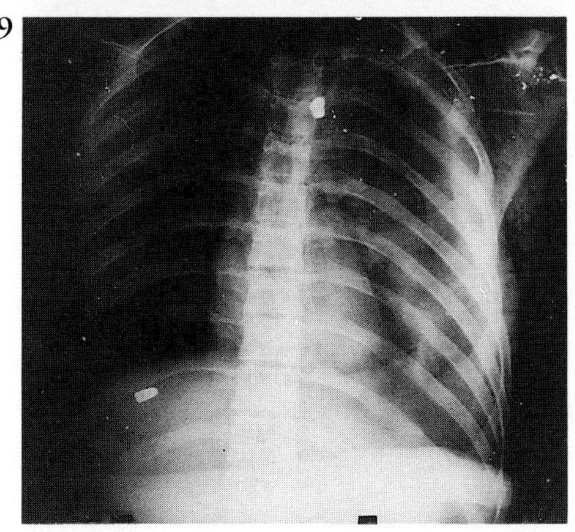

59 **Small-bore bullet injuries to the chest in a 23 year-old woman.** The cranially situated bullet was deformed after striking the left scapula. Lead fragments are also visible in the X-ray.

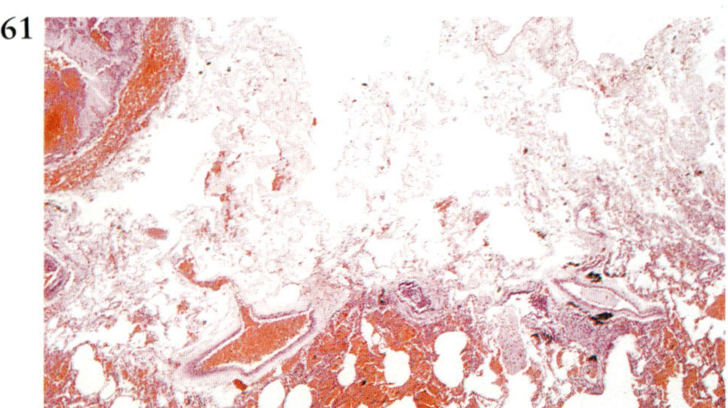

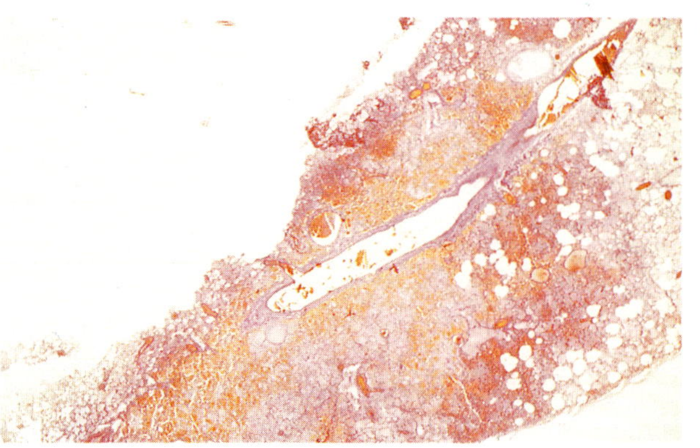

61   Lung. Gunshot wound from a 7.65 mm (0.32 inch) pistol. Diffuse haemorrhage is seen in alveoli, as well as intra- and peri-bronchially. There is extensive parenchymal disruption. (*H&E ×15*)

62   Lung. Haemorrhagic infarct in the lung parenchyma adjacent to the bullet track, caused by a 7.65 mm (0.32 inch) pistol. (*H&E ×10*)

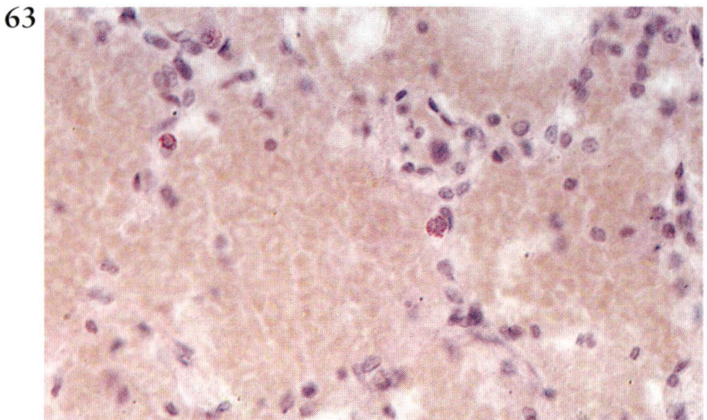

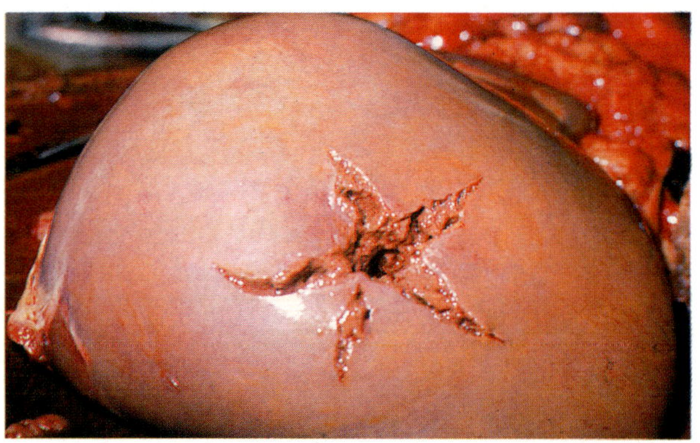

63   Lung. Material from the lung parenchyma adjacent to the bullet track, showing alveoli filled with erythrocytes. Gunshot wound from a 6 mm (0.243 inch) pistol. (*H&E ×640*)

64   Liver. Entry wound caused by a 7.65 mm pistol. Note the stellate laceration of the capsule caused by expanding gases which follow the bullet into the parenchyma.

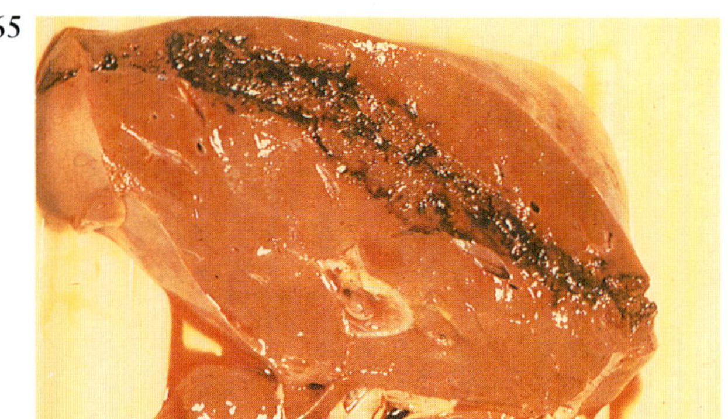

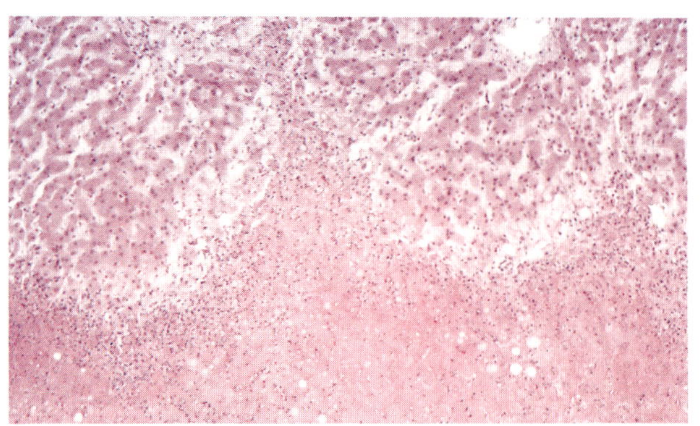

65   Liver. Bullet channel (pistol) traversing the liver.

66   Liver. Perforating gunshot wound, 7.9 mm (0.323 inch) pistol. The edge of the bullet channel is shown, with intact liver parenchymal cells (above) and an area of liver cell necrosis (below). The beginning of leucocytic demarcation between necrotic zone and normal parenchyma can be seen. Post-traumatic survival time: 24 hours. (*H&E ×100*)

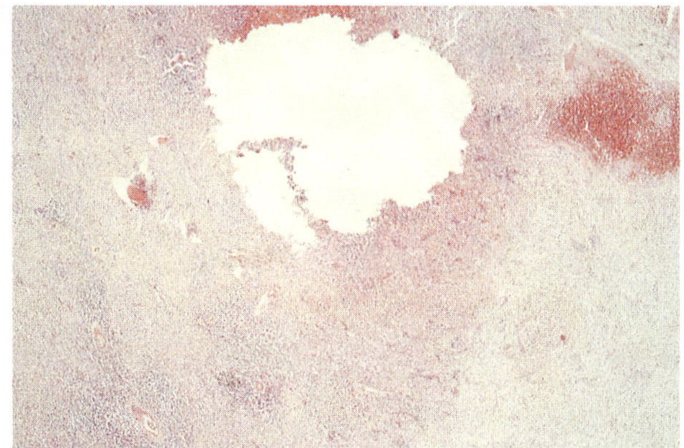

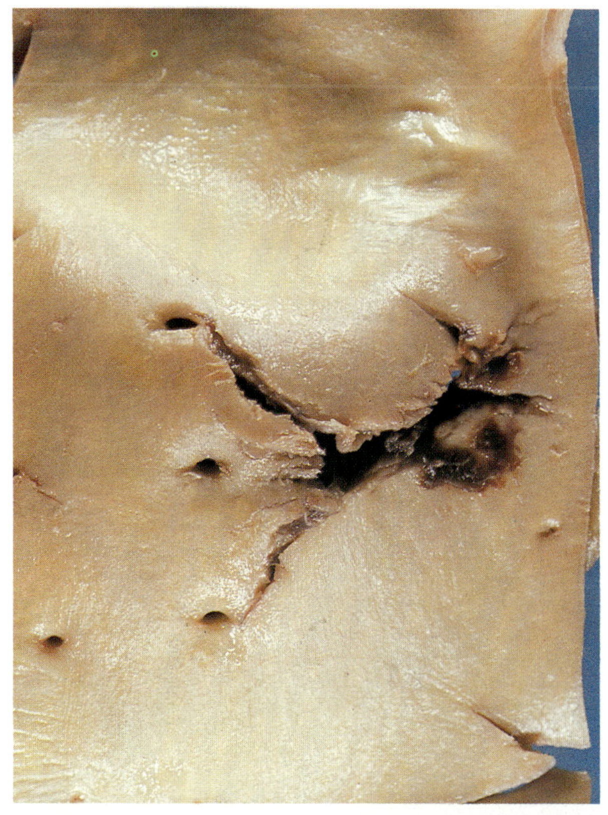

67 Spleen. Perforating abdominal gunshot wound, 7.65 mm (0.32 inch) pistol. The bullet channel is clearly seen with areas of haemorrhage in the splenic parenchyma around it. Death was almost immediate and therefore no cellular reaction took place. (*H&E ×12*)

68 Gunshot wound to the thoracic aorta caused by a 7.65 mm pistol.

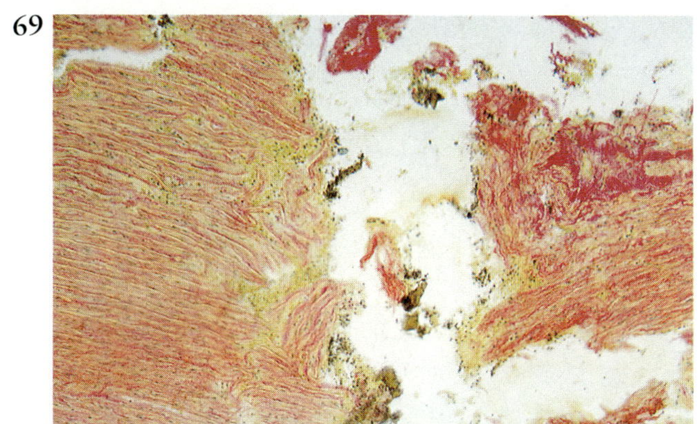

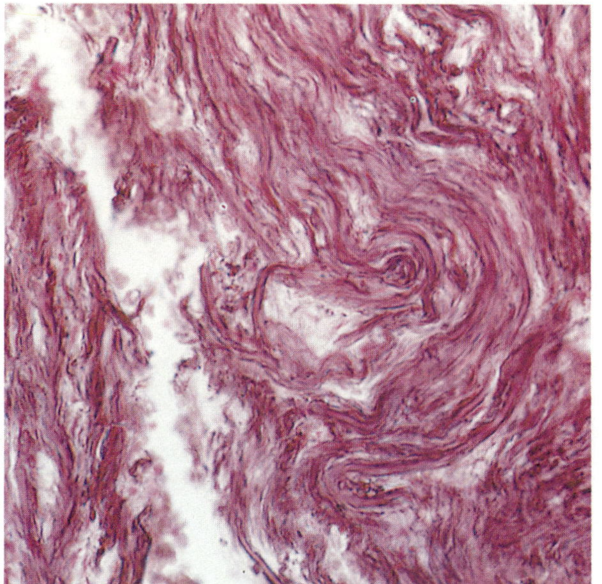

69 Aorta. Perforating abdominal gunshot wound, 6 mm (0.243 inch) pistol. Important features are the complete disruption of aortic continuity (bullet channel, middle) and the presence of foreign material and non-aortic tissue in the bullet channel and its edges. Material from a 10 year-old girl who died immediately. (*van Gieson ×80*)

70 Aorta. Same as **69**. The picture shows the disruption of the aortic elastic fibres, which have assumed a whorled appearance. This alteration was caused by blast injury to the aorta adjacent to the bullet channel. (*Elastic stain: resorcin–fuchsin ×500*)

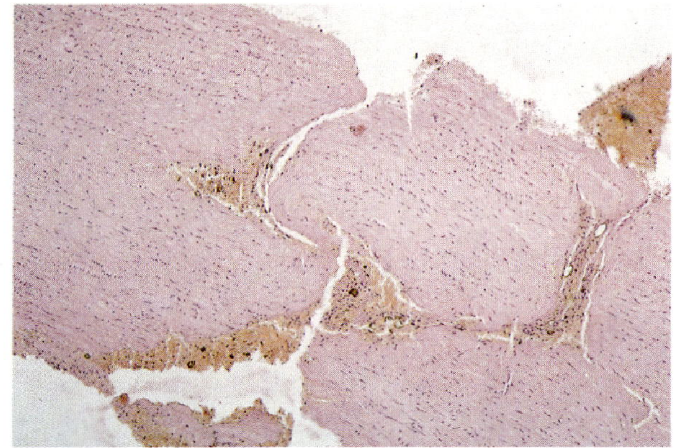

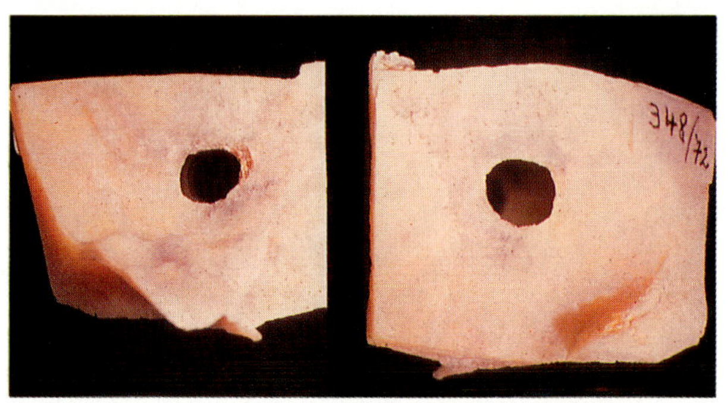

71 Aorta. Abdominal gunshot wound, 7.65 mm (0.32 inch) pistol. Disruption of the aortic wall with haemorrhage, caused by a bullet striking the aorta tangentially. Material from a 26 year-old male. The dark colouration in the area of haemorrhage is formalin pigment. (*H&E ×80*)

72 Skull segment. Two views of the same entrance gunshot wound caused by a 7.65 mm pistol. The external table (right) shows clearly demarcated edges while the internal table (left) shows a terrace-shaped deformity (or bevel). This is definite evidence that the bullet struck the external table first and confirms that it is an entrance wound to the skull (see **74**, which shows an exit wound from the skull).

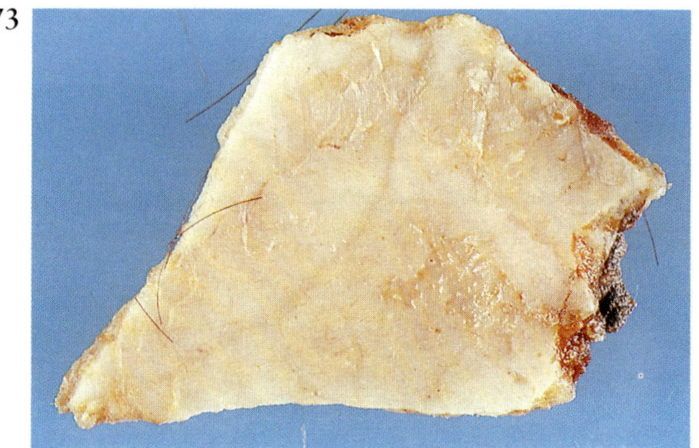

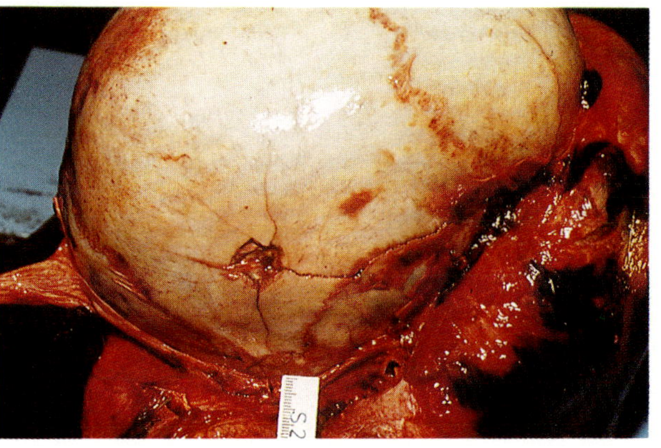

73 Inner surface of the parietal bone. Note the terrace-shaped (or bevel) defect at the lower right corner.

74 Exit wound (pistol) in the posterior region of the right parietal bone. Note the terrace-shaped avulsion of the bone with radiating fracture lines. Extensive haemorrhage in the neighbouring soft tissue of the scalp and exit wound in the skin (lower left).

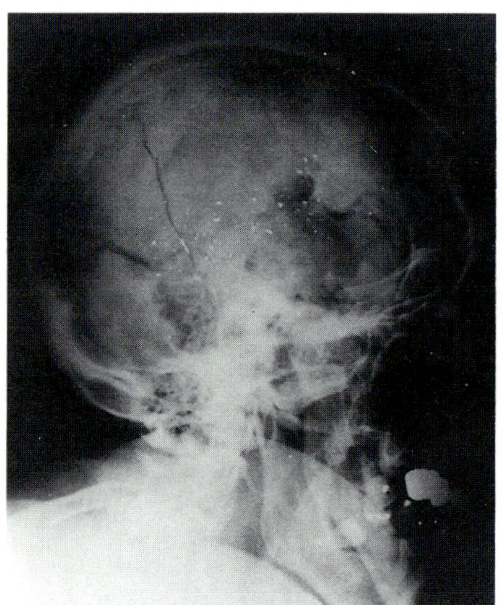

75 Fracture of the skull following a small-bore gunshot injury (6.35 mm) to a 22 year-old woman. The X-ray shows multiple lead particles from the bullet.

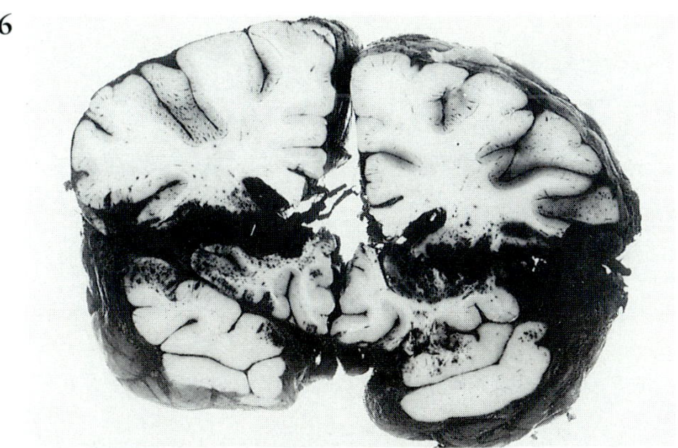

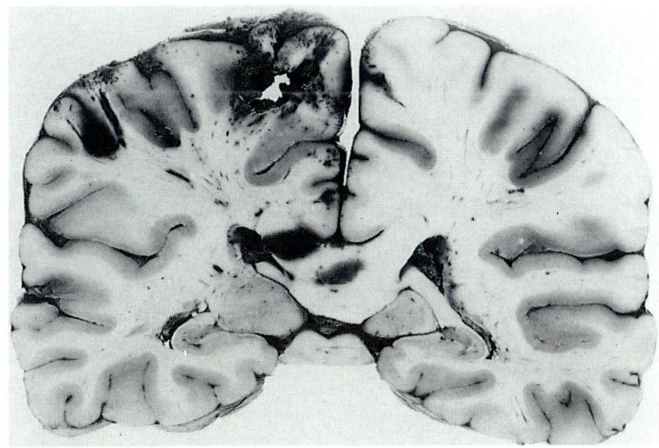

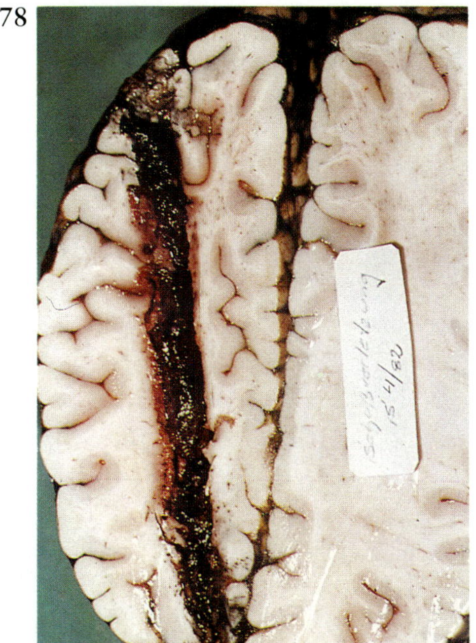

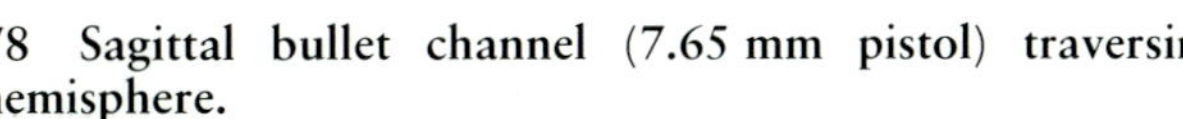

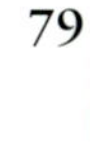

76   Bullet injury to the brain by a 7.62 mm rifle. The bullet channel is wide and the adjacent cerebral tissue is haemorrhagic. To the right of the picture a funnel-shaped defect in both grey and white matter can be seen (exit wound).

77   Bullet wound (7.65 mm pistol) to the left parietal region of the brain. Note the areas of haemorrhage in the surrounding tissue as a result of blast injury.

78   Sagittal bullet channel (7.65 mm pistol) traversing a cerebral hemisphere.

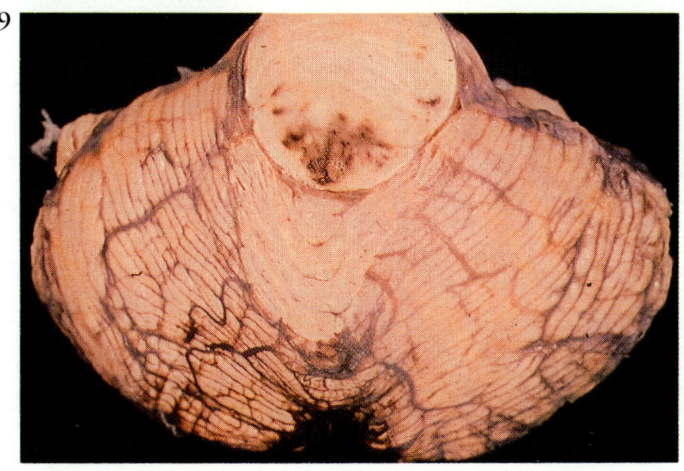

79   **Perforating gunshot wound to the skull.** Pontine haemorrhage as a result of pressure waves. These haemorrhages occur with severe craniocerebral wounds — for example with military weapons. The pressure waves can extend to the spinal cord.

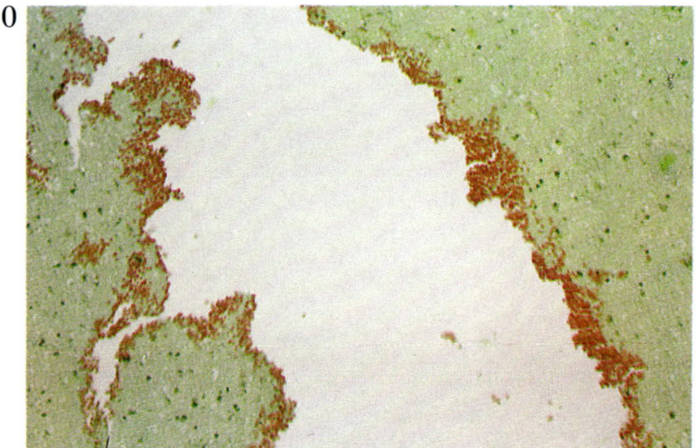

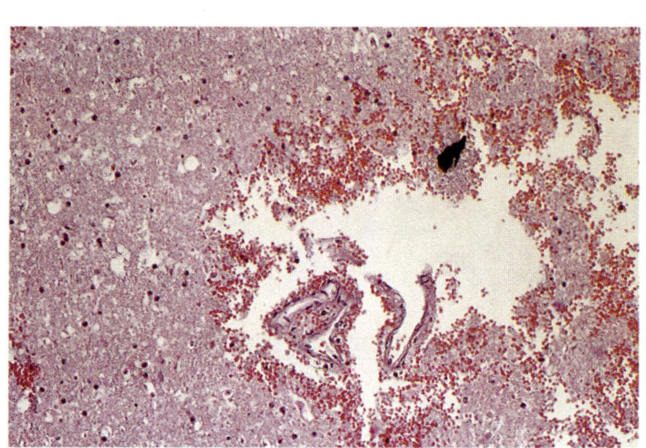

80 Cerebrum. Penetrating gunshot wound from a 7.65 mm (0.32 inch) low-velocity pistol (spherical bullet). The patient died 24 hours after injury. The bullet channel is shown with areas of haemorrhage and the formation of tissue clefts. (*H&E ×40*)

81 Cerebrum. Same as **80**, showing splitting of the parenchyma along the bullet tract, haemorrhage, torn blood vessels and the presence of powder residue. (*H&E ×40*)

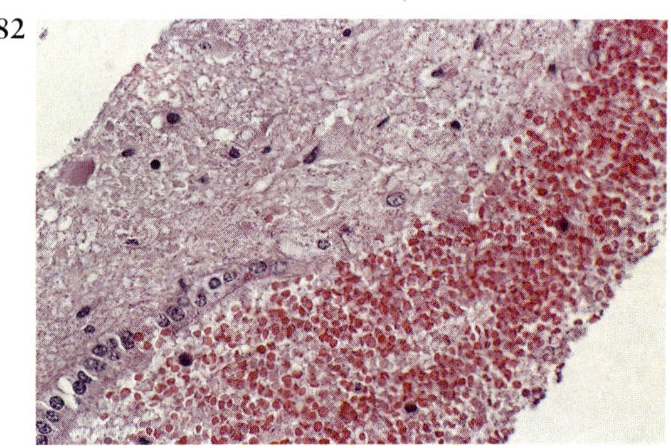

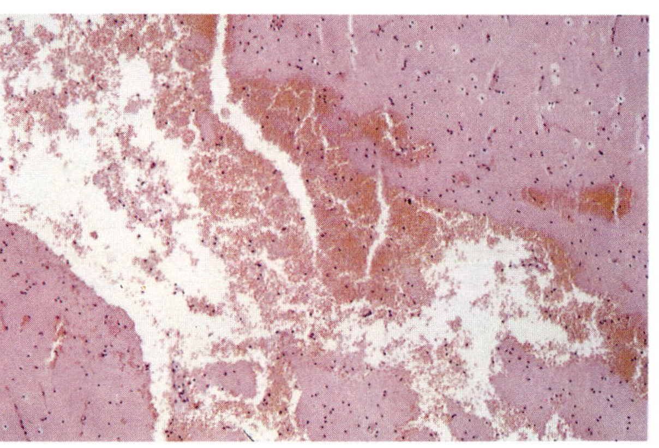

82 Cerebrum. Same case as in **72**, showing the effects of blast injury caused by the penetrating bullet. Haemorrhage is evident in the region of the partially intact ependyma. (*H&E ×250*)

83 Cerebrum. Penetrating gunshot wound, 6 mm (0.243 inch) pistol. The cerebral parenchyma is extensively disrupted and shows fissures penetrating into the parenchyma from the bullet channel. Haemorrhage in the bullet channel and the adjacent tissue. Material from a 21 year-old male. Instantaneous death. (*H&E ×100*)

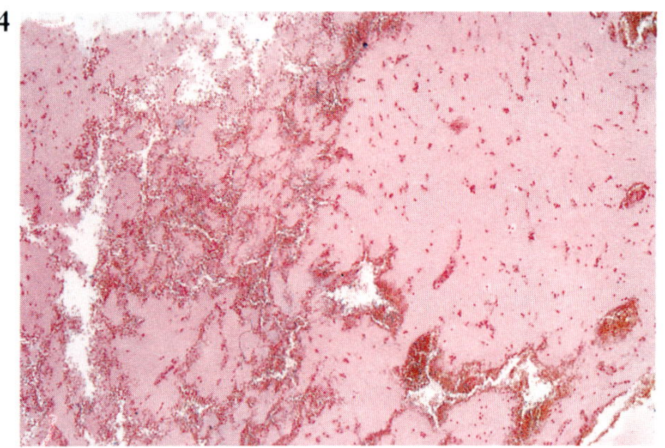

84 Cerebrum. Penetrating gunshot wound, as in **83**. The picture shows the cerebral parenchyma adjacent to the bullet channel and contains multiple areas of haemorrhage as a result of the blast injury. (*H&E ×100*)

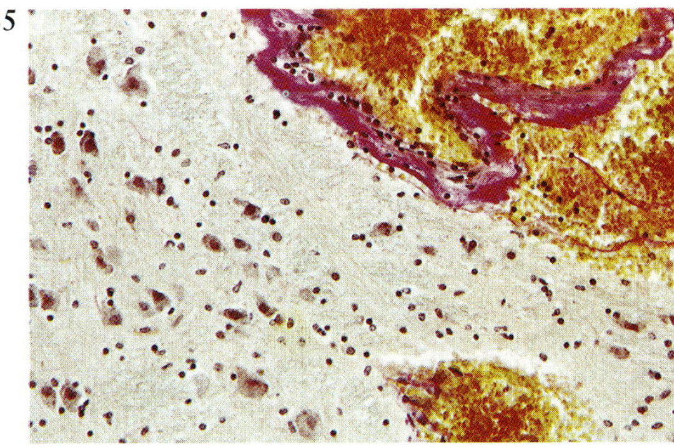

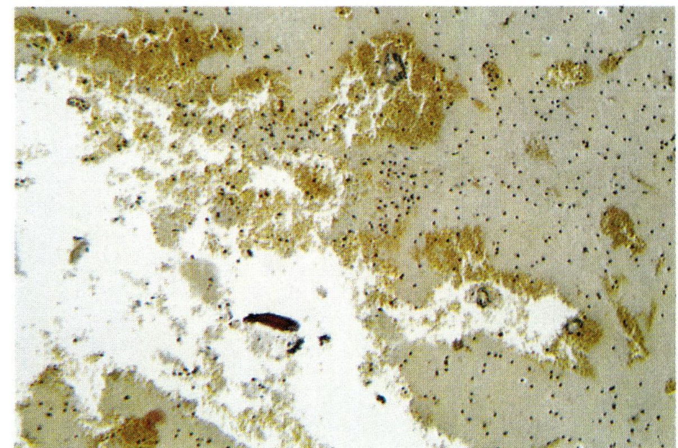

85 Cerebrum. Penetrating gunshot wound, 6 mm (0.243 inch) pistol. Note the perivascular haemorrhage around a larger blood vessel (upper right), as well as a smaller area of parenchymal haemorrhage (below) near ganglion cells. Effects of blast injury are shown in the neighbourhood of the bullet channel. Material from a 63 year-old male. Instantaneous death. (*van Gieson ×250*)

86 Cerebrum. Penetrating gunshot wound from a 6 mm (0.243 inch) pistol, showing the bullet channel containing bone fragments from the skull. Note also the small 'recessus' branching from the bullet channel and areas of haemorrhage. Material from a 21 year-old male. (*van Gieson ×100*)

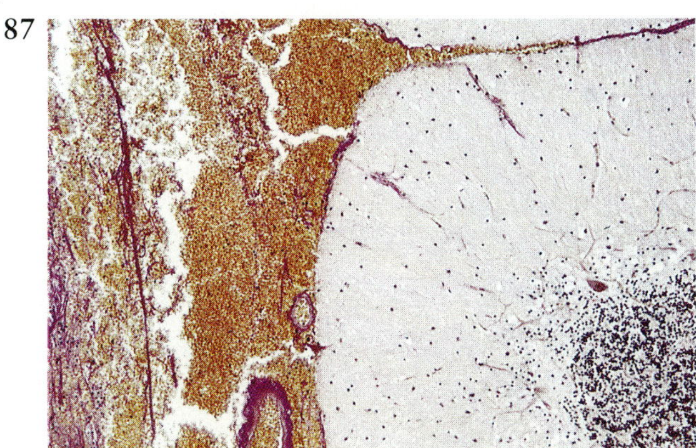

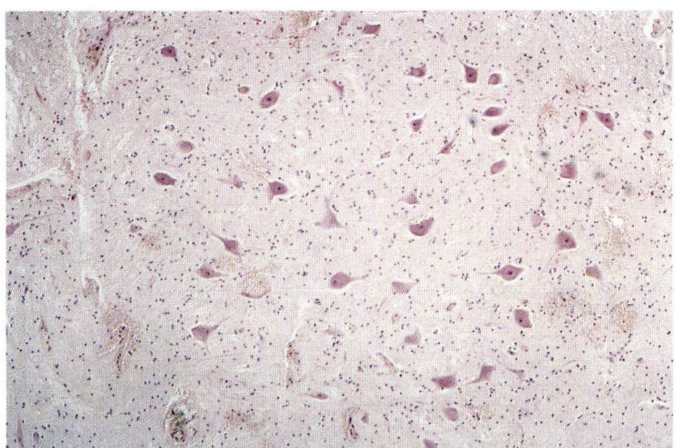

87 Cerebellum. Penetrating gunshot wound from a 6 mm (0.243 inch) pistol. The important feature is the massive subarachnoid haemorrhage (right) arising from the blast injury. (*van Gieson ×100*)

88 Medulla oblongata (caudal region). Penetrating gunshot wound from a 6 mm (0.243 inch) pistol. The picture shows an area of ganglion cells with mutliple foci of haemorrhage because of the kinetic energy acting on the tissue adjacent to the bullet channel. Material from a 24 year-old male. (*H&E ×640*)

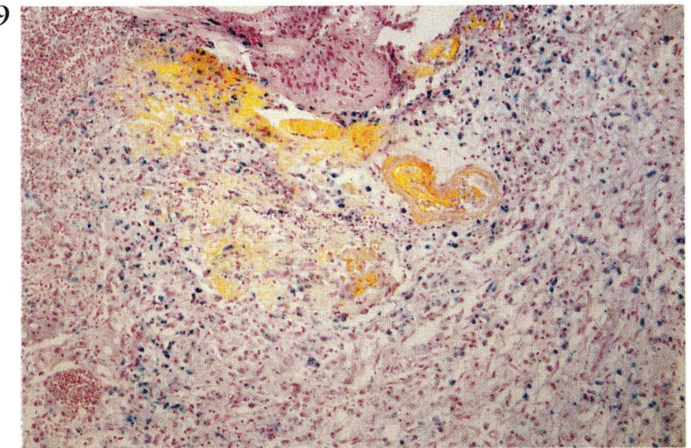

89 Cerebrum. Injury resulting from shrapnel 39 years prior to death. The parenchymal defect has been replaced by proliferation of glial tissue. Evidence for previous haemorrhage is provided by the presence of marked deposits of haemosiderin (blue) and haematoidin (orange–yellow). (*Prussian blue ×100*)

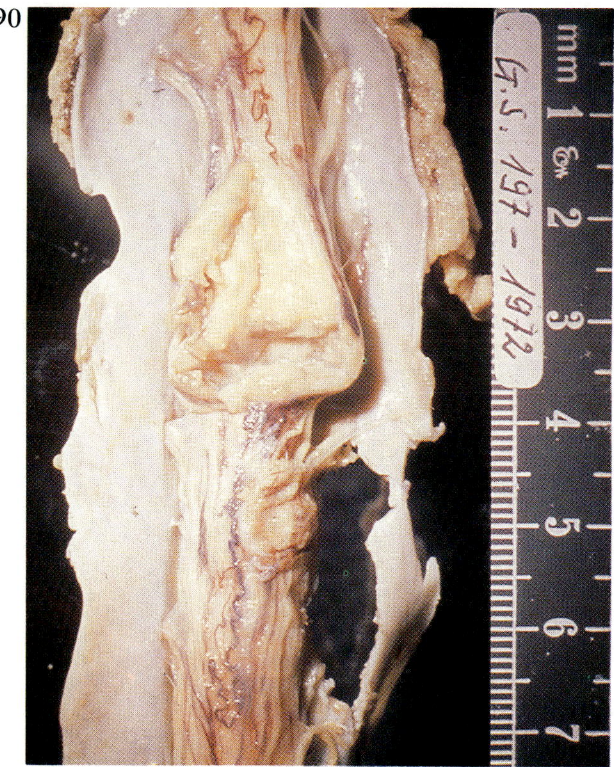

90 **Spinal cord.** Penetrating gunshot wound producing a transection of the spinal cord.

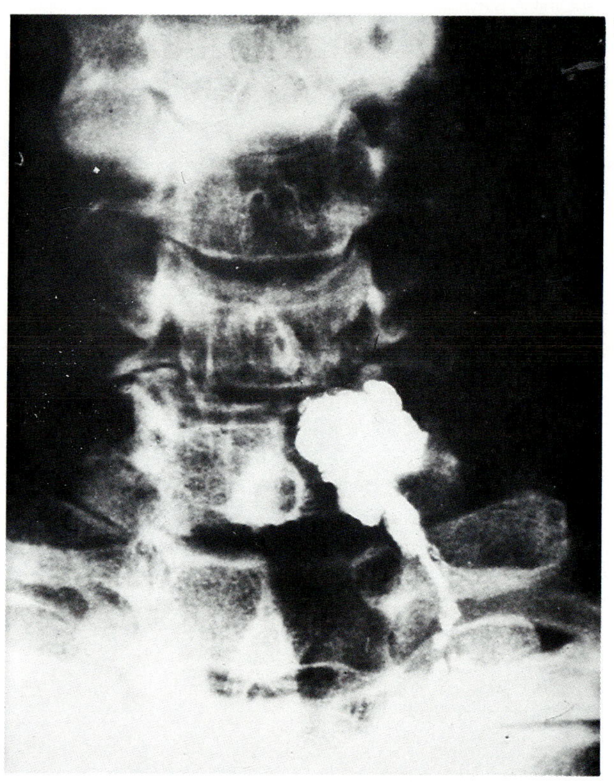

91 **Neck.** A deformed lead bullet in the cervical region with lead particles removed by the lymphatic system. The patient was shot 27 years previously. Lead serum level not known.

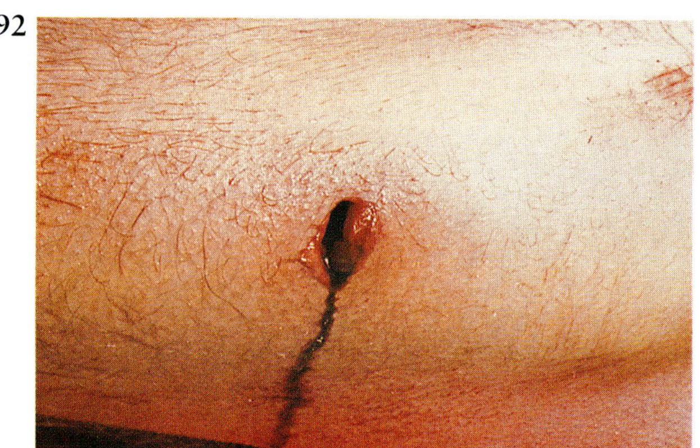

92 **Exit wound in the left thigh** caused by a rapid-fire bullet (7.62 mm). Soft-tissue injury only. Poor blood coagulation, with sudden death. There was haemorrhage from the wound in the femoral artery.

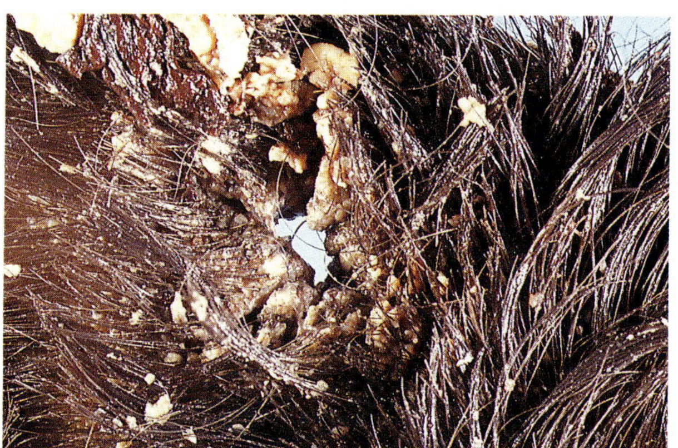

93 **Exit wound in the scalp,** caused by a 9 mm pistol. Note the star-shaped laceration of the surrounding tissue, which also contains fragments of brain tissue, and the considerable tissue destruction. (*Formalin-fixed tissue*)

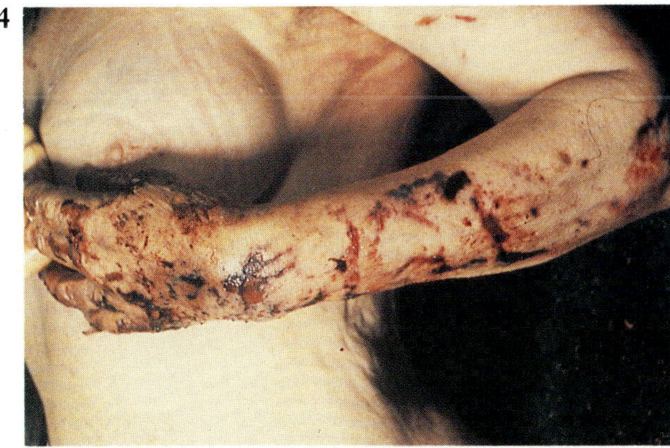

94 Multiple incisions and lacerations caused by shrapnel from a bomb explosion. There is also dirt infiltration.

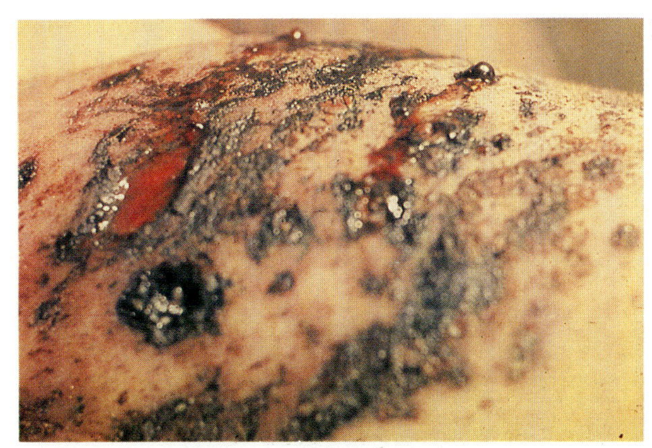

95 Multiple shrapnel injuries with powder infiltration.

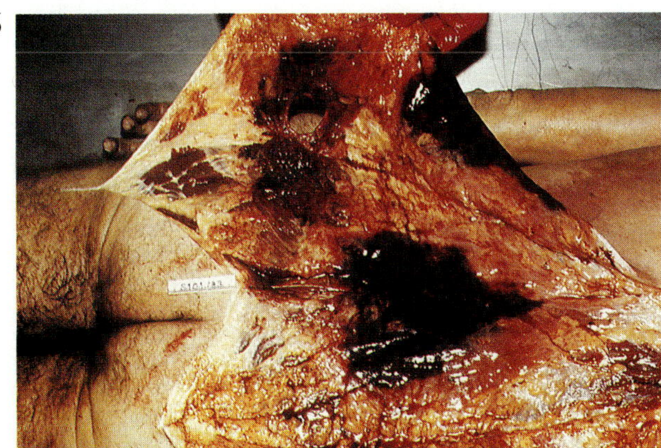

96 Injury to the buttock and pelvis caused by mortar fragments (12 cm). Massive haemorrhage in the wounds and surrounding tissue. Abdominal position. The skin has been removed from the sacral area.

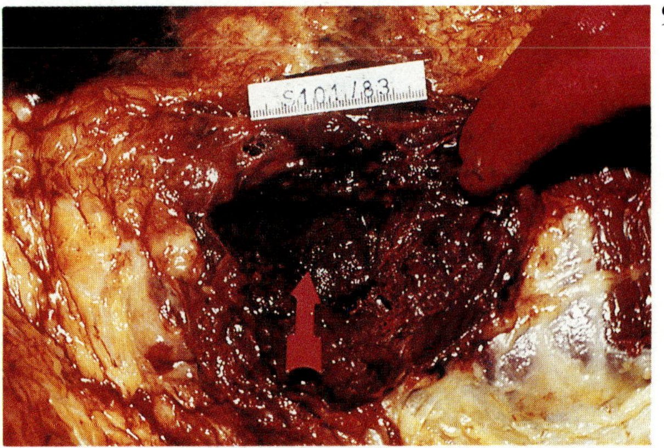

97 Same as **96**. Close-up view showing cavitation in muscle and pelvic bone.

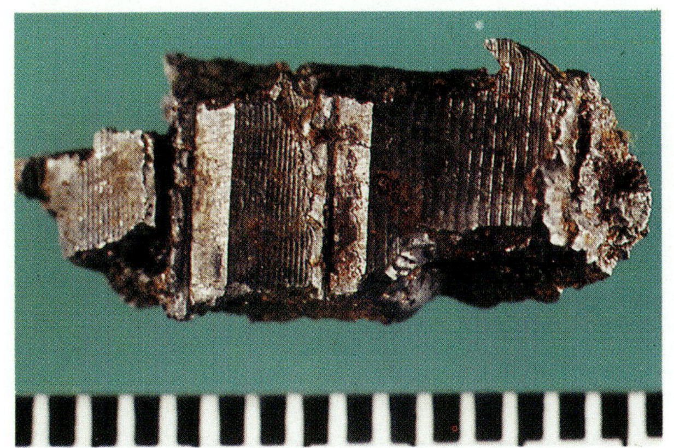

98 Same as **96**, showing the sharp, irregular edge of the mortar fragments.

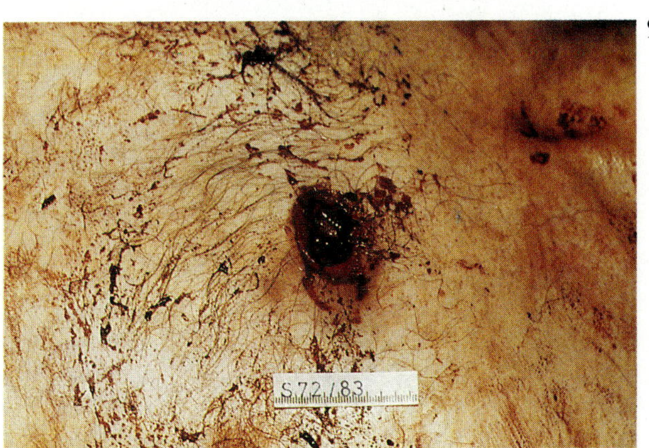

99 Wound to the anterior thorax caused by a shotgun fired at point-blank range, but *not* with the weapon in contact with the skin. Some of the expanding gases may have escaped in the space between the end of the muzzle and the skin. Thus, there are no radial lacerations from the central wound.

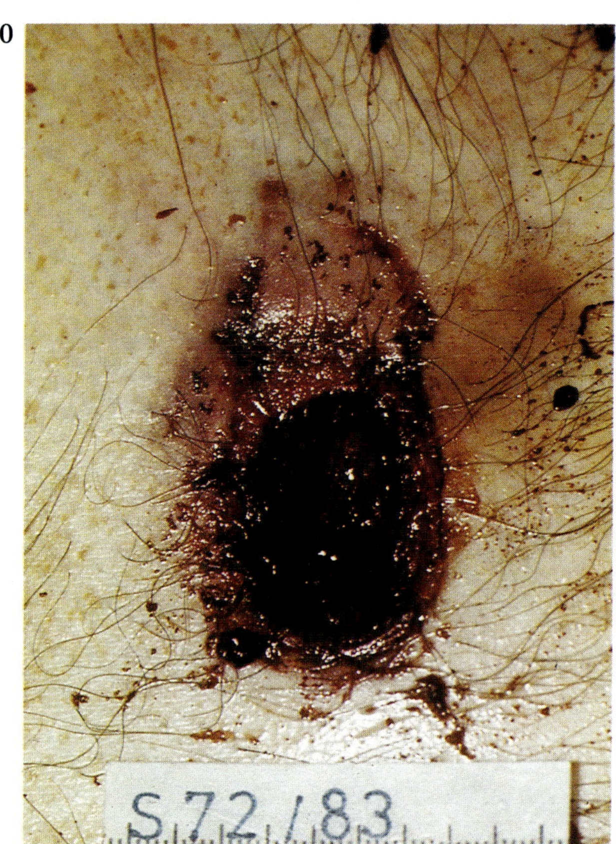

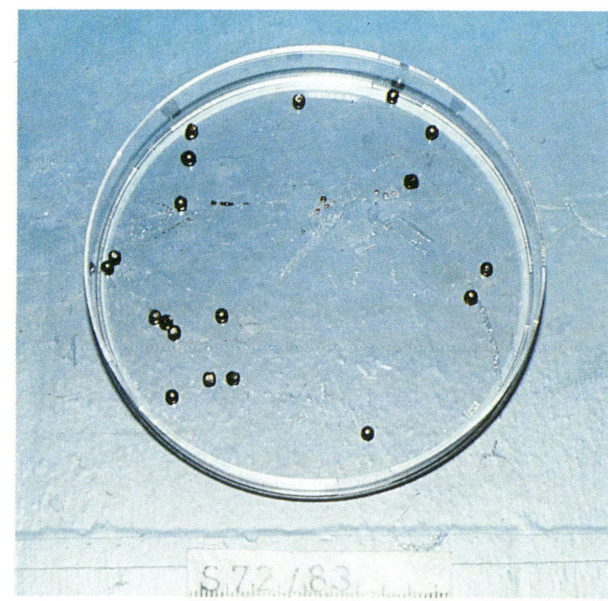

100   Same as **99**. Close-up view. Some gases have entered the skin and expanded, forcing the skin into hard contact with the muzzle, thus leaving an imprint of the other (unfired) barrell of the shotgun above the entrance wound.

101   Same as **99**, showing some pellets recovered from the wound.

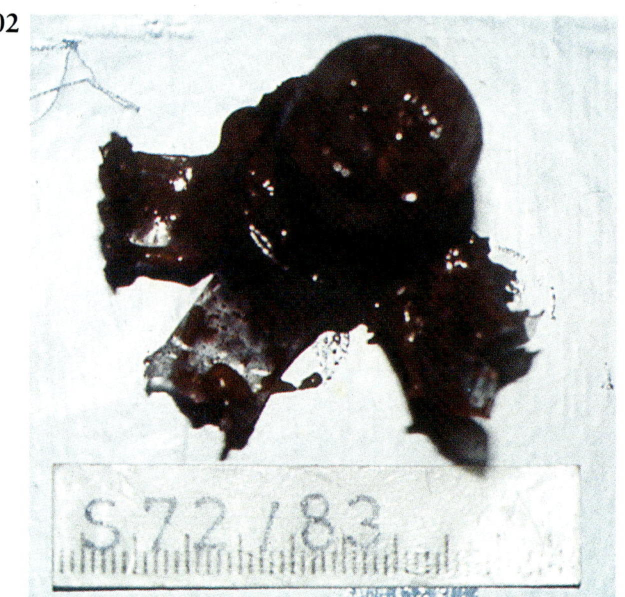

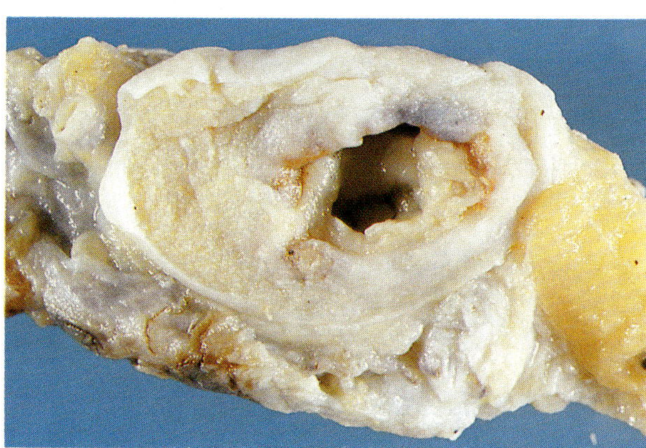

103   **Injury to the testis** caused 38 years previously by grenade shrapnel. Traumatically induced cavities show haemorrhage residues and a moderate fibrosis. (*Formalin-fixed tissue*)

102   Same as **99**. Note the presence of torn plastic shot carrier from the shotgun shell in the wound.

4 Blunt injuries

The spectrum of injuries caused by blunt force is very broad. The type and extent of injury depend largely on whether the blunt force is *generalised*, as when a body falls from a height, or *localised*, for example, as a result of striking the head with a blunt object. What must be borne in mind, both by the pathologist and the clinicians, is that the extent of the internal injuries caused by a blunt force may be considerably greater than the visible lesions on the body surface. A typical example is injury due to kicking.

Abrasions are caused by the tangential application of force to the skin resulting in removal of part of the superficial epidermis. Portions of dermis and even subcutaneous tissue may also be removed. Haemorrhage is usually of a punctate nature. The presence of particles of dirt predisposes to infection.

Contusions or **bruises** vary greatly in size and form, depending on the area of contact between the body and the applied object. The continuity of the skin surface is unbroken, the pathological changes occurring in the subcutaneous tissue as a result of rupture of blood vessels with extravasation into the neighbouring tissues.

Lacerations of the skin involve a break in the continuity of the skin. The wound edges are typically irregular and the depth of the wound variable. The extent of haemorrhage depends on the number and type of blood vessels injured. Lacerations of the skin arise particularly frequently over bone or bony prominences, for example, in the scalp and knee regions, but can be located anywhere. Most confusing is a laceration that appears to be a straight line. If examination with a hand lens reveals that the fine hair follicles are intact, *i.e*, entirely on one or the other side of the wound, then it is clear the skin has been torn, rather than cut (in which case the follicles will be cut).

Crush injuries to the skin are caused by pinching or squeezing of the skin between two blunt surfaces. A good example is the bite wound caused by animals with blunt teeth, such as horses, cattle or pigs. Tissue destruction, haematoma formation and the impairment of the blood supply to the crushed tissue all contribute to the development of post-traumatic infection. Crush injuries may, of course, be much more severe, causing life-threatening damage to vital internal organs. This is typically the case in severe road traffic accidents, in which crush injury may lead to rupture of the hollow viscera or even cause rupture of the abdominal wall with subsequent evisceration.

In road traffic accidents, *crushing* or pressure forces are frequently accompanied by *traction* forces, which may lead to stripping of large areas of skin and subcutaneous tissues, including muscle, from limbs and trunk (décollement), or to complete avulsion of a limb. The application of such traction forces to soft tissues causes the formation of blood filled cavities in remaining subcutaneous tissue and muscle.

Discussion of the severe forms of blunt injury leads inevitably to the term *polytrauma* – injury to more than one system or region of the body. Thus a severely traumatised patient may have a combination of injuries to the limbs, trunk and head. It is evident that such a constellation poses major medical problems for the physicians and surgeons responsible for the medical care of such victims.

Traction and rotational forces applied to the body can cause *distorsion* (sprain) or *dislocation* of joints. In the former case a temporary abnormal movement between the articular surfaces results in a stretching of the joint capsule, whereas in the latter, parts of the joint capsule are usually torn and the joint assumes an abnormal anatomical position.

The term subluxation is used to describe less marked forms of dislocation. The combination of dislocation and fracture of the bones involved is termed *fracture–dislocation*.

A fracture is a break in the continuity of a bone and can assume various forms depending on the type of bone involved, for example, long bones, skull and vertebral bodies. The opening of the bone marrow cavity leads to bleeding and paves the way for fat embolism, or, more rarely, bone marrow embolism.

It is not the purpose of this book to detail the various forms of fracture, such as transverse, spiral, impacted, simple and compound fractures, infraction, etc. However, the pathologist needs to bear in mind that fractures often accompany trauma, and they may be easily overlooked, as the greenstick fracture or fractures of the base of the skull. The possibility of localised or generalised infection as a result of compound fractures, in which a skin wound directly communicates with the fracture, is important. It is also worth remembering that not only objects, but also blows from a fist, may cause fractures.

Blunt injury to the head may be life threatening, either as a result of primary trauma or secondary circulatory disturbances. Among the variety of injuries are subarachnoid, subdural and epidural haemorrhage, cerebral cortical contusion, subependymal haemorrhage, as well as haemorrhage in the corpus callosum and cortical white matter. It is particularly important to remember that severe trauma to the head may cause not only a contusion at the site of impact, but also the so-called contre-coup injury to the surface of the brain diametrically opposite the impact injury.

Injuries that result from blunt-instrument violence are encountered as lacerations, abrasions and contusions, of internal organs as well as of the skin. Skin defects are also to be found among these injuries.

In every case tissue is destroyed, with the disruption of blood vessels leading to the formation of a haematoma. Apart from the tissue defect, various features can be seen as a tissue reaction to the trauma:

- Haemorrhage with extravasation of fibrin and leukocytes and the release of disrupted collagen and elastic fibres.
- Oedema and plasma exudation.
- Capillary dilatation.

A series of biological processes representing the body's reaction to trauma is set in motion to remove cell detritus and restore tissue integrity. The course of wound healing is governed by basic biological principles, although certain differences exist between various tissues.

In an investigation of subcutaneous haemorrhage, Berg & Ebel (1969) observed polymorphonuclear cells after 9 hours, haemosiderin normally after 90 hours and haematoidin as early as 9 days. The development of granulation tissue was only rarely observed. The tissue reaction to trauma will be delayed by severe impairment of vital functions, a point which must always be borne in mind when tissue reaction is absent.

An exact differentiation between recent congestive haemorrhage or haemorrhage resulting from asphyxia and post-mortem lividity is impossible, as is a clear differentiation between supravital and vital changes. Reactive changes in the edges of the wound, as well as the deposition of fibrin, permit a diagnosis of ante-mortem reaction. However, the absence of fibrin is not necessarily proof of a post-mortem injury. In cases of tissue desiccation, particularly in the skin, a shrivelling of tissue components with masking of the normal tissue structure is seen (for example, loss of stratification of the epidermis).

Orsós (1935) used a Mallory stain to study mechanical, chemical and thermal injury to connective tissue and was able to demonstrate a red staining reaction of the collagen fibres, which normally stain blue.

In cases of cardiac concussion and contusion, myocardial as well as subepicardial haemorrhages can be seen along the small and medium-sized branches of the coronary vessels. Damage to the blood vessel walls covers a spectrum from intimal lesions to aneurysms and focal areas of thrombosis. Subendocardial haemorrhages have also been observed (Parmley *et al.*, 1958; Rajs & Jakobsson, 1976; Rajs, 1977; Froede *et al.*, 1979).

In brain lesions it is important to distinguish between two forms:

Primary. These lesions arise simultaneously with and as a direct consequence of the application of force. They are localised and often multifocal. An example is the formation of erythrocyte cuffs around blood vessels. If the survival time is short, cell changes tend to be minimal. Necrosis manifests itself after several hours.

Secondary. These lesions arise from circulatory disturbances as a result of hypoxic or anoxic processes (incomplete and complete traumatic necrosis, diapedetic haemorrhage and cerebral oedema):

(a) Ischaemic cell necrosis or ischaemic cell change (disappearance of the Nissl substance, loss of demarcation of the nuclear membrane, contraction of the cytoplasm and nucleus, eosinophilia of the cytoplasm). In the Purkinje cells the essential feature is cloudy swelling.

(b) Partial or elective parenchymal necrosis (neuronal death with, however, preservation of the glial cells and the connective tissue of the blood vessels. Glial cells which have proliferated demonstrate phagocytosis, the so-called neuronophagia).

(c) Proliferation of the microglial cells and transformation to compound granular corpuscles (or gitter cells).

(d) Total parenchymal necrosis. Here there is absence of nuclear stainability of neurons, glial cells and connective tissue cells of the blood vessels (Unterharnscheidt, 1972).

In the brain, differentiation between ante-mortem ischaemic ganglion cell alterations and post-mortem degeneration is extremely difficult, if not impossible. Early changes, such as chromatolysis and cloudy swelling, are to be found in each.

Courville (1965) attempted to describe an approximate time scale for histological findings:

- *Death after 3 hours following injury* – capillary hyperaemia.
- *Death after 2 days* – glial swelling.
- *Death after 4 days* – leucocytic infiltration and glial mobilisation.
- *Death after 6 days* – phagocytosis of haemosiderin.
- *Death after 10 days* – formation of capillary sprouts.
- *Death after 15 days* – presence of cerebral macrophages (compound granular corpuscles).

According to Peters (1970), the important traumatic alterations in the spinal cord are:

(a) Principal foci or spinal cord contusions, consisting of haemorrhage followed by complete or incomplete necrosis, reparation and organisation.
(b) Cysts with necrotic content (secondary focus). These are sharply demarcated areas of necrosis which tend to be localised to the dorsal tracts.
(c) Focal vacuolisation or spongioid foci in the white matter and predominantly localised in the peripheral regions of the spinal cord.
(d) Secondary degeneration in the ascending and descending spinal tracts.

Recent injury to the spinal cord shows histopathologically as dissociation of the grey matter along with destruction of tissue infiltrated with blood. Here the nerve cell bodies and fibres may be wholly or partially destroyed. The next step is the infiltration into the necrotic area of cells of microglial origin. These cells phagocytose and remove the necrotic tissue. Finally, an area of irregular scar tissue is produced by glial activation. Cystic change can also occur in the adjacent tissue.

In the early stages of spinal cord compression, the picture is dominated by oedema, with complete or partial destruction or swelling of the myelin sheaths. An inflammatory cell reaction can be observed later. At first the ganglion cells are swollen and may demonstrate chromatin loss, as well as a shift of the cell nucleus to a more peripheral position as a result of ischaemia. A complete or partial disruption and pyknosis of the ganglion cells arise later; some may even appear as ghost cells (Minckler, 1971).

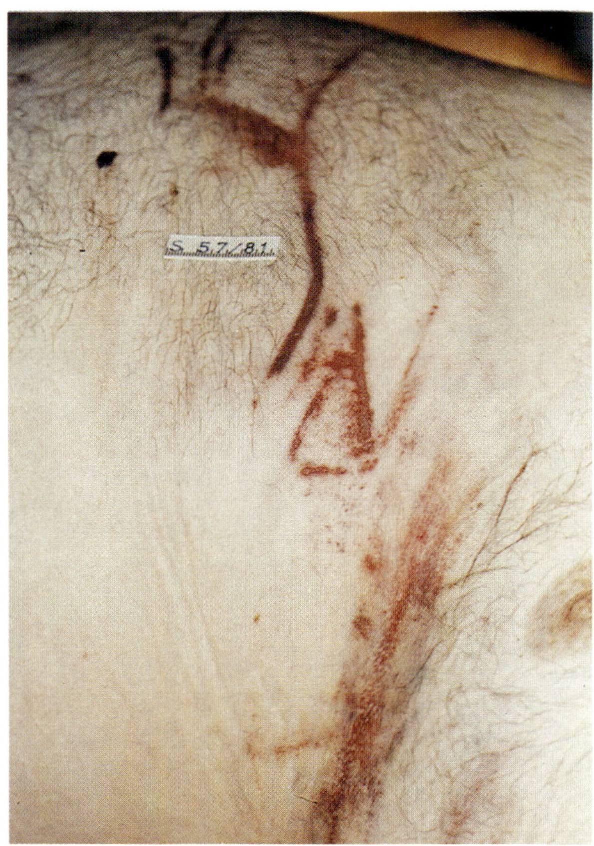

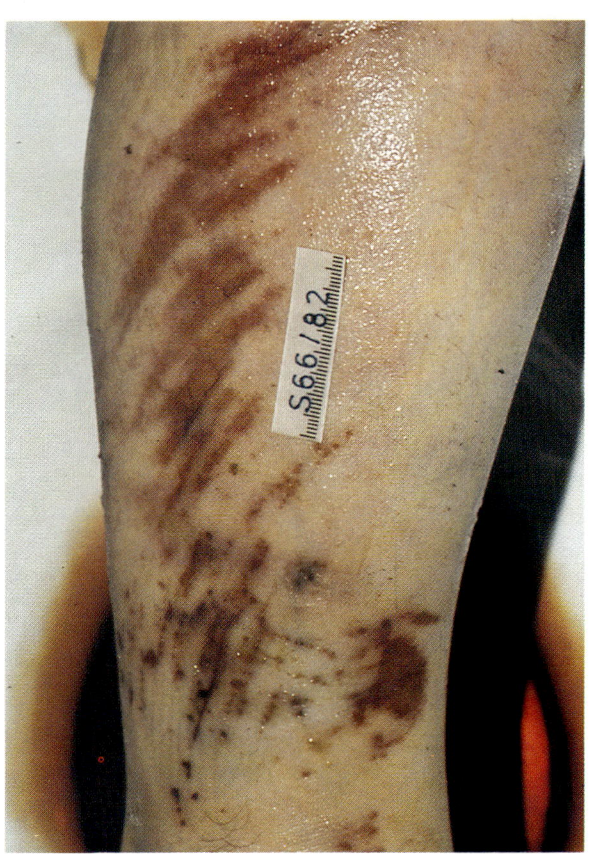

104 Superficial skin abrasions caused by a safety belt are the diffuse injuries just below the nipple. The sharply defined injuries central and beneath this area were caused by the body striking something, probably the steering mechanism in this case of a high speed car crash.

105 Severe abrasions on the right thigh as a result of a fall from a motorcycle.

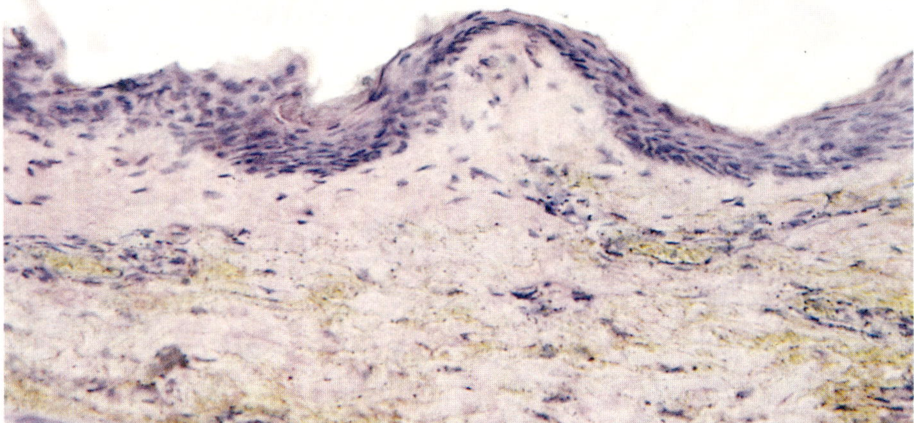

106 Skin (chin). Superficial epidermal defect caused by a fall. Shedding of the horny layer and the upper cell layers of the stratum spinosum, resulting in localised thinning of the epidermis. Diffuse bleeding in the dermis (*H&E* ×63).

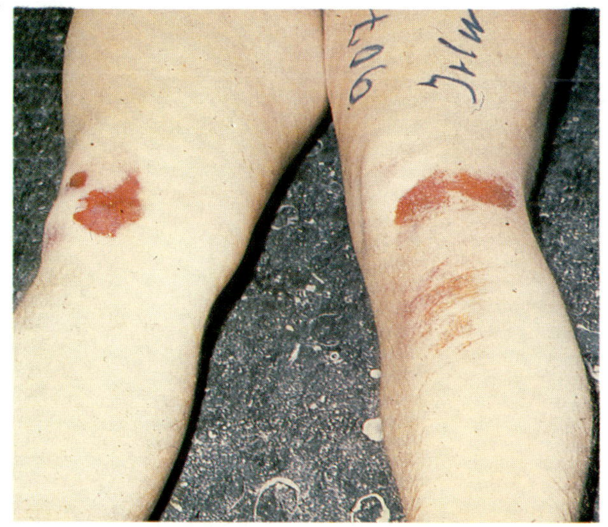

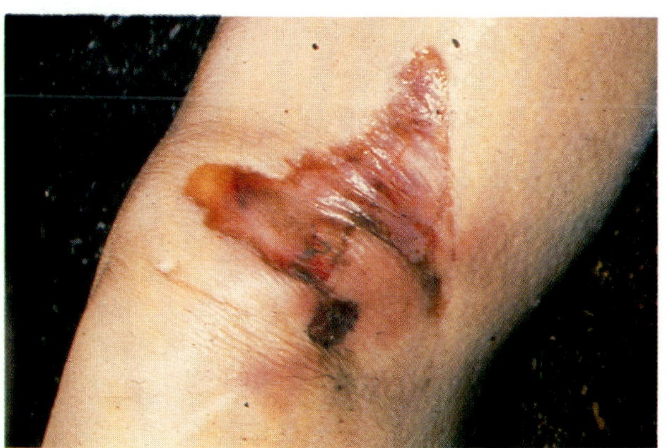

108 Abrasion and contusion on the right knee with haemorrhage in the surrounding tissue (dashboard injury).

107 Superficial abrasions on both knees and the left shin caused by impact against the dashboard.

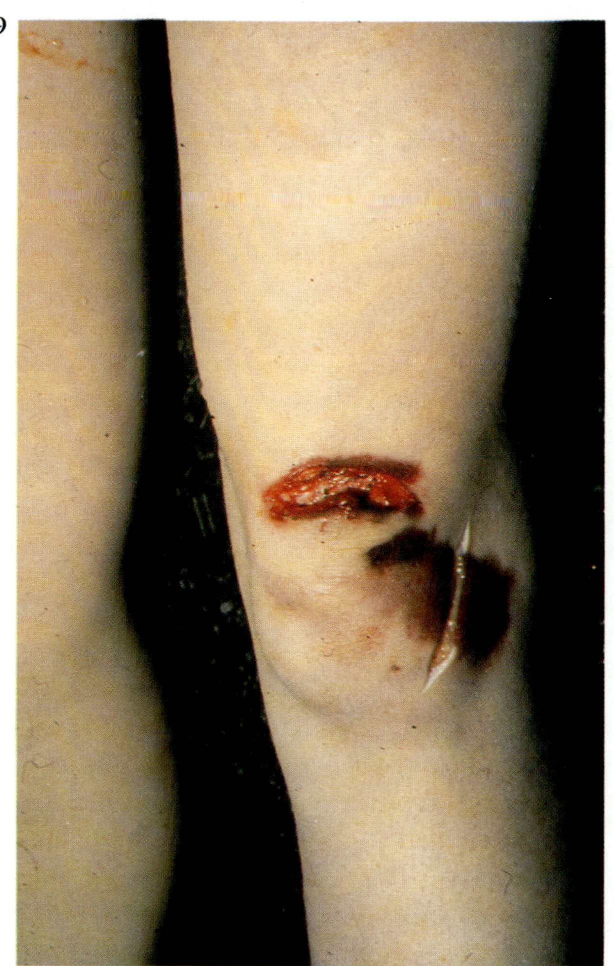

109 Transverse laceration above the left patella with haematoma on the lateral aspect, and effusion. (There is a post-mortem incision on the lateral aspect to demonstrate the extent of the haematomas.)

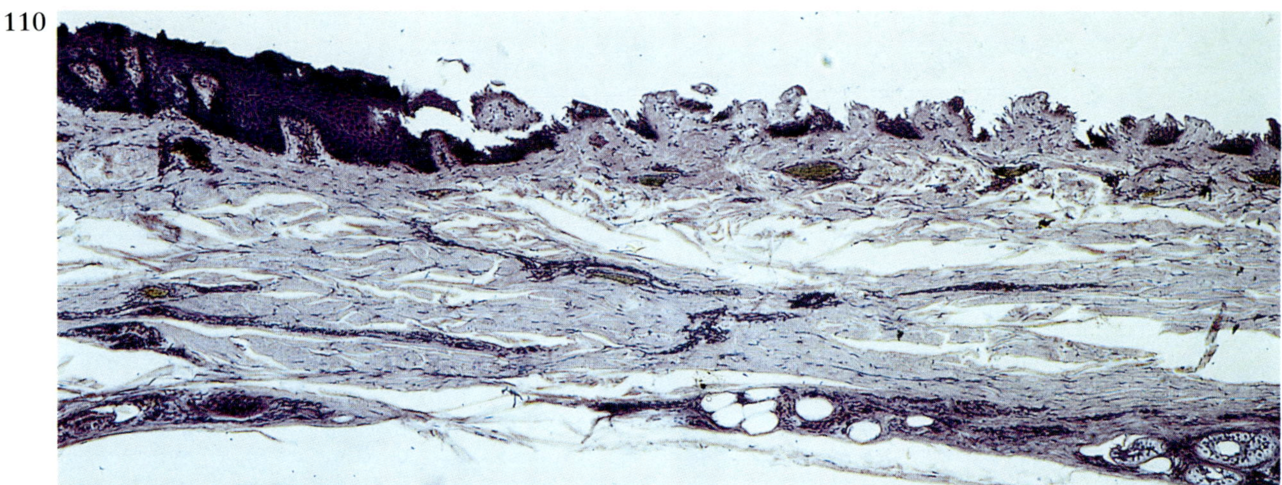

110 **Skin.** Recent scratch or abrasion with extensive loss of the epidermis. Papillary bodies are still intact. Hyperaemia of the dermis is to be seen beneath the defect. To preserve the structure of the torn tissue a thick section was necessary. (*H&E ×16*)

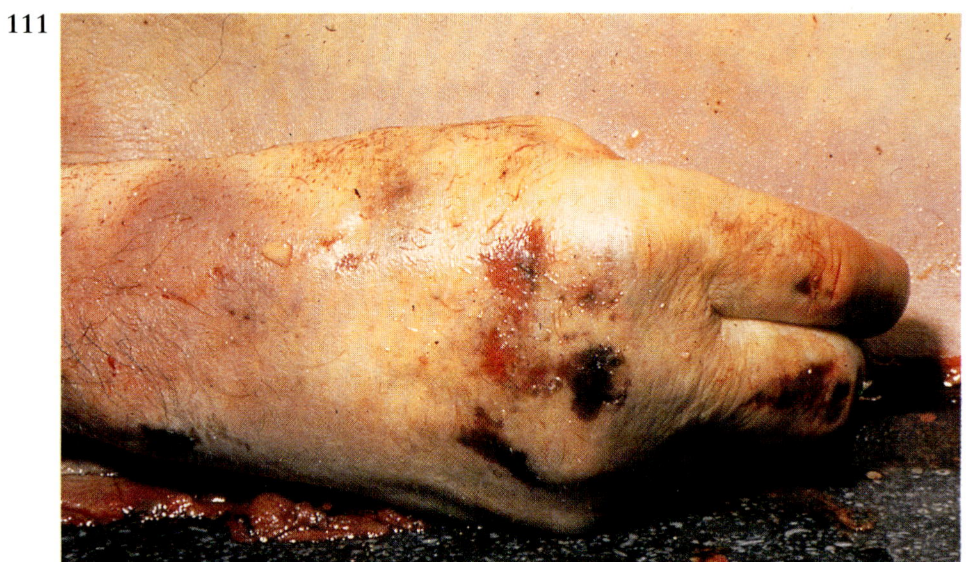

111 **Abrasions, scab formation and haematoma on the right hand** of a pedestrian who was run over by a lorry.

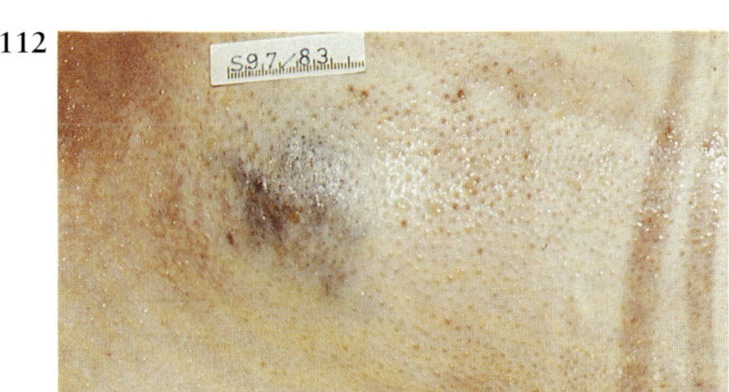

112 **Subcutaneous haematoma** as a result of blunt injury.

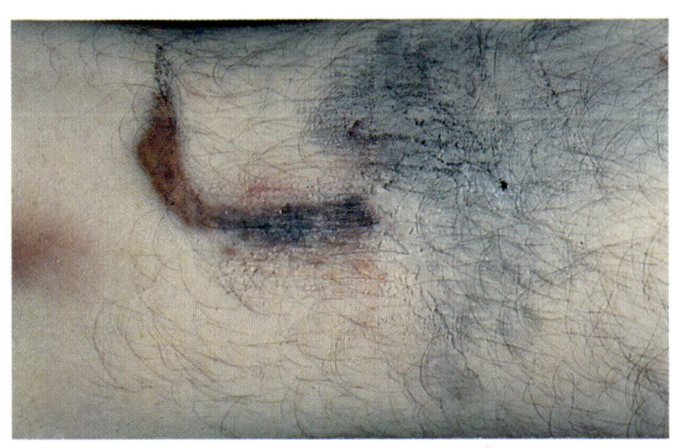

113 **Abrasions on the forearm** with contamination of the lesions with dirt.

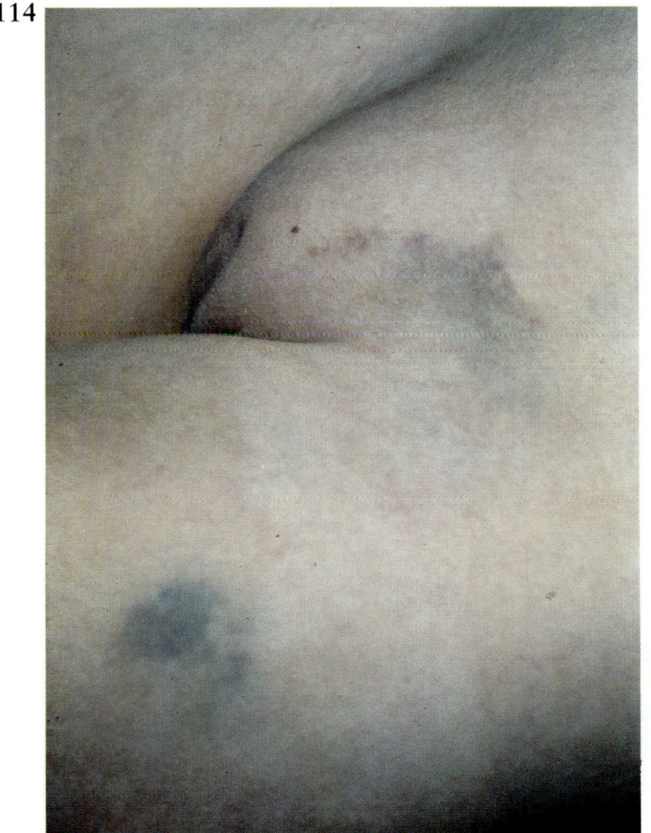

114 **Haematoma on the thigh and pubic region** of a young girl who was battered 3 days previously.

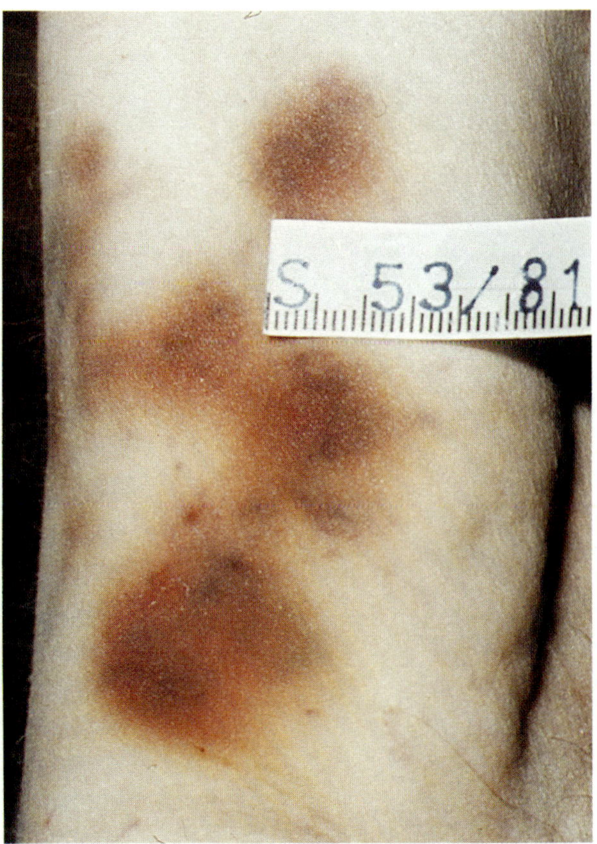

115 **Partially confluent haematoma,** a few days old (post-mortem photograph).

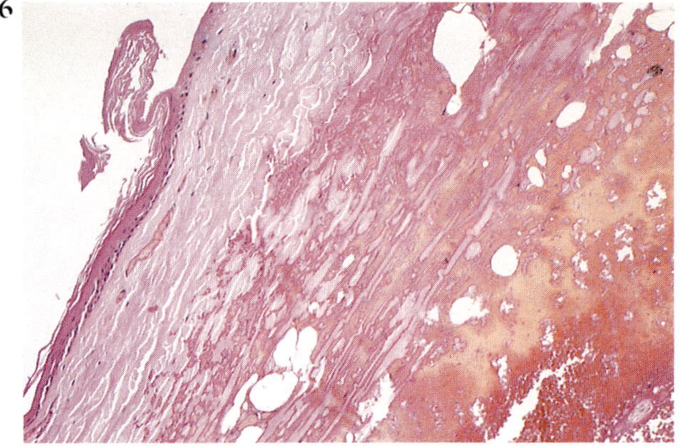

116 Skin. Superficial abrasion following a blow to the leg. Important features are the elevation of part of the epidermis, and massive diffuse bleeding in the dermis and subcutaneous tissue. Note also the marked gas formation caused by bacterial activity in the necrotic wound. Material obtained by wound debridement. (*H&E* ×63)

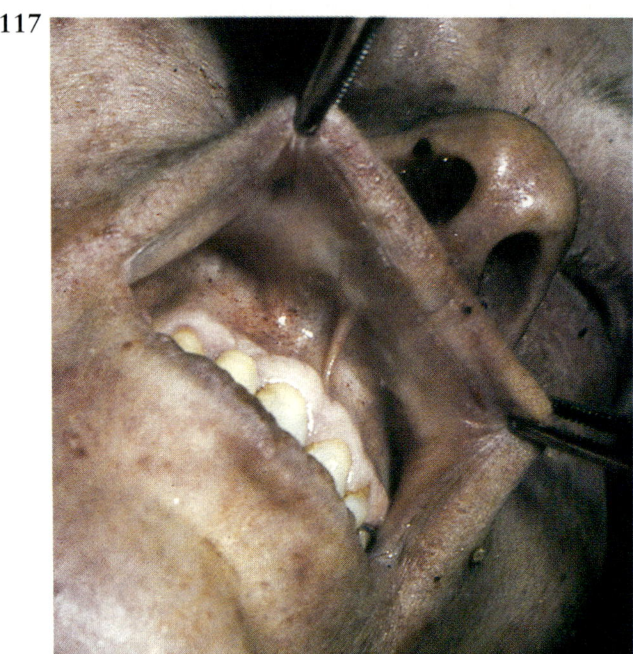

117 Haematoma in the region of the upper lip caused by a blow to the mouth.

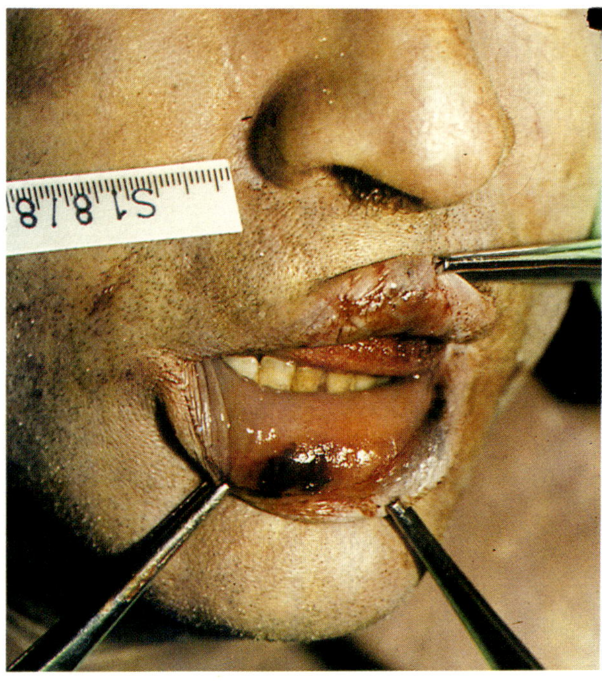

118 Haematoma in both lips. A laceration of the upper lip was caused by forcible contact between the lip and the upper teeth.

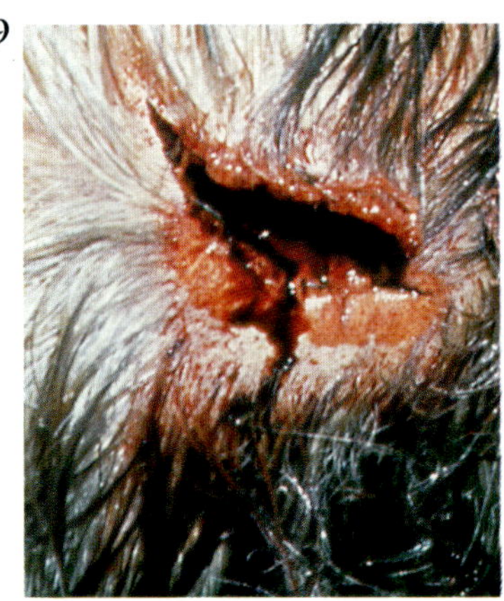

119 Gaping wound in the scalp, with extensive stripping of soft tissue.

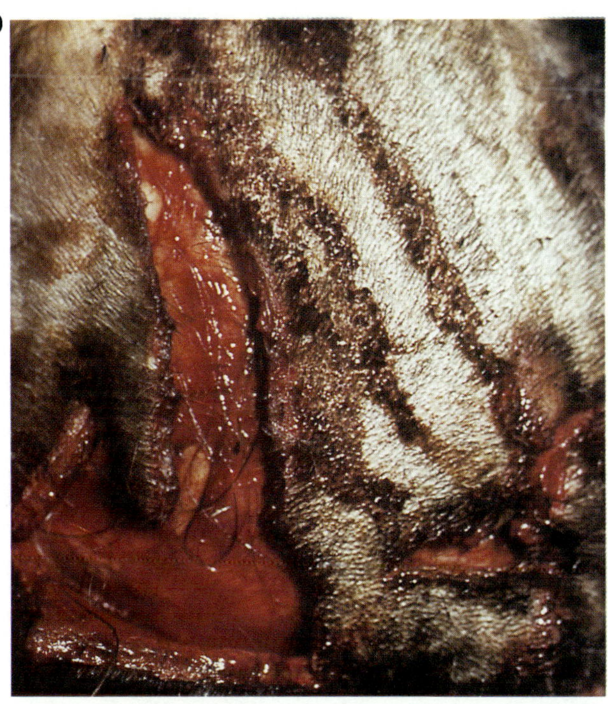

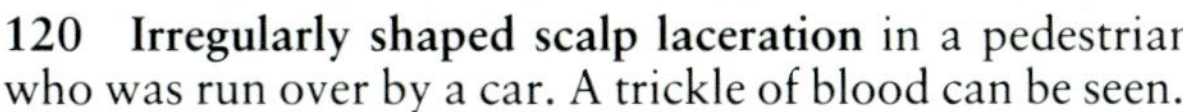

120   Irregularly shaped scalp laceration in a pedestrian who was run over by a car. A trickle of blood can be seen.

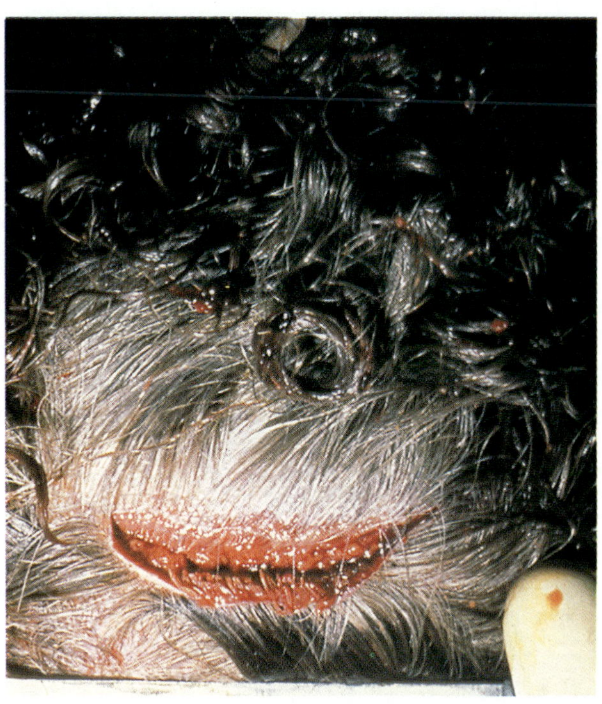

121   Scalp laceration in the parieto-occipital region as a result of impact of the head on the roof of a car. The pedestrian was struck by the car.

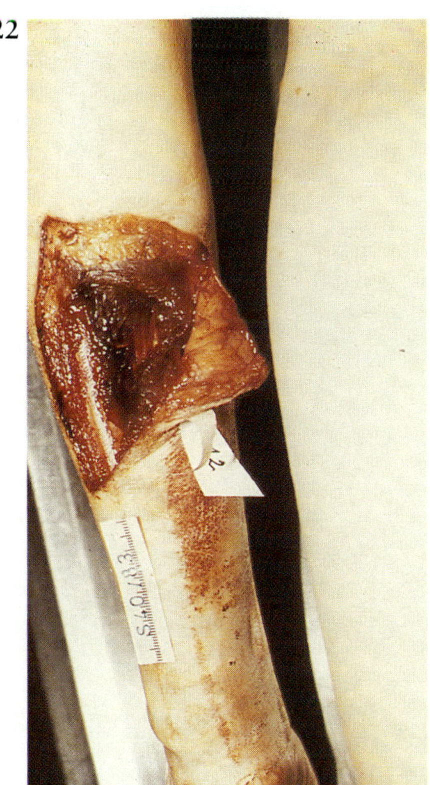

122   Impact injury to the posterior part of the left leg with extensive bleeding into the muscles. The pedestrian was hit from behind by a car.

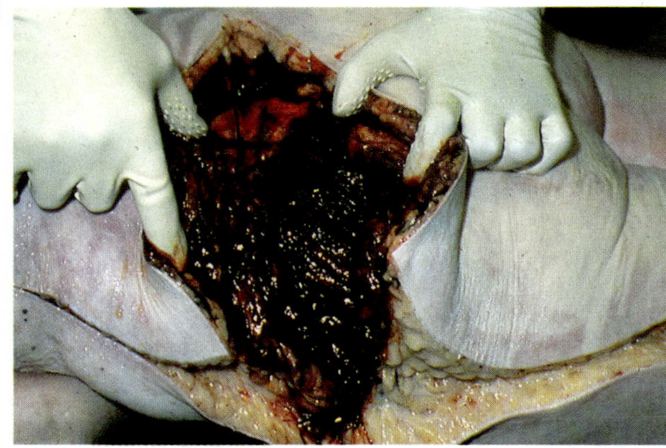

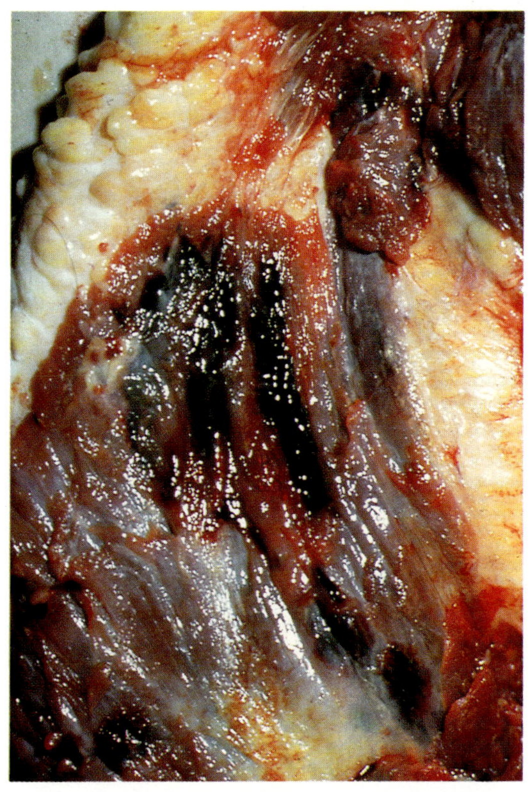

123 and **124** **Impact injury above the buttock** of a female pedestrian run over by a car. Note the extensive stripping of the soft tissues (décollement) with massive haemorrhage.

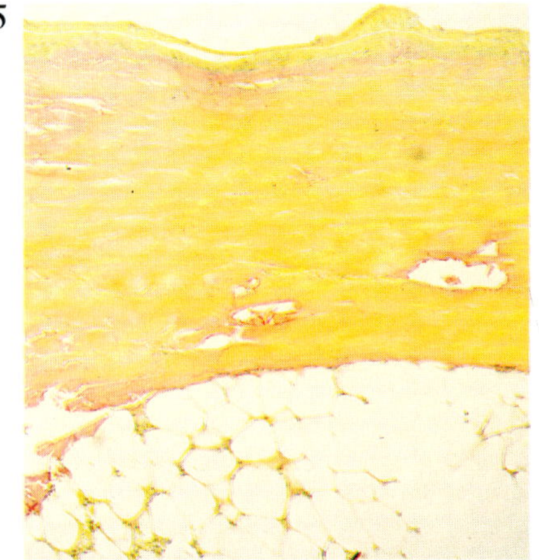

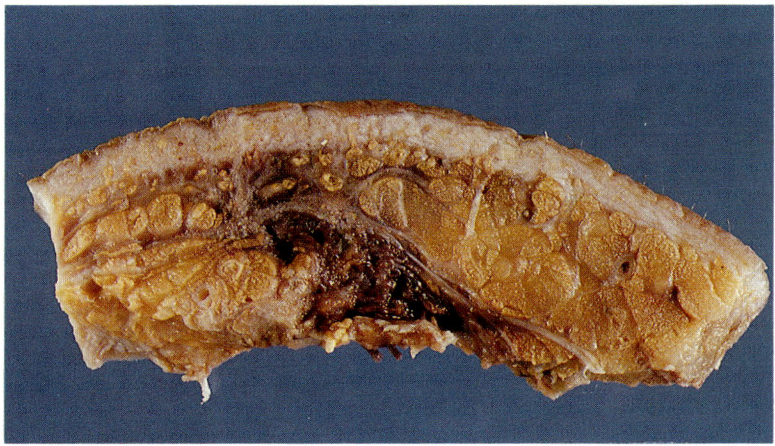

125 Skin (thigh). Impact injury caused by a car bumper. Note the thinning of the epidermis as a result of compression, and swelling of the dermis accompanied by an alteration in the staining reaction of the collagenous connective tissue (metachromasia) and the nuclei of the epidermal cells (poorly stained). (*van Gieson ×25*)

126 Skin and subcutaneous tissue from an impact injury without décollement. Strip-like areas of haemorrhage in the subcutaneous tissue.

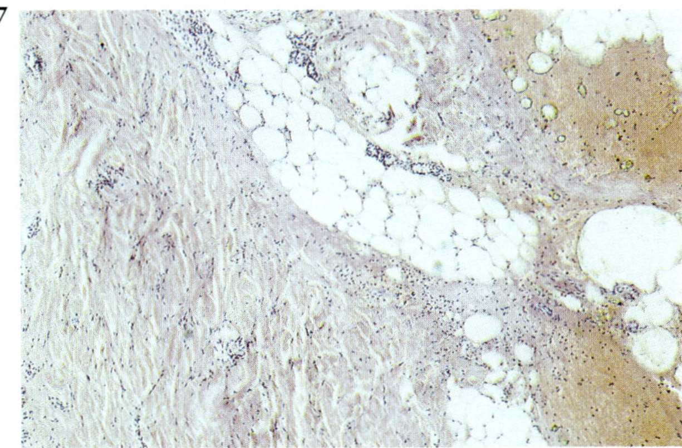

127 Skin. Acute bleeding into the subcutaneous tissue (right). Note that the remaining dermis is free of haemorrhage. An artefactual feature in the area of haemorrhage is the presence of formalin pigment, precipitated during routine tissue processing. (*H&E ×16*)

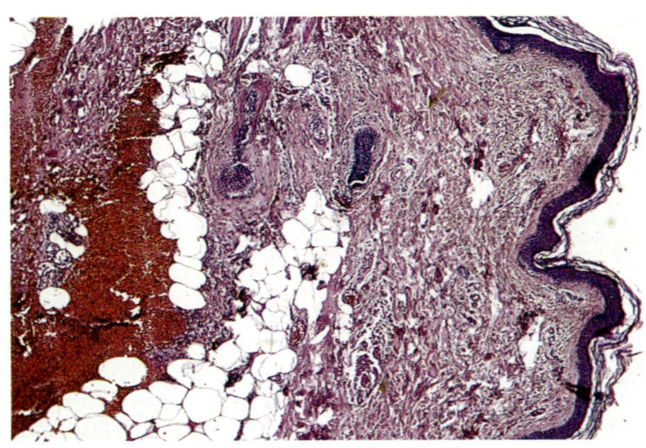

128 Skin and subcutaneous tissue. Blunt injury caused by beating with the fist. Note the extensive haemorrhage in the subcutaneous adipose tissue. Epidermis and dermis show no evidence of injury. Material from a 28 year-old woman. (*H&E ×40*)

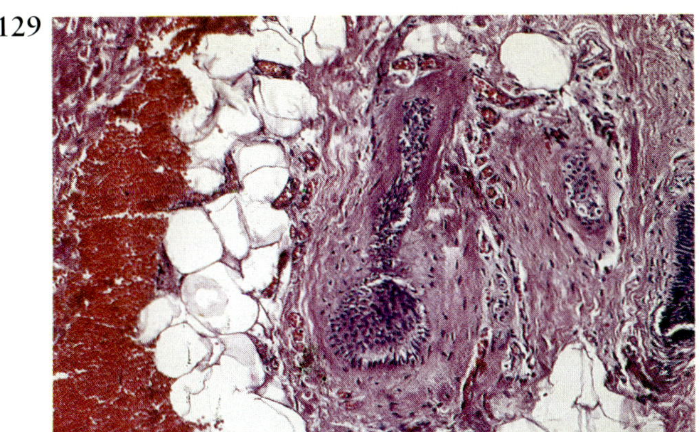

129 Same case as in **128**, but higher magnification (×250).

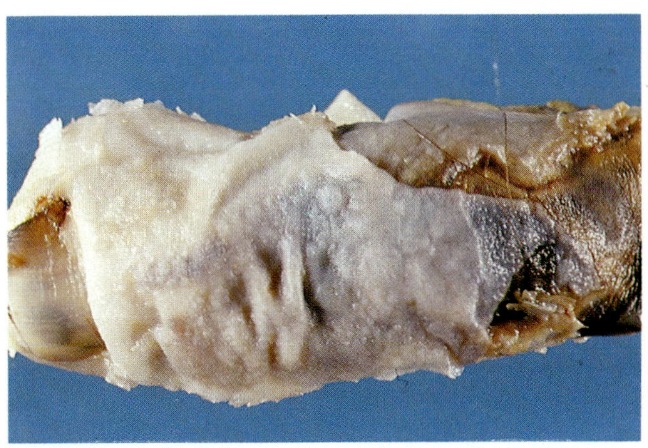

130 Severely crushed toe after amputation, with necrosis and removal of the skin.

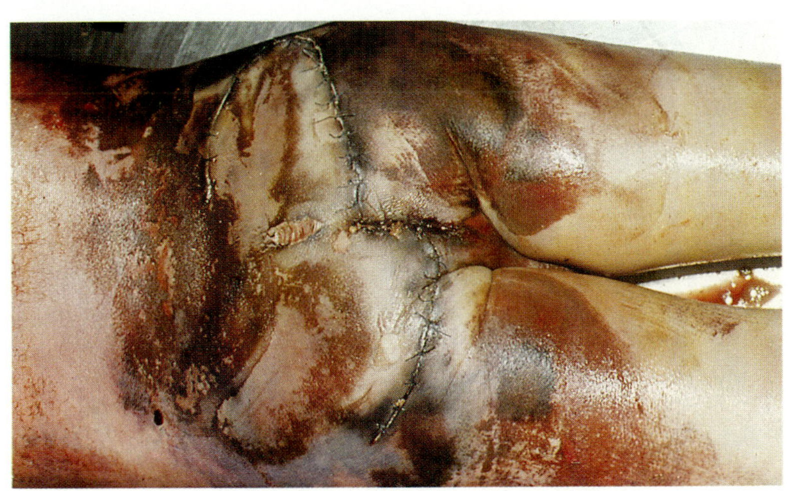

131 Severe contusion and laceration of the skin in the buttock region of a 6 year-old boy run over by a lorry (crush injury). The sutures are from surgery after the injury.

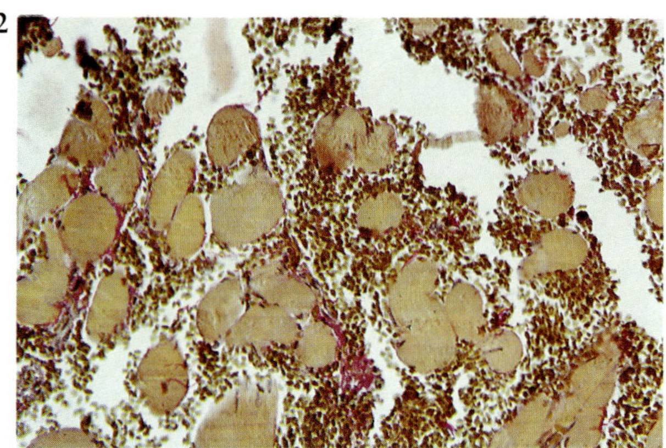

132 Skeletal muscle. Acute haemorrhage with dissociation of the muscle bundles. The characteristic striation pattern of the individual muscle cells is for the most part intact. (*van Gieson ×63*)

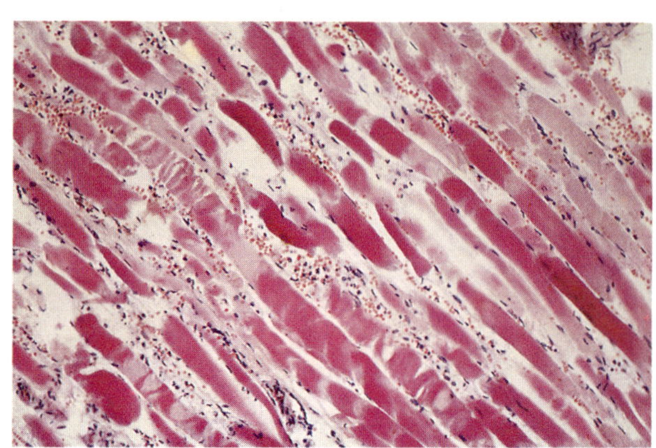

133 Skeletal muscle. Crush injury to the thigh muscles as a result of a road traffic accident. One sees the reduced stainability of portions of the partially disrupted muscle fibres as well as erythrocytes between the fibres. Material from a 6 year-old boy who died 2 days following the accident. (*H&E ×25*)

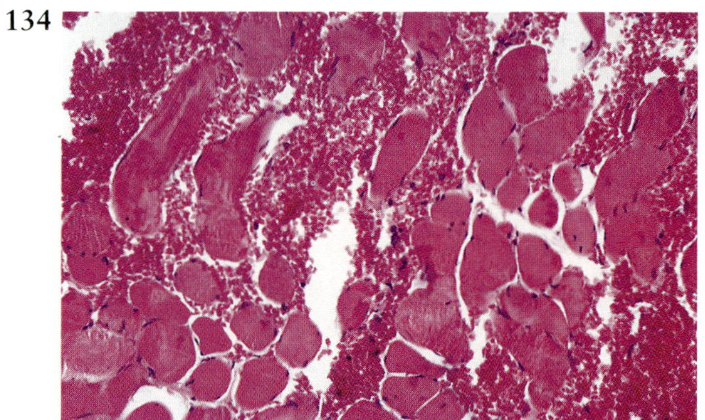

134 Skeletal muscle. Acute injury with haemorrhage between the muscle cells. (*H&E ×25*)

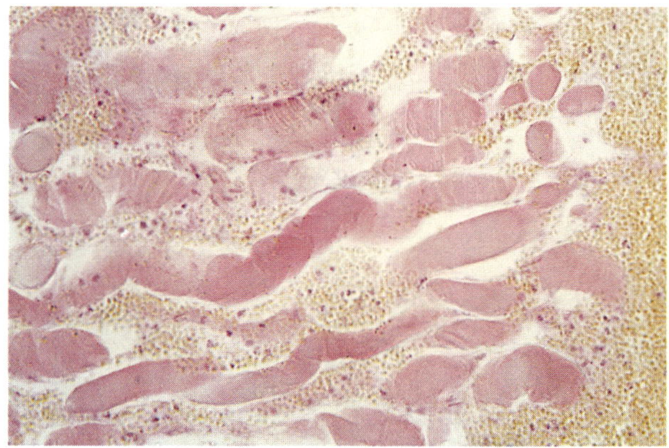

135 Skeletal muscle. 4 day-old injury with haemorrhage and disruption of the structure of the muscle bundles. Marked necrosis is evident from the loss of striation pattern and decreased staining reaction of the myocyte nuclei. (*H&E ×63*)

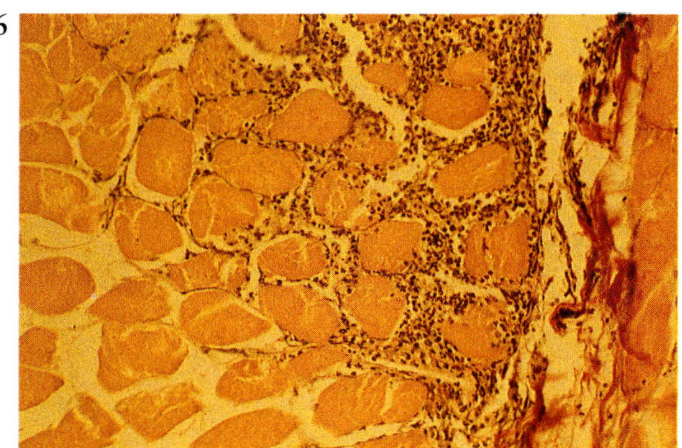

136 Skeletal muscle. Purulent inflammation (3 days after injury) with numerous polymorphonuclear granulocytes at the periphery of an area of necrosis caused by a crush injury to the muscle of the thigh. Dissociation of the connective tissue (red) caused during sectioning. (*H&E ×63*)

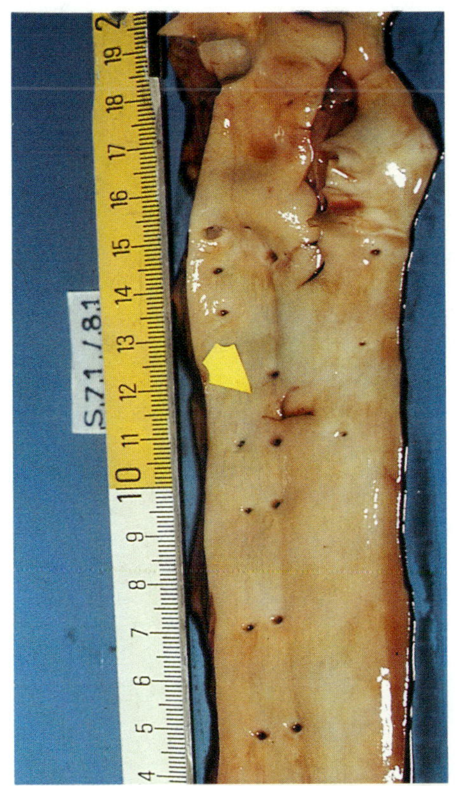

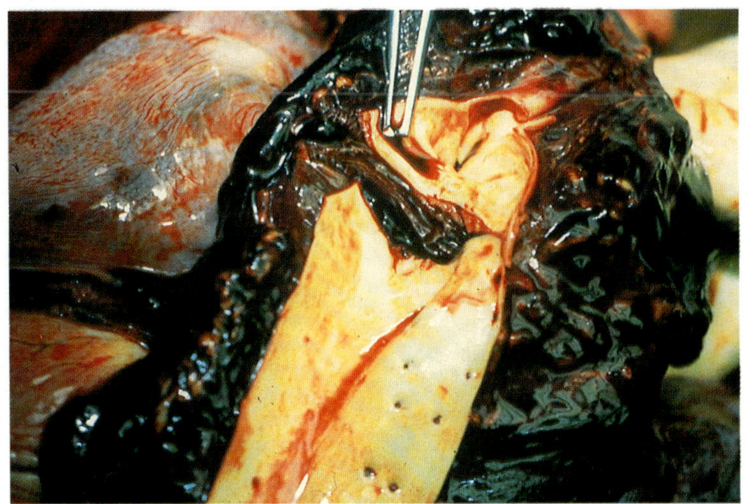

137   Thoracic aorta. Rupture (arrow) caused by severe blunt injury to the thorax of a driver of a car involved in a road traffic accident.

138   Thoracic aorta. Transverse rupture at a characteristic site, namely the origin of the descending part. Severe blunt injury to the thorax of a passenger in a vehicle in an accident.

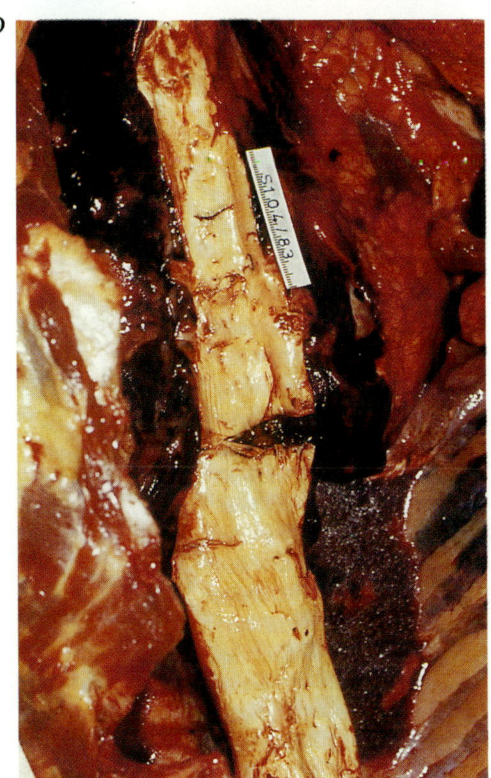

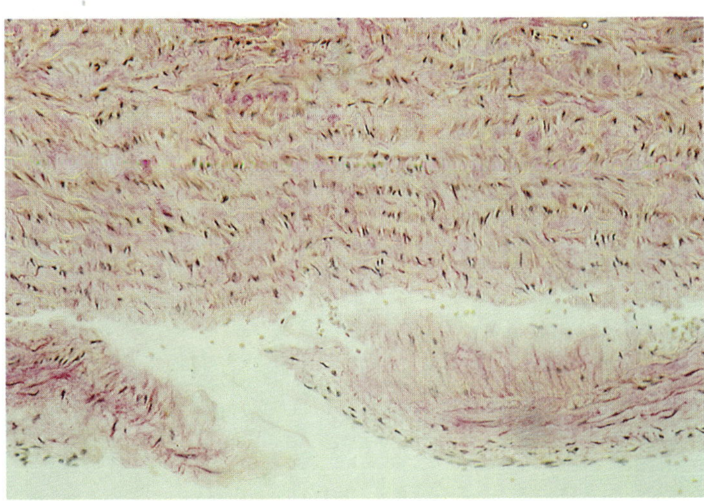

139   Thoracic aorta. Multiple tears as a result of a severe crush injury to the thorax in a pedestrian run over by a car.

140   Thoracic aorta. Dilatation of the intima following an accident in which the victim was run over by a train. As death was instantaneous there is no inflammatory reaction. (*van Gieson ×50*)

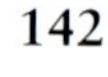

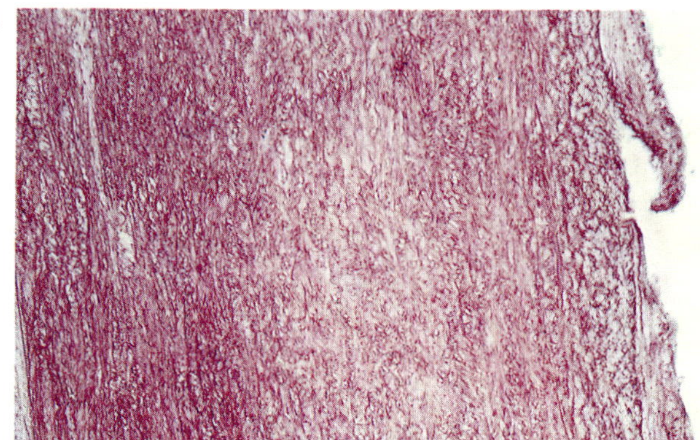

141 Thoracic aorta. Intimal tear (right) with involvement of the tunica media in a 38 year-old male following a road traffic accident. Instantaneous death, therefore no inflammatory reaction. (*H&E ×25*)

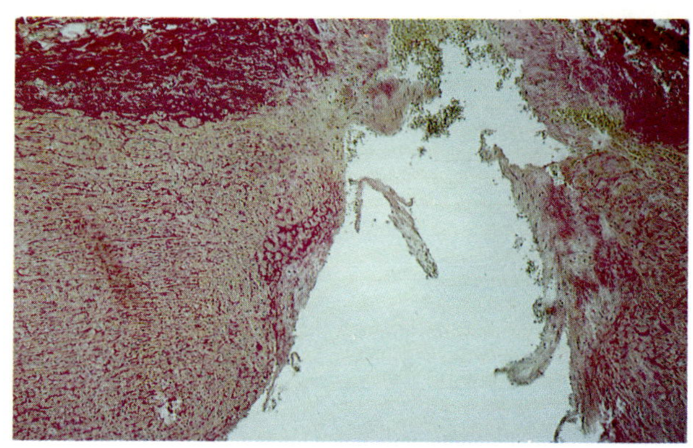

142 Thoracic aorta. Crush rupture of the aorta caused by a vertebral body as a result of thoracic compression. The rupture edges show disintegration of the intimal tissue. Further features are the disruption of the adventitial connective tissue (red) and the presence of erythrocytes (green). Material from a young male who died instantly in a road traffic accident. (*van Gieson ×20*)

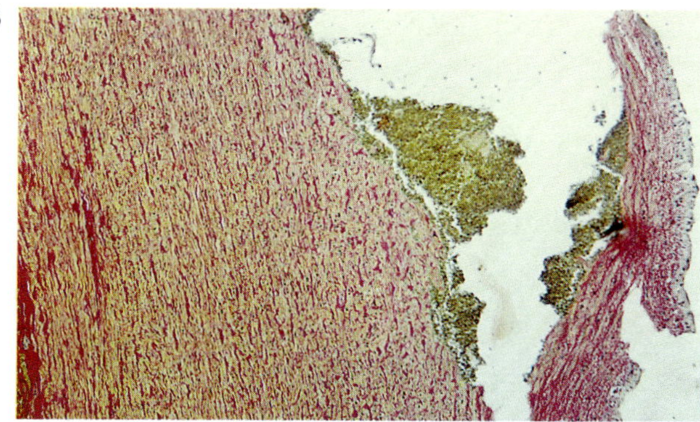

143 Thoracic aorta (proximal part of the aortic arch). Partial rupture caused by a road traffic accident. Erythrocytes (green) are seen in the rupture cleft. Death occurred 3 hours after injury. (*van Gieson ×25*)

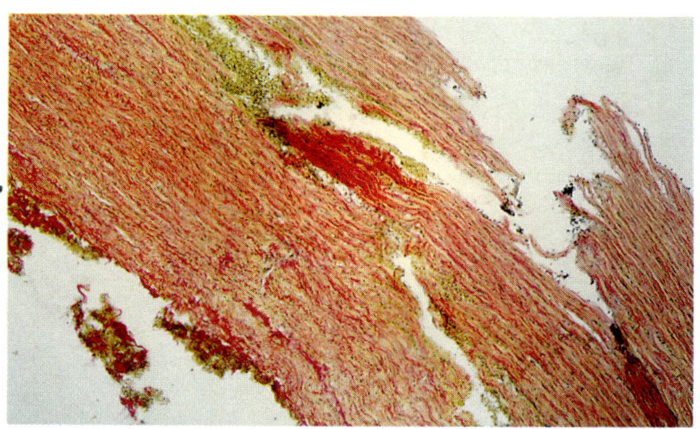

144 Thoracic aorta (proximal part of the aortic arch). Rupture with disruption of the structure of the aortic wall and haemorrhage in the rupture clefts (erythrocytes stained green). Death occurred within minutes of injury. (*van Gieson ×25*)

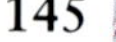

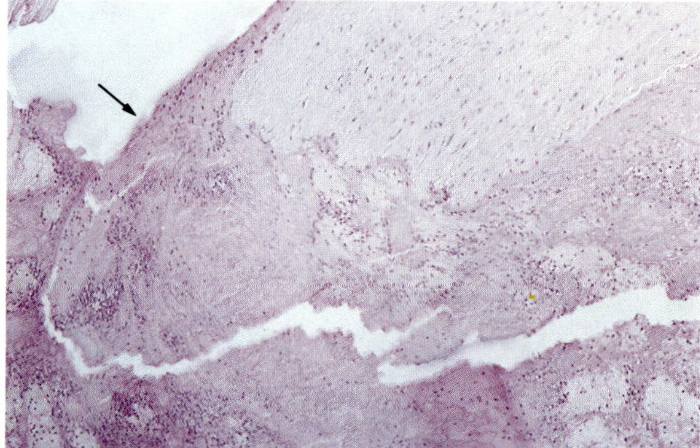

145 and 146 Thoracic aorta. Partial rupture caused by a road traffic accident. Material from a 35 year-old female who lived for 4 days after the accident. Between the

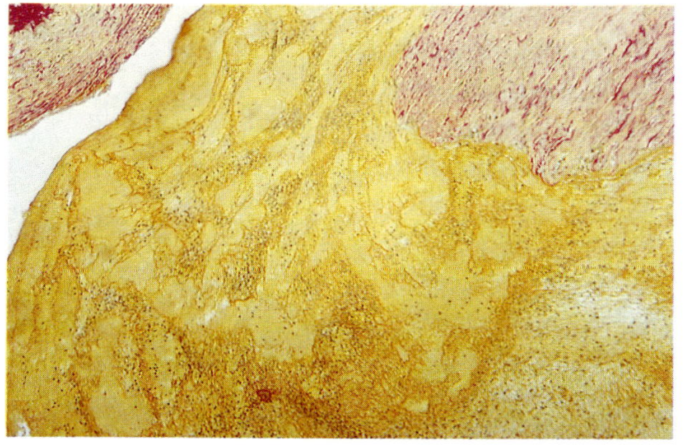

partially necrotic edges of the aortic rupture (arrow) lie large amounts of fibrin containing numerous leucocytes. (*H&E and van Gieson ×25*)

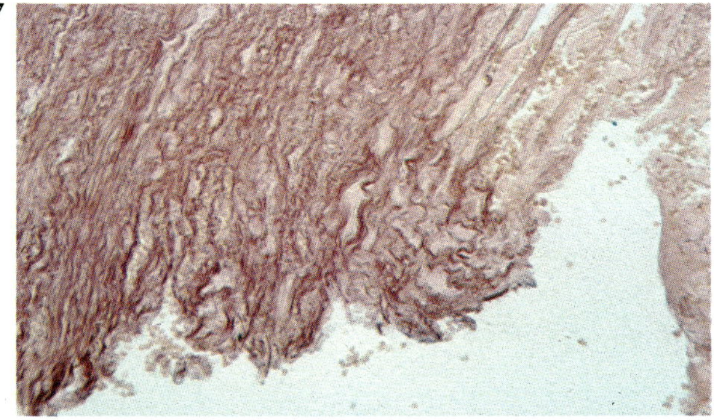

147 Thoracic aorta. A recent complete rupture of the thoracic aorta as a result of blunt injury to the thorax. The autopsy was performed 3 days after death, hence the autolytic changes. The structure of the elastic fibres is recognisable. (*Elastic stain: resorcin–fuchsin ×63*)

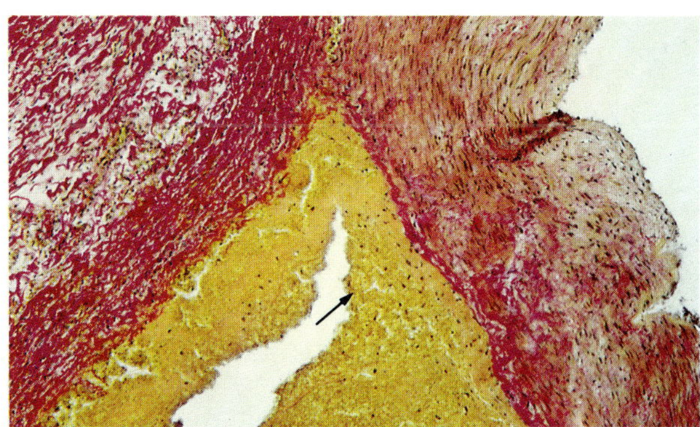

148 External carotid artery. Subintimal haematoma (arrow) following a blow to the neck with the fist. The patient survived the trauma for 8 days. (*van Gieson ×25*)

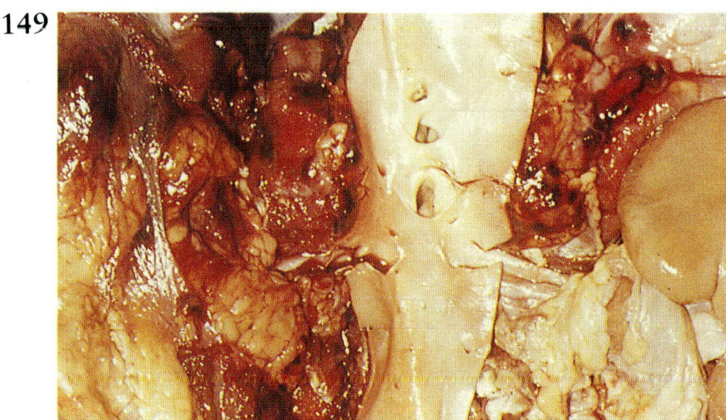

149 Traumatic rupture of the abdominal aorta at the level of the superior mesenteric artery with haemorrhage into the para-aortic tissue. Material from a 19 year-old man, who was run over by a car. Death was instantaneous.

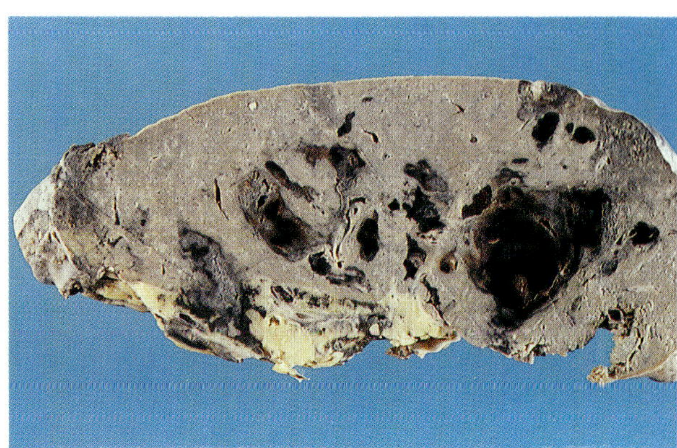

150 Spleen. Multiple capsule tears and areas of haemorrhage in the parenchyma caused by blunt upper abdominal injury in a road traffic injury. (Formalin-fixed operative specimen)

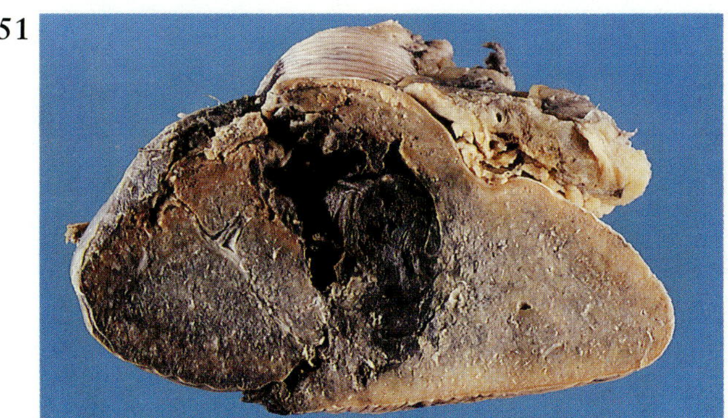

151 Spleen. Extensive crushing with massive haemorrhage in a road accident victim. (Formalin-fixed specimen)

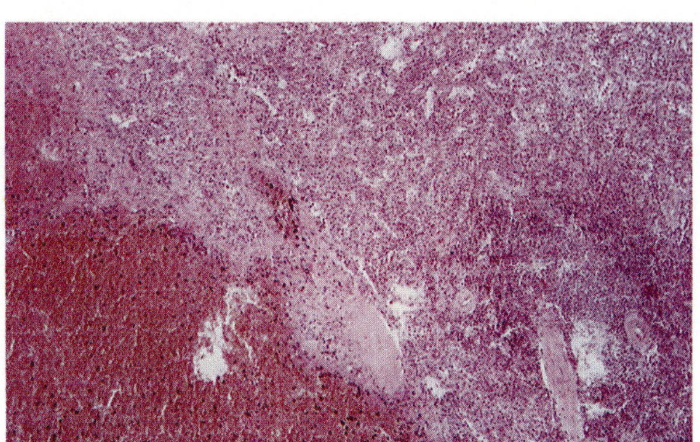

152 Spleen. Fresh rupture with massive haemorrhage (bottom left) and dissociation of the parenchyma. Note the artefactual formalin pigment in the area of haemorrhage. Operative removal of the ruptured spleen in a 20 year-old male. (*H&E ×25*)

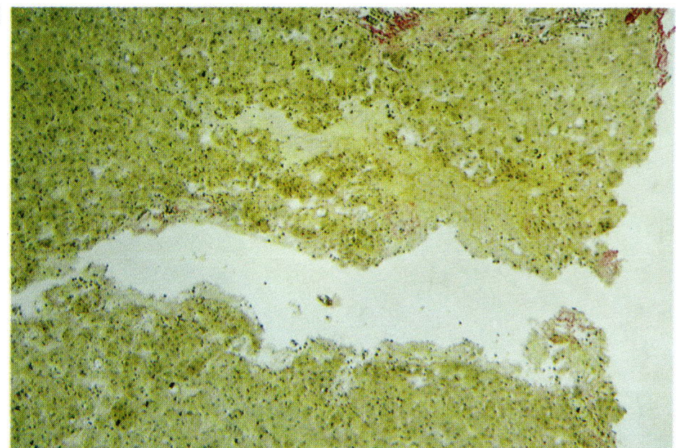

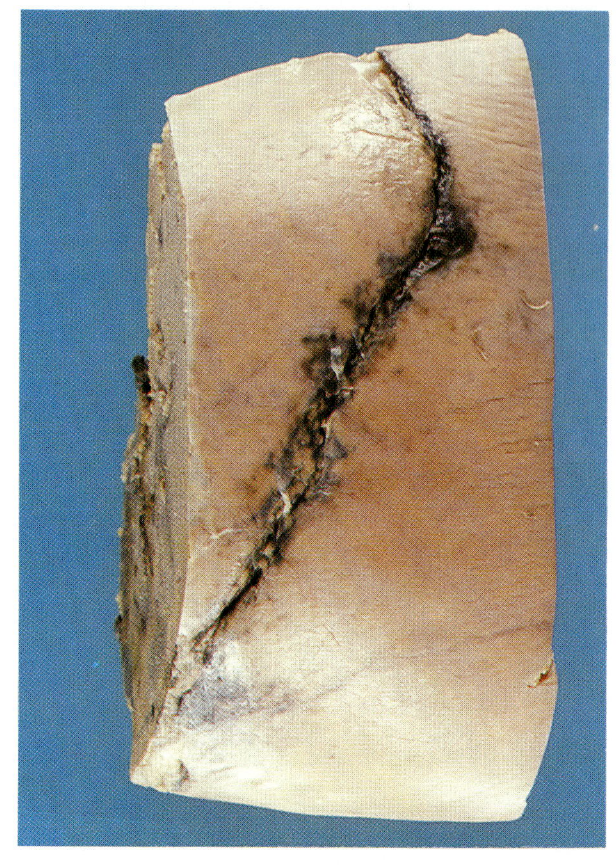

153 Spleen. Fresh rupture of the splenic capsule with dissociation of the adjacent parenchyma and haemorrhage. (*van Gieson ×25*)

154 Liver. Deep laceration with intrahepatic haemorrhage caused by blunt injury to a driver involved in a road traffic accident. (*Formalin-fixed operative specimen*)

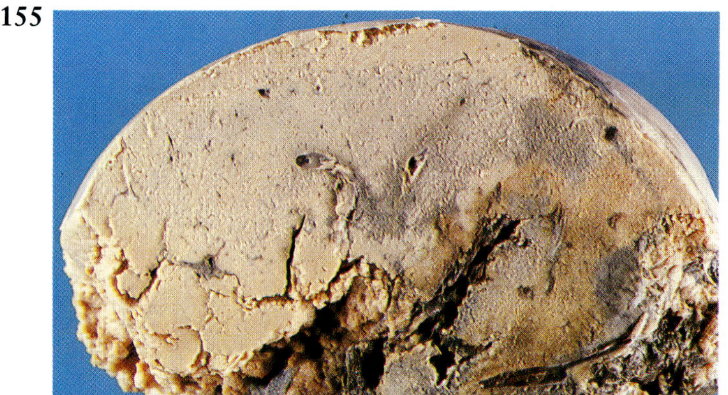

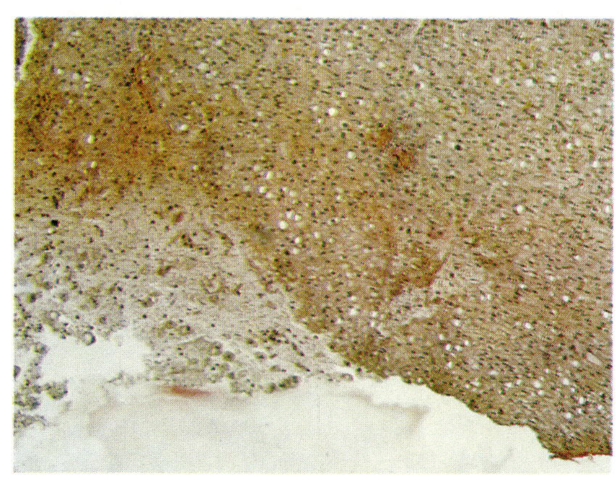

155 Same as **154**. Lateral view showing the laceration and parenchymal haemorrhage.

156 Liver. Extensive superficial parenchymal injury to the liver, which shows fatty change. At the bottom left, individual disrupted hepatocytes may be seen together with fibrinous material and cell debris. Survival time after injury: 20 hours (*van Gieson ×25*)

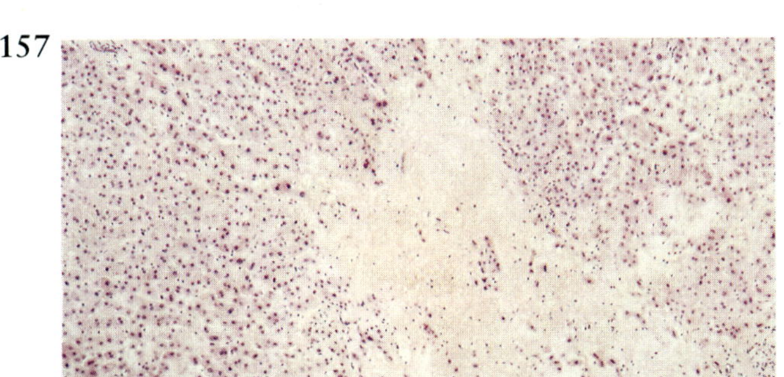

157   Liver. Recent contusion of the liver with central laceration of the hepatic parenchyma and haemorrhage (centre). At the bottom right, a non-specific cellular infiltrate in a periportal region — an incidental finding unrelated to the trauma. (*H&E ×25*)

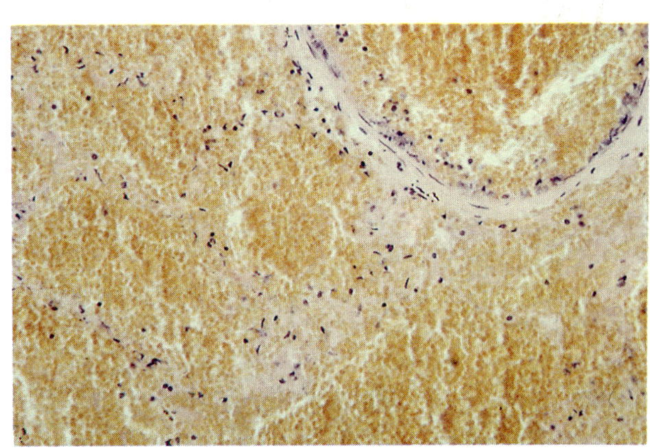

158   Liver. Laceration of the liver. Important features are the presence of blood, fibrin and disrupted liver parenchymal cells in the region of the rupture. The patient survived for 30 minutes after the injury. (*H&E ×25*)

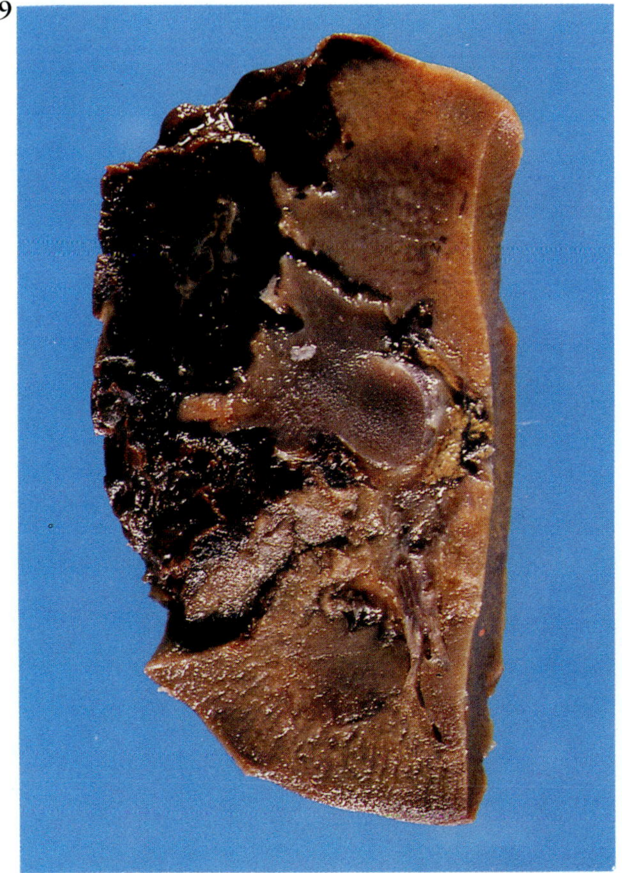

159   Kidney. Severe blunt injury to the kidney with parenchymal laceration and massive haemorrhage in the medullary region. Injuries sustained in a road traffic accident.

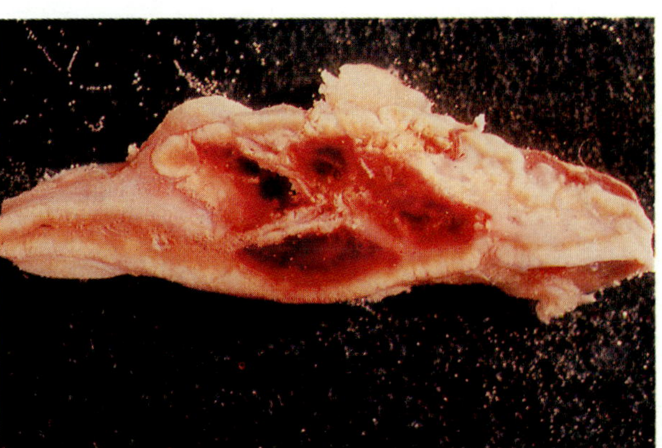

160   Adrenal gland. Severe haemorrhage in the adrenal medulla caused by blunt injury to the abdomen.

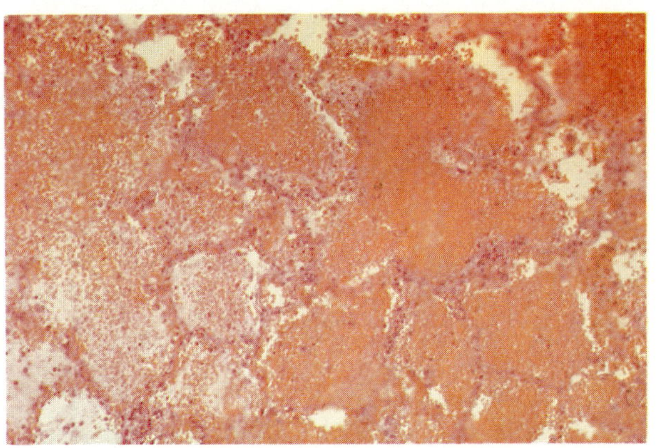

161   Lung. Intra-alveolar haemorrhage following thorax contusion. A dilated blood vessel is also seen (upper right). Autolysis is beginning (the autopsy was performed 36 hours after death). (*H&E ×60*)

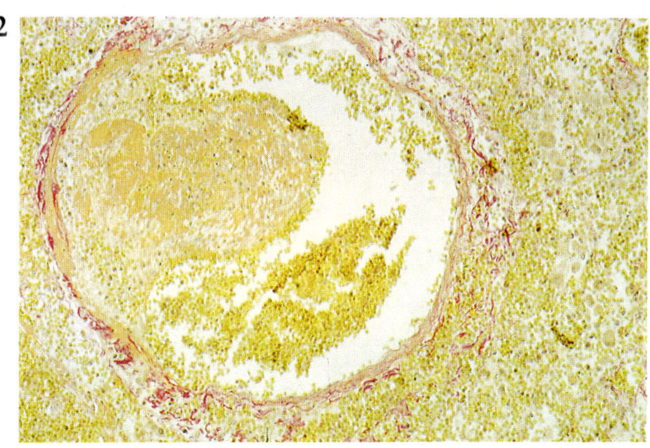

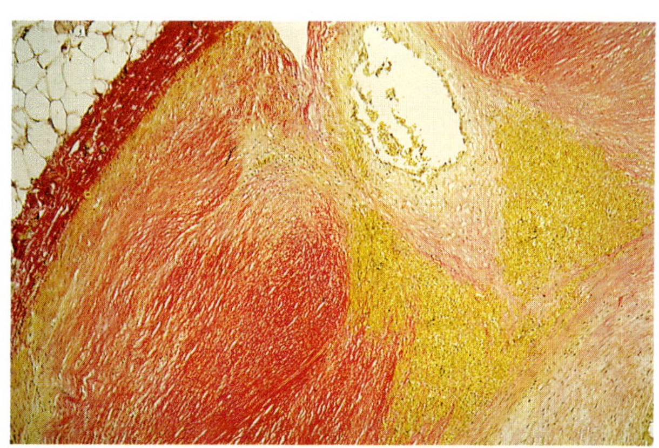

162 Lung. Thrombus in a branch of the pulmonary artery caused by pulmonary contusion. Post-traumatic survival time: 3 days. (*van Gieson ×40*)

163 Heart. Arteriosclerosis of the descending branch of the left coronary artery. Of traumatological interest is the acute haemorrhage (yellow–green) in the arterial wall as a result of cardiac contusion. (*van Gieson ×20*)

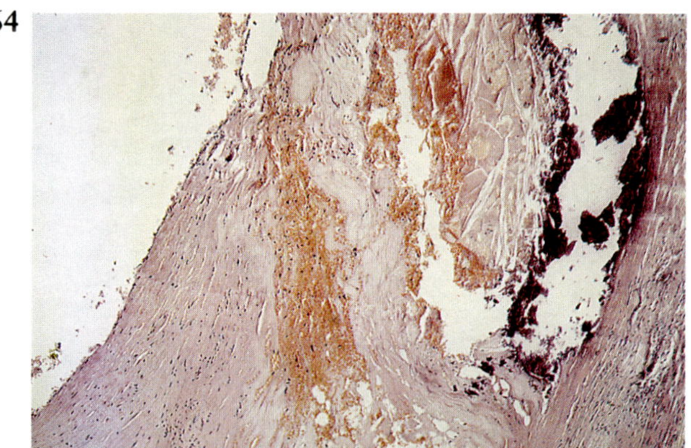

164 Ascending branch of the left coronary artery. Haemorrhage into the arteriosclerotic wall following cardiac bruising. The horizontal bands were caused during sectioning by the calcium deposits (violet, right) present in the arterial wall. (*van Gieson ×20*)

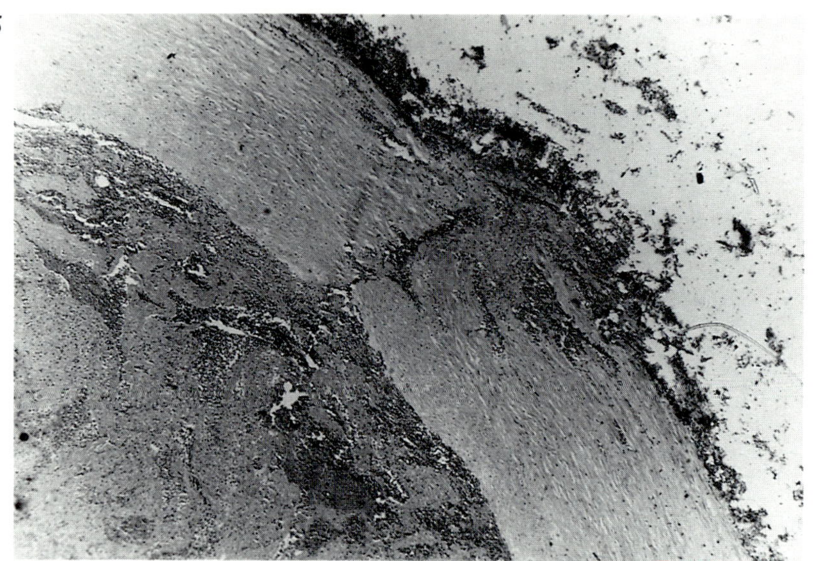

165 Common carotid artery. Traumatic thrombosis and rupture of the artery following a road traffic accident with whiplash injury. The 76 year-old victim survived for 3 days. (*H&E ×16*)

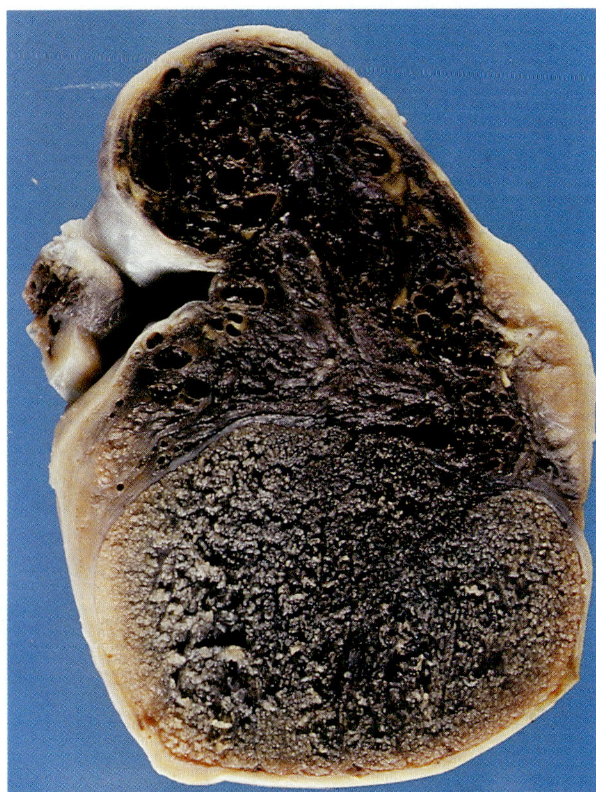

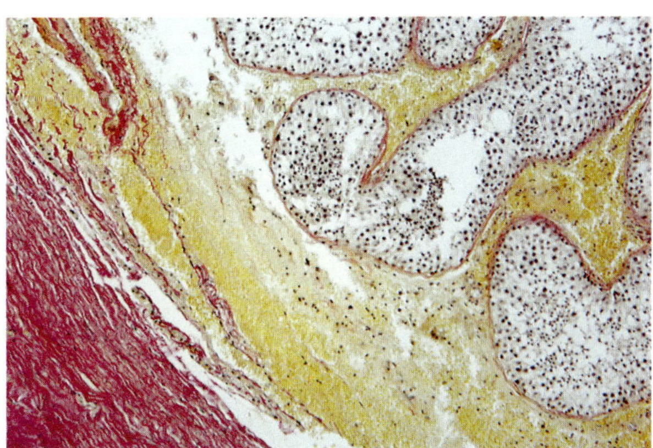

167 Testis. Subcapsular and interstitial haemorrhage, appearing yellow–orange in the van Gieson stain. Thick bands of collagenous connective tissue of the testicular capsule (red) can be seen on the left. (*van Gieson ×25*)

166 Testis and epididymis. Severe haemorrhage and infarction as a result of blunt injury. (*Formalin fixed*)

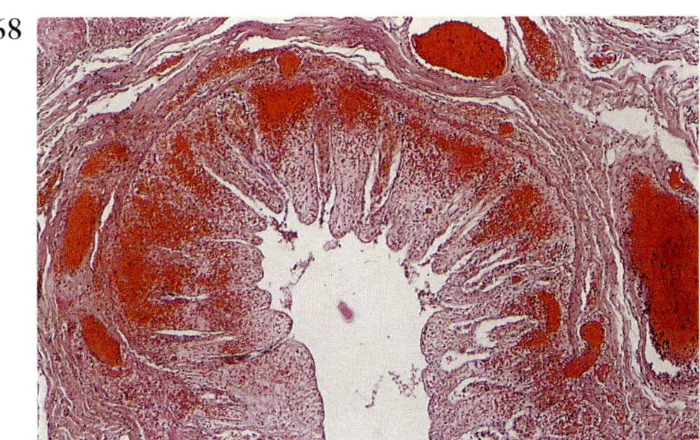

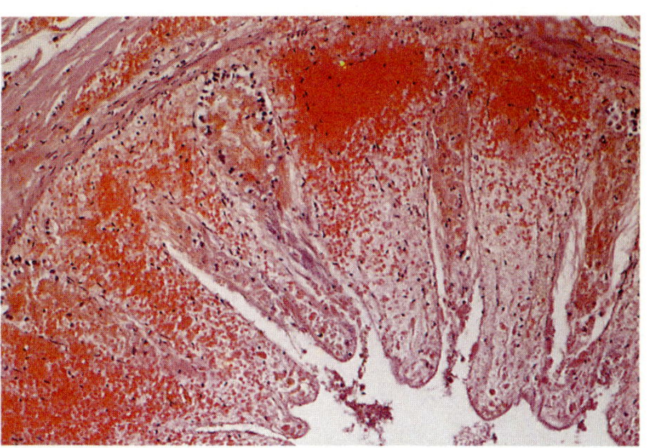

168 Colon. Crush injury to a 6 year-old boy who was run over by a bus. Post-traumatic survival: 2 days. Note the diffuse mucosal haemorrhage, dilatation and hyperaemia of the submucosal vessels and the loss of epithelial components. (*H&E ×100*)

169 Colon. As in **168**. The loss of the epithelial cell layer is evident, as is mucosal necrosis (middle) (*H&E ×250*)

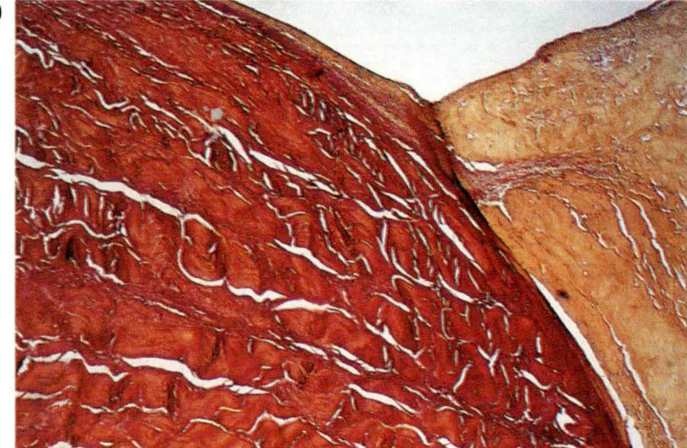

170 Tendon (from the foot). Rupture of the tendon. Note the fibrinoid deposit (right). (*van Gieson ×25*)

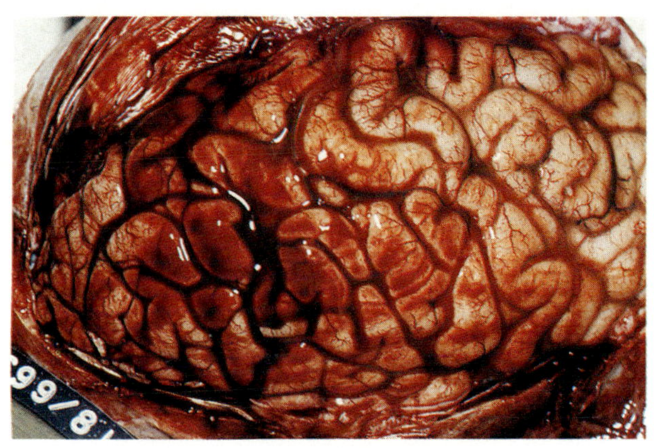

171 Day-old subarachnoid haemorrhage in the right occipital region due to blunt trauma.

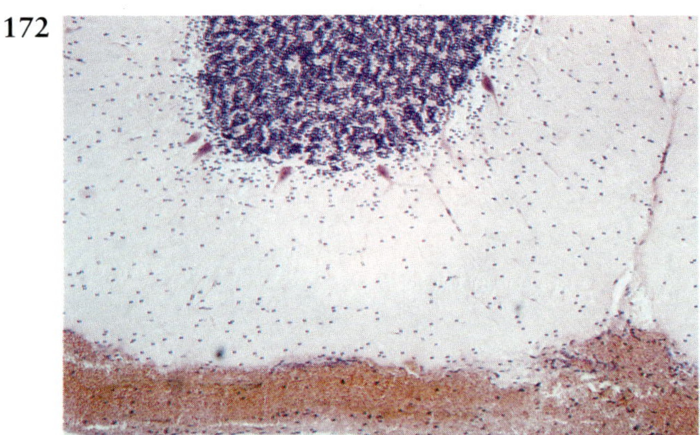

172 Cerebellum following a closed head injury. A recent subarachnoid haemorrhage can be seen (bottom). Note the normal structure of the granular layer and the Purkinje cells. (*H&E ×25*)

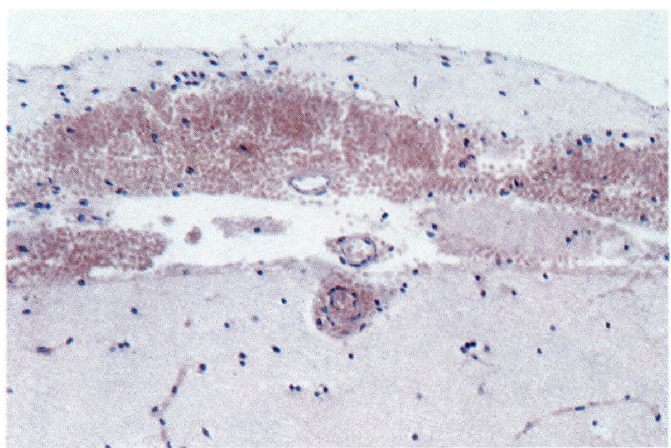

173 Cerebrum. Acute subarachnoid haemorrhage in a 43 year-old female who was beaten to death. A small area of intracerebral haemorrhage can be seen. (*H&E ×60*)

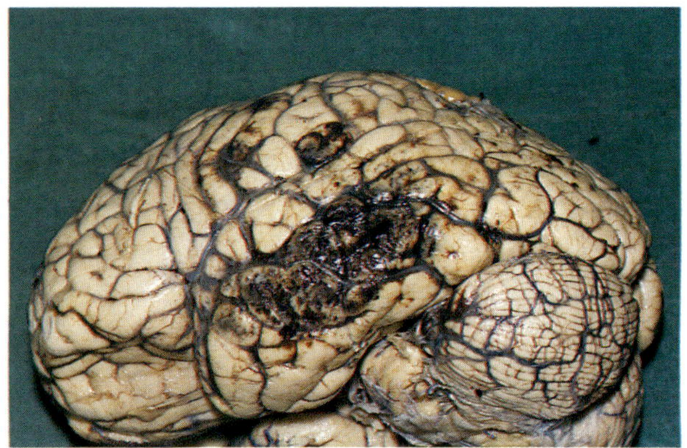

174 Cortical contusion of the left temporal lobe of the brain with haemorrhage in necrotic areas. (*Formalin-fixed brain*)

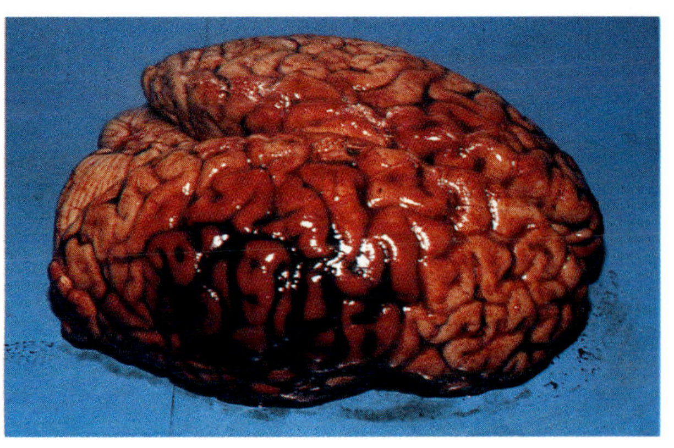

175 Extensive subarachnoid haemorrhage over the right parietal lobe, in particular in the sulci. Focal contusion of the cerebral cortex with oedema.

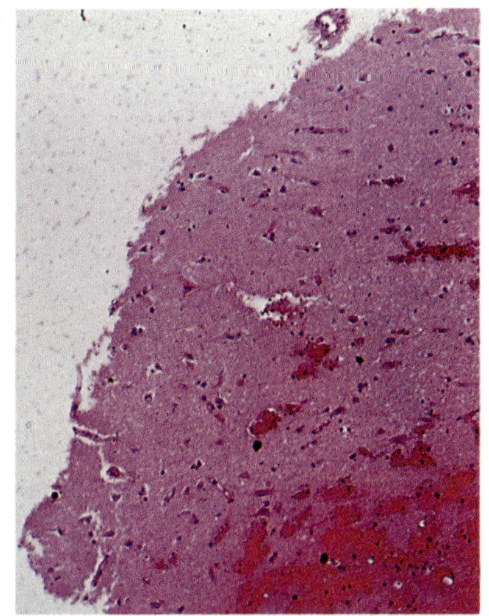

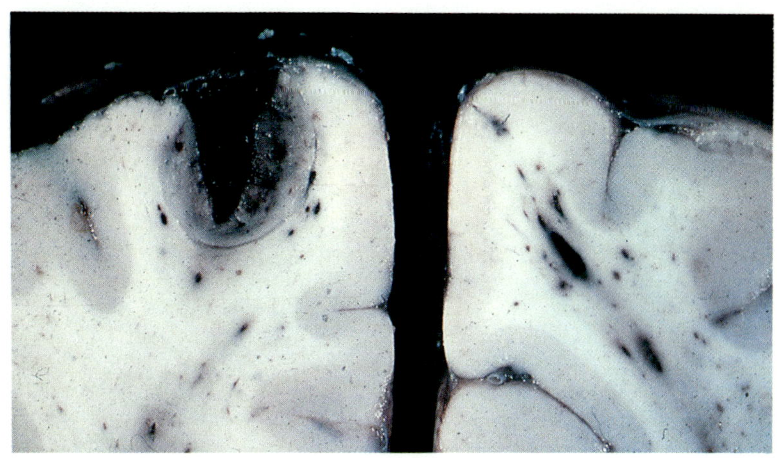

177 Circumscribed contusion of the cerebral cortex. Punctate and streak-like areas of haemorrhage in the white matter.

176 Cerebral cortex. Contusion of the cerebral cortex, showing multiple, partially confluent areas of haemorrhage. Note separation of the leptomeninges (artefact) and the presence of formalin pigment. From a 19 year-old man who survived for 10 hours after a road accident. (*H&E ×63*)

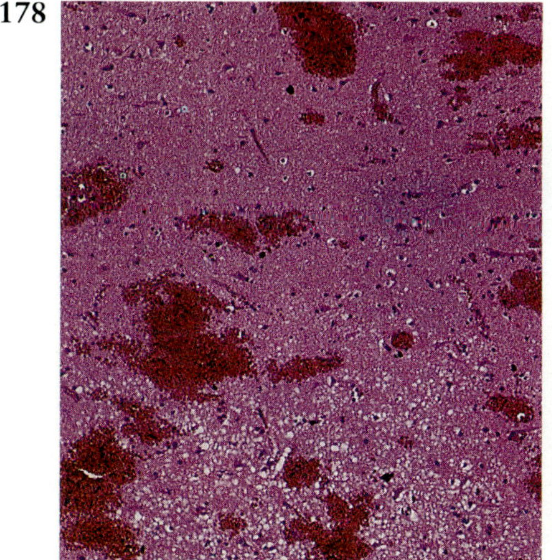

178 Cerebral cortex. As in **176**, showing the recent cerebral contusion containing numerous areas of haemorrhage with focal oedema. Note the absence of a glial reaction, evidence that the lesion is of recent origin. (*H&E ×60*)

179 Cerebrum. Acute haemorrhage (erythrocytes yellow) in the cortical layer, showing absence of degenerative change in the ganglion cells (large cells). Almost instantaneous death. (*van Gieson ×60*)

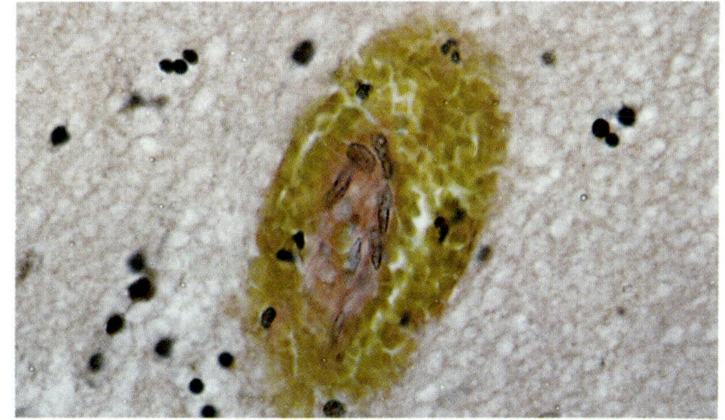

180 Cerebrum. Perivascular haemorrhage ('annular' haemorrhage) with perifocal oedema in a 43 year-old woman who was beaten to death. (*van Gieson ×160*)

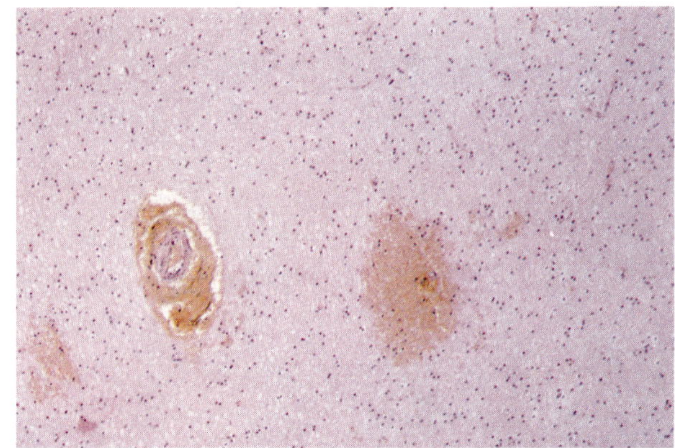

181   Cerebrum. Annular and ball-like haemorrhages (circumscribed areas of haemorrhage in the parenchyma) in a 25 year-old man following a fall from a bicycle. Survival time: 15 minutes. (*H&E ×25*)

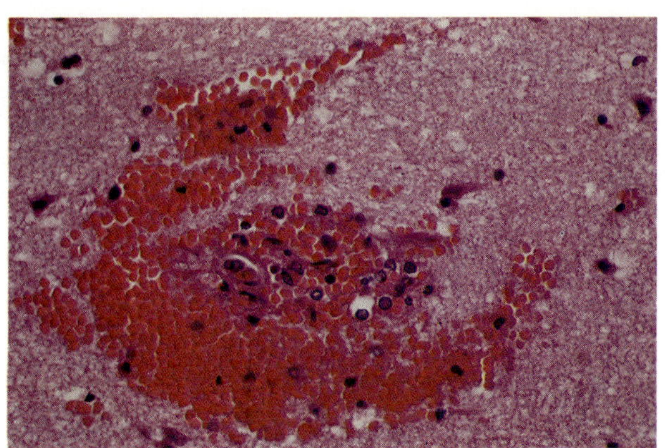

182   Cerebral cortex. Acute haemorrhage in the region of a focus of cerebral contusion. Note the presence of perifocal oedema. (*H&E ×100*)

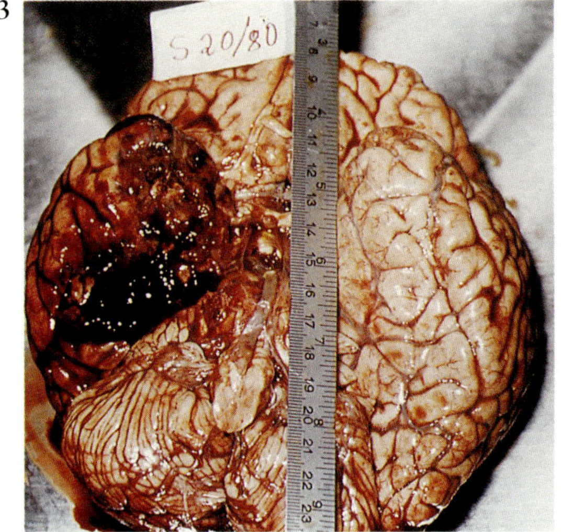

183   Areas of cerebral cortical contusion on the base of the right temporal lobe with haemorrhagic softening.

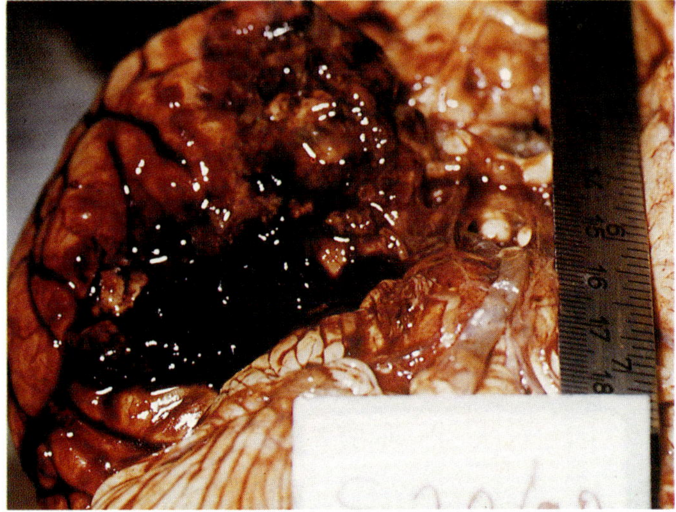

184   Closer view of **183**.

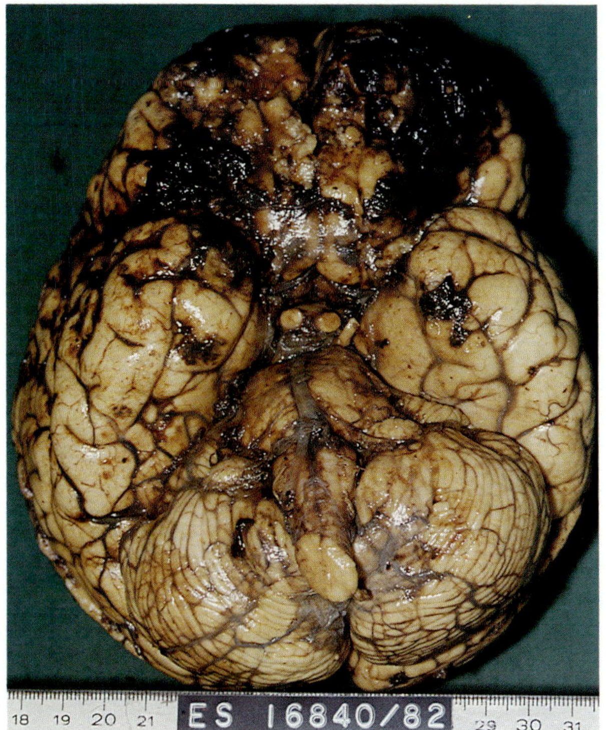

185 **Foci of cerebral cortical contusion** with haemorrhagic necrosis at the base of both frontal lobes. Less marked changes in both temporal lobes. (*Formalin-fixed brain*)

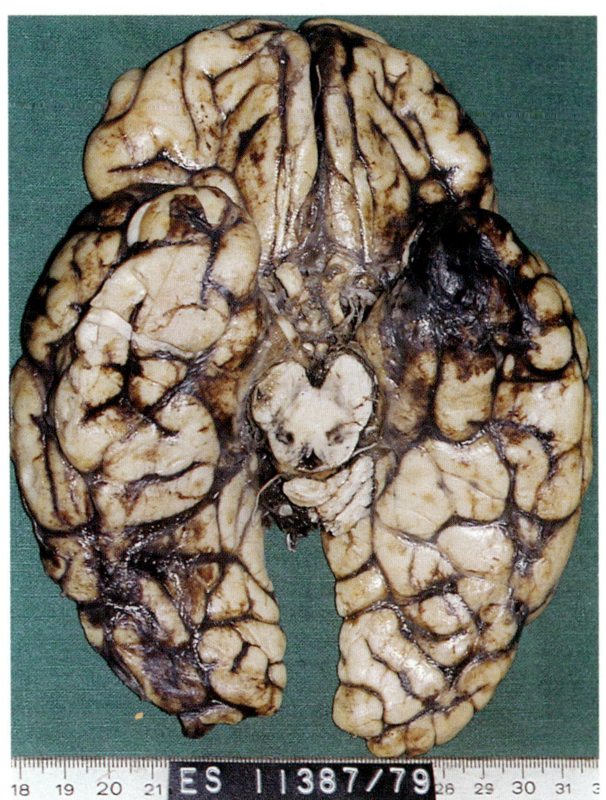

186 **Subarachnoid haemorrhage in a region of severe cortical contusion** at the base of the left temporal lobe of the brain. Contre-coup injury to the base of the right occipital lobe. (*Formalin-fixed brain*)

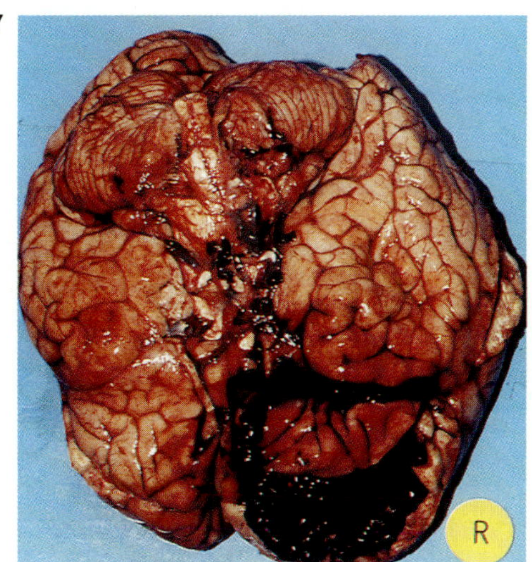

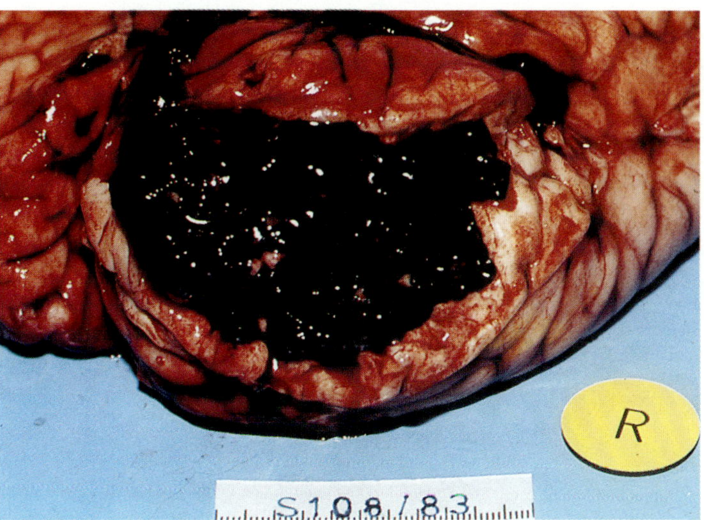

187 and 188 **Severe blunt injury to the head.** There are haemorrhage and necrosis in the base of the right frontal lobe, haemorrhage in the region of the pituitary stalk and pons, and contusion of the base of both occipital lobes, especially on the left side. **188** shows a closer view.

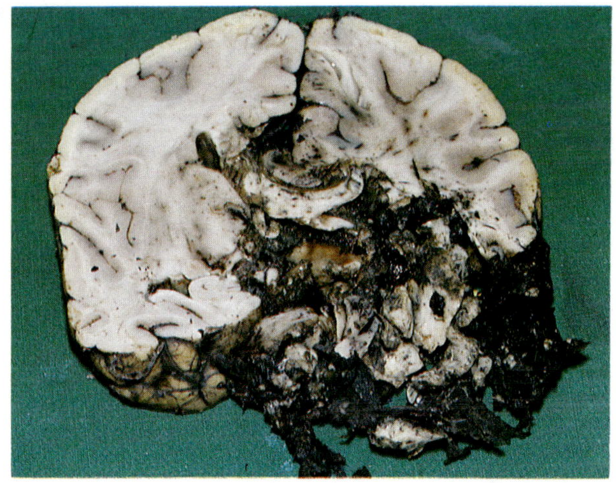

189 **Severe laceration of the right temporal lobe and adjacent occipital lobe of the brain** caused by blunt head injury with compound fracture of the skull. (*Formalin-fixed brain*)

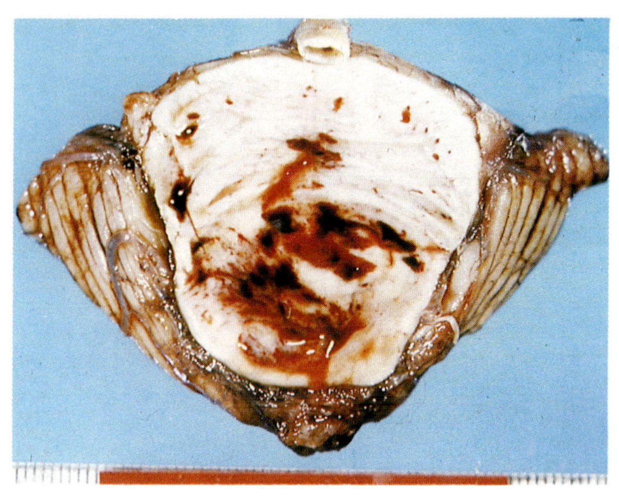

190 **Medulla oblongata.** Fresh haemorrhage caused by severe blunt injury to the head and neck. The victim was run over by a car.

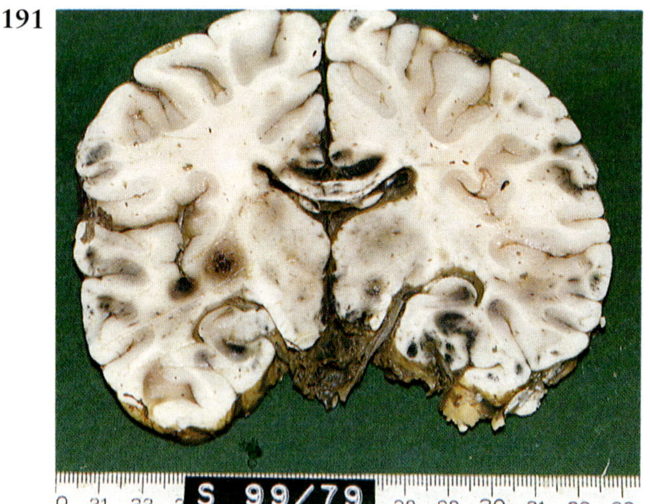

191 **Cortical contusion** and areas of intracerebral haemorrhage following a blunt head injury. (*Formalin-fixed brain*)

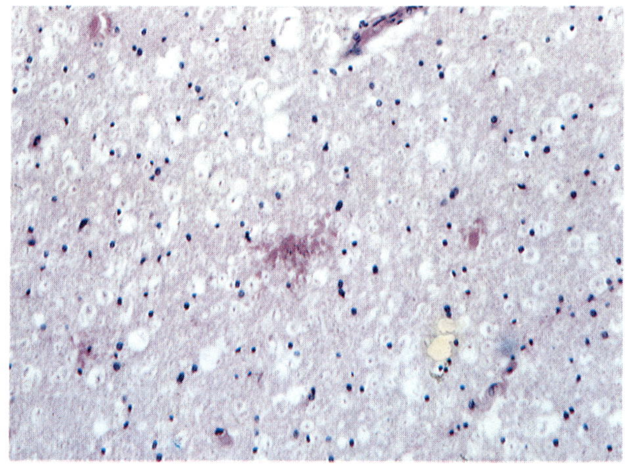

192 **Cerebrum.** Closed head injury 3 days before death. Important features are the microhaemorrhages in the presence of marked cerebral oedema, as well as minimal activation of the glial structures. (*H&E ×25*)

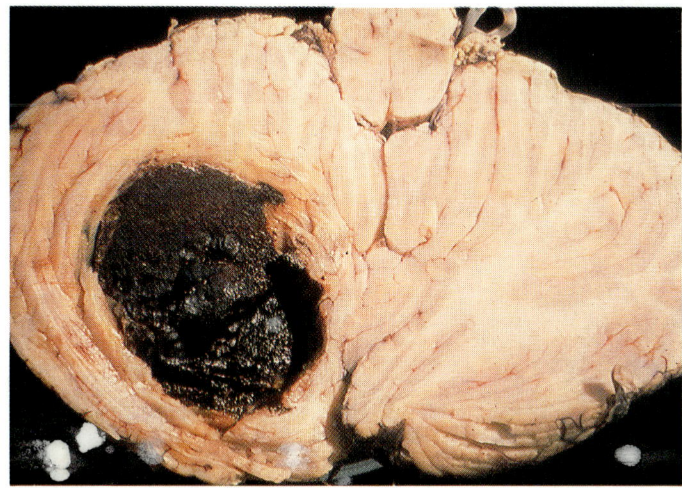

193 Massive haemorrhage in a cerebellar hemisphere.

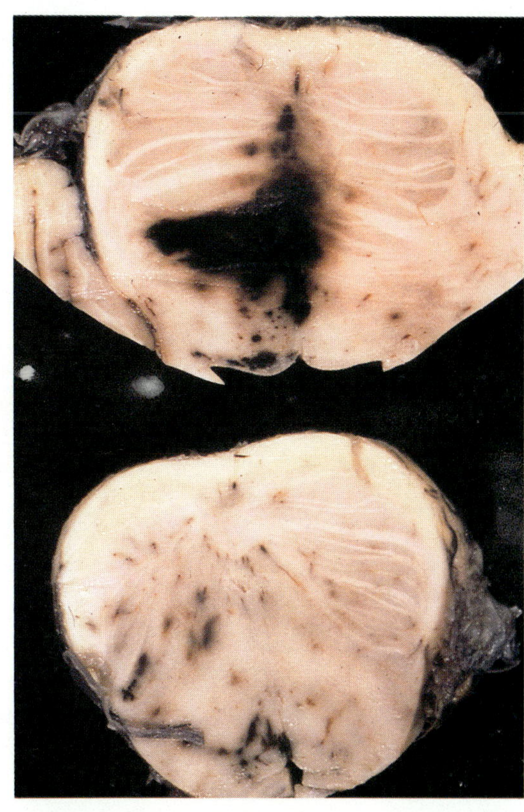

194 **Areas of haemorrhage in the pons** as a result of severe head injury.

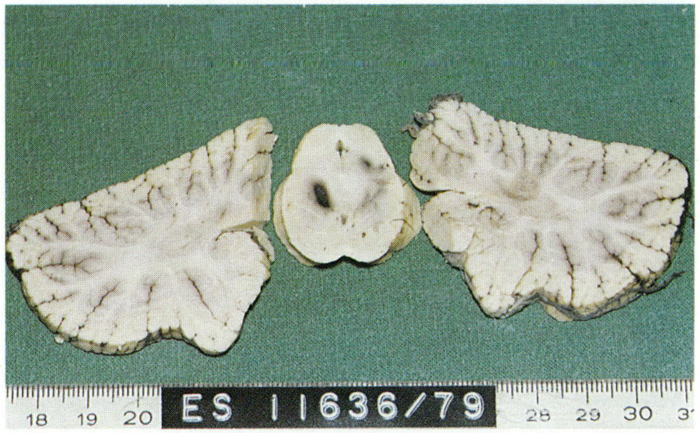

195 **Horizontal section through the midbrain** and cerebellum, showing haemorrhage in the pons, a result of blunt head injury. (*Formalin-fixed brain*)

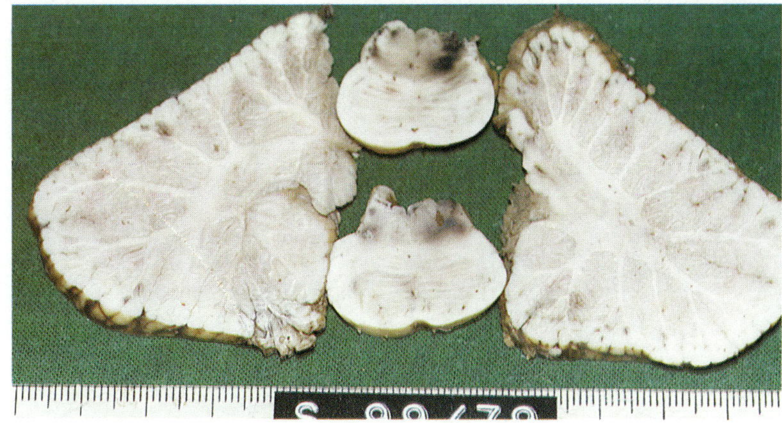

196 **Punctate haemorrhage in the cortex of the cerebellum** and areas of haemorrhage in the midbrain. A case of severe blunt head injury. (*Formalin-fixed brain*)

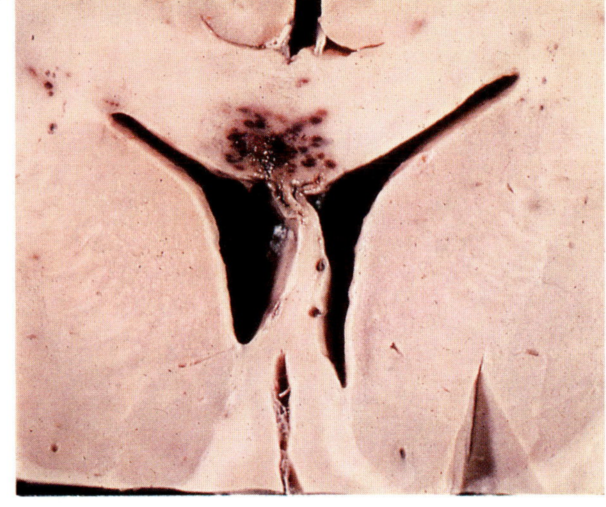

197   Areas of haemorrhage in the corpus callosum.

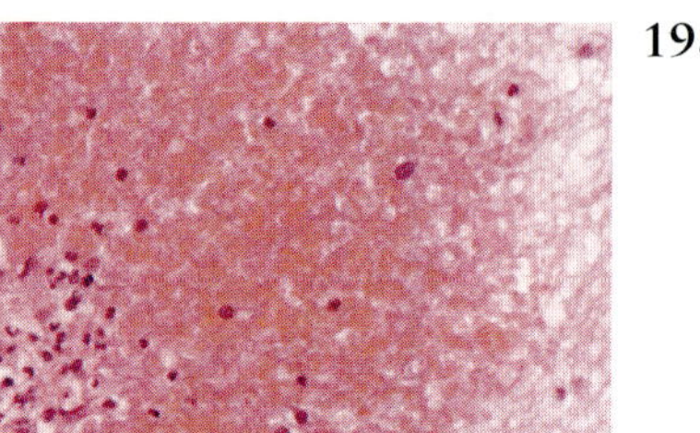

198   Cerebral medullary layer. Perivascular haemorrhage and marked oedema (upper right). Note the presence of a leucocytic reaction. Material from a 31 year-old female who survived a road traffic accident for 4 days. (*H&E ×60*)

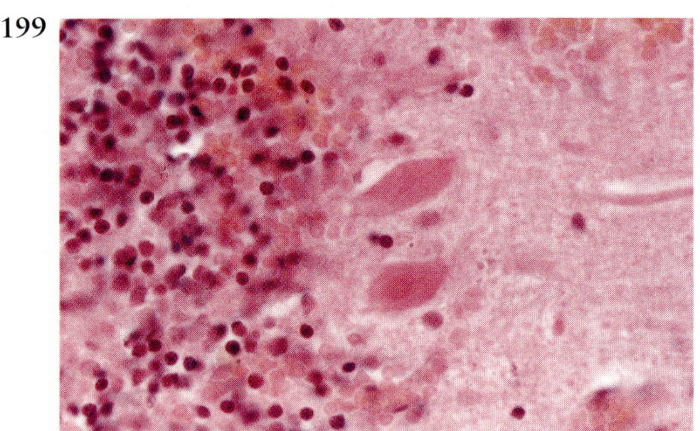

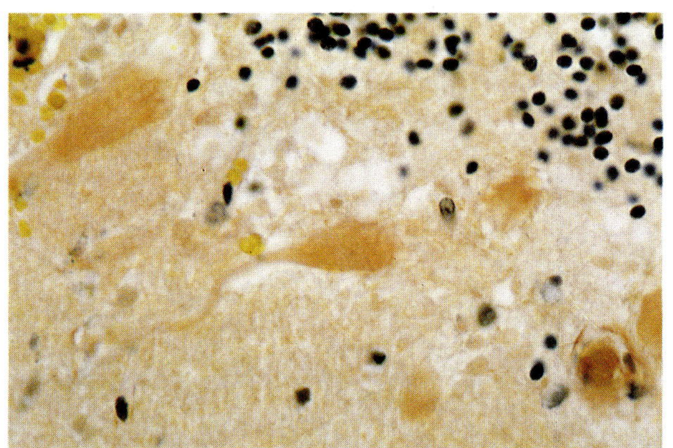

199 and **200   Cerebellum.** Disseminated haemorrhages, cell necrosis in the stratum granulare (left, **199**) and hypoxic changes in the Purkinje cells with surrounding oedema (**200**). Material from a 31 year-old female who survived a road traffic accident for 4 days. (*H&E and van Gieson ×160*)

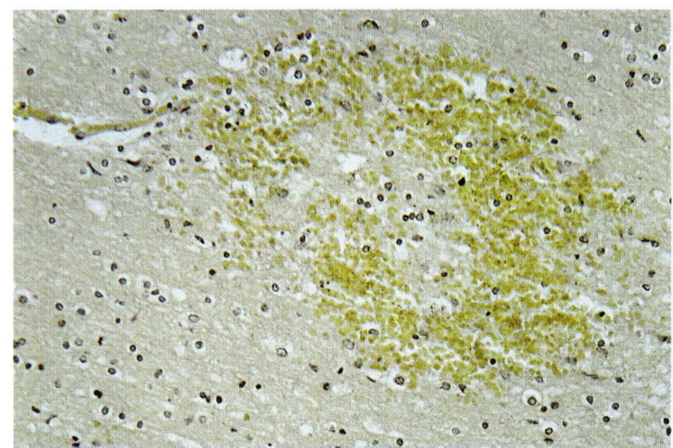

201   Cerebrum. Annular haemorrhage around an area where necrosis is starting. Material from a 20 year-old male who died 8 days after a road traffic accident. (*van Gieson ×60*)

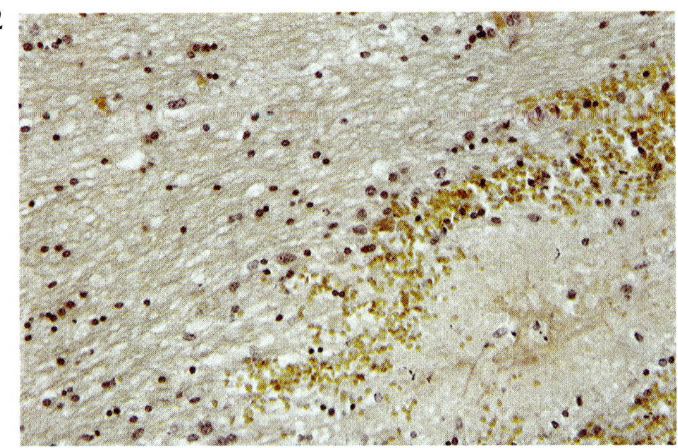

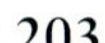

202 Cerebral medullary layer. Annular haemorrhage around a necrotic area. Note the minimal glial reaction (left side of the picture). Material from a 20 year-old male who died 6 days after a road traffic accident. The histopathological appearance can also be seen in cases of fat or air embolism (see **208**). (*van Gieson ×63*)

203 Cerebrum. Closed head injury as a result of blows with the fist. Note the cell cuff around a blood vessel, as well as a glial reaction. Material from a 19 year-old male who died 8 days after the trauma. (*H&E ×50*)

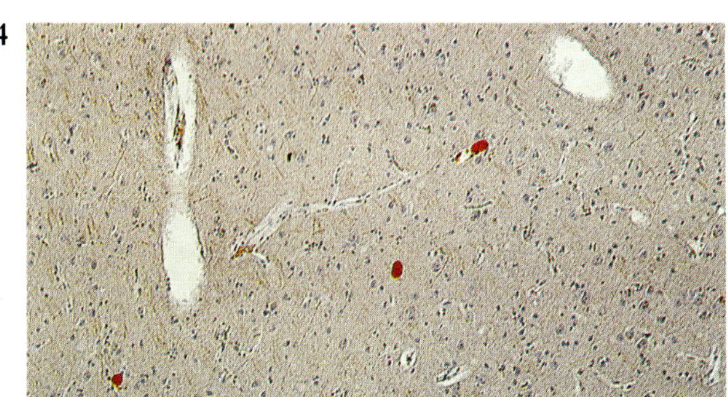

204 Cerebral medullary layer. Fat embolism (red) as a result of polytrauma with multiple fractures. An important feature is the absence of a local tissue reaction. Death occurred 5 days after injury. (*Sudan ×20*)

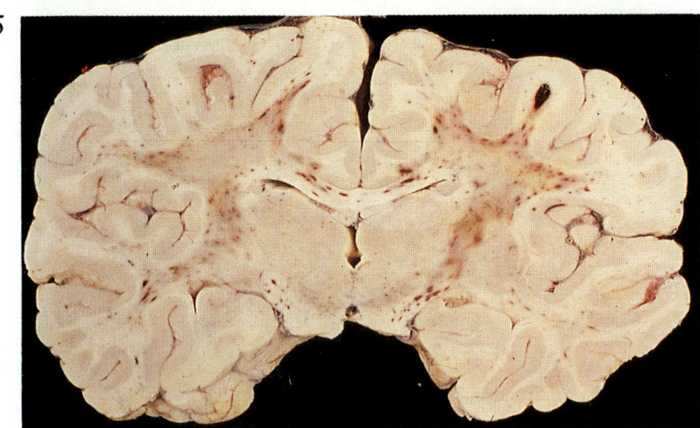

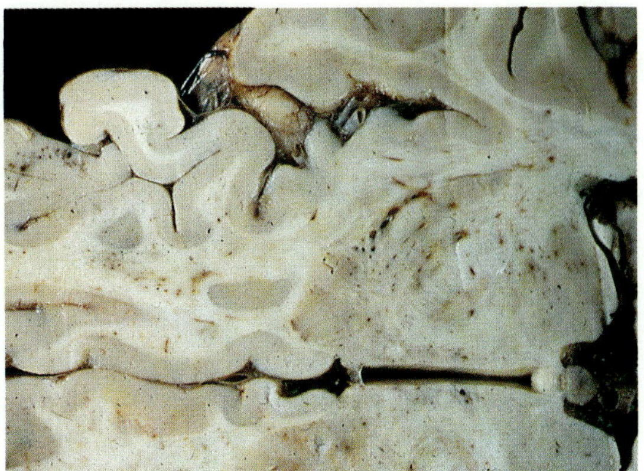

205 Multiple punctate haemorrhages (petechiae), principally in the white matter of the cerebral hemispheres. 'Cerebral purpura' caused by fat embolism.

206 Closer view of **205**.

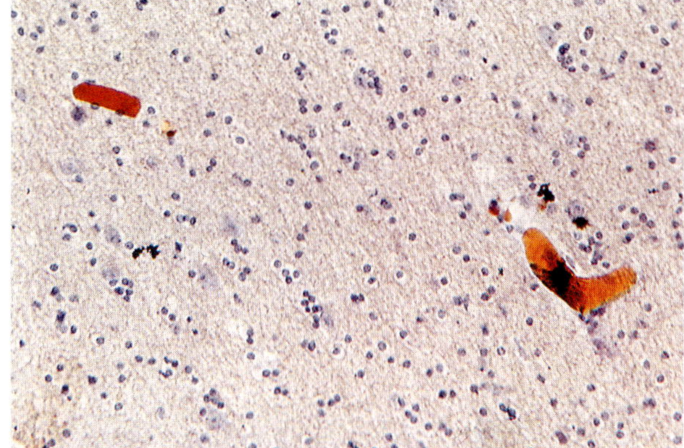

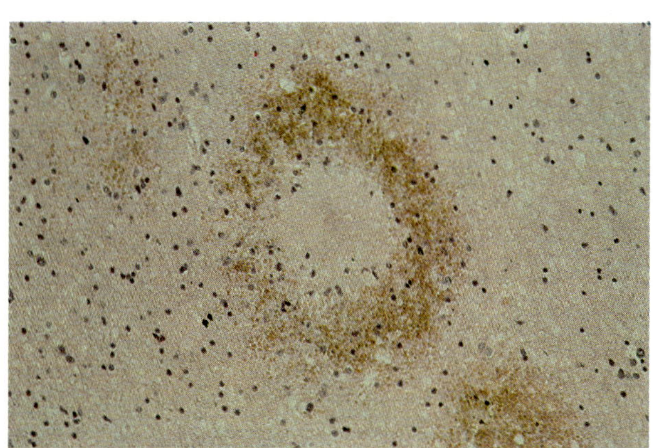

207 Cerebral medullary layer. Fat embolism. Death occurred 24 hours after osteosynthesis (intramedullary nail) of a simple femur fracture. (*Sudan ×60*)

208 Cerebral medullary layer. Annular haemorrhage with an area of central necrosis in a case of fat embolism following a fracture of the femur (with polytrauma). Post-traumatic survival time: 6 days. (*H&E ×50*)

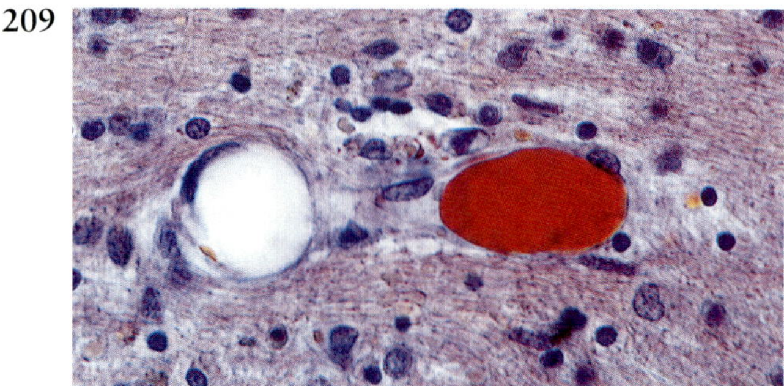

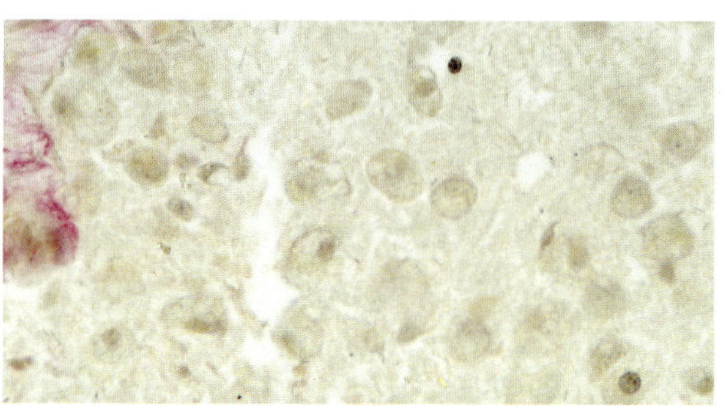

209 Cerebral medullary layer. Fat embolism with injuries received during a fight. Post-traumatic survival time: 11 days. (*Sudan stain ×160*)

210 Medulla oblongata from a 21 year-old male who died 25 days after a road traffic accident. Macrophages (gitter cells or compound granular corpuscles) are visible in an area of necrosis. In **211**, iron is visible in these macrophages. (*van Gieson ×160*)

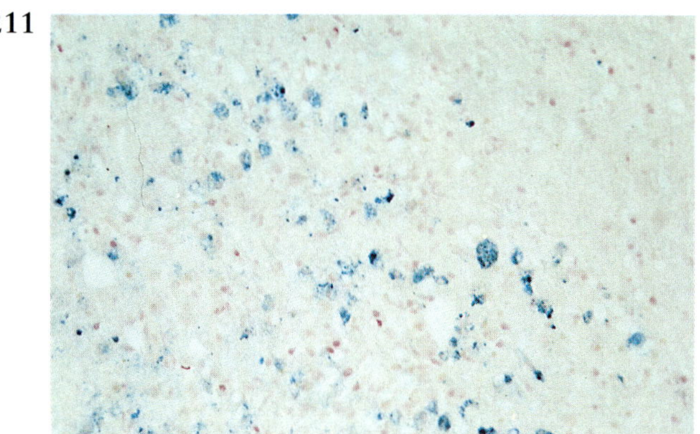

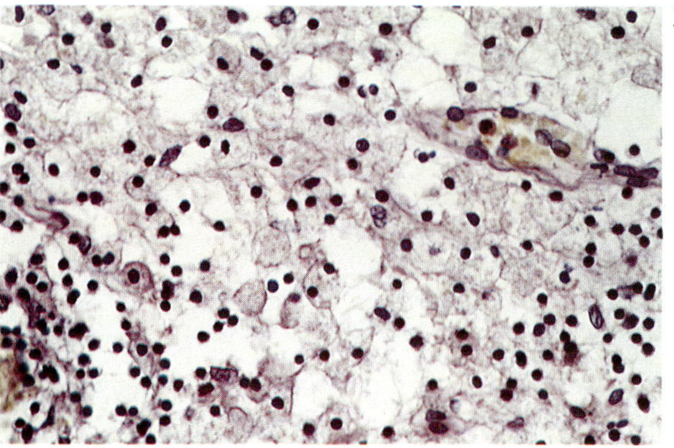

211 As in 210. (*Prussian blue ×60*)

212 Cerebrum from a patient who lived for 6 weeks following a closed head injury. Numerous macrophages can be seen in a continuous lesion. An activation of the glial cells (small dark cells) is also a feature. (*H&E ×125*)

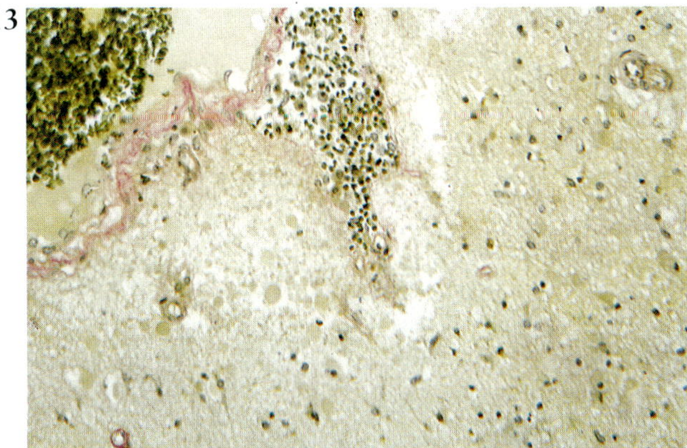

213   Cerebrum. An old area of cortical contusion with marked disruption of the interstitial tissue. Several corpora amylacea are visible. (*van Gieson ×63*)

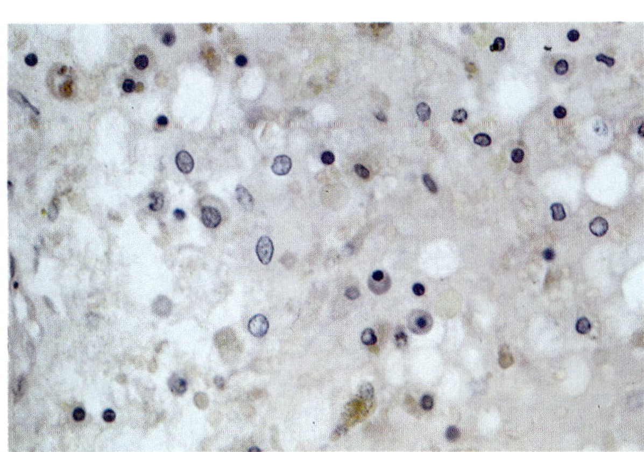

214   Cerebrum. Oedematous loosening in an old focus of cortical contusion. Note the macroglial cells (cells with large nuclei) and haemosiderin pigment (brown) as a result of haemoglobin degradation. (*H&E ×160*)

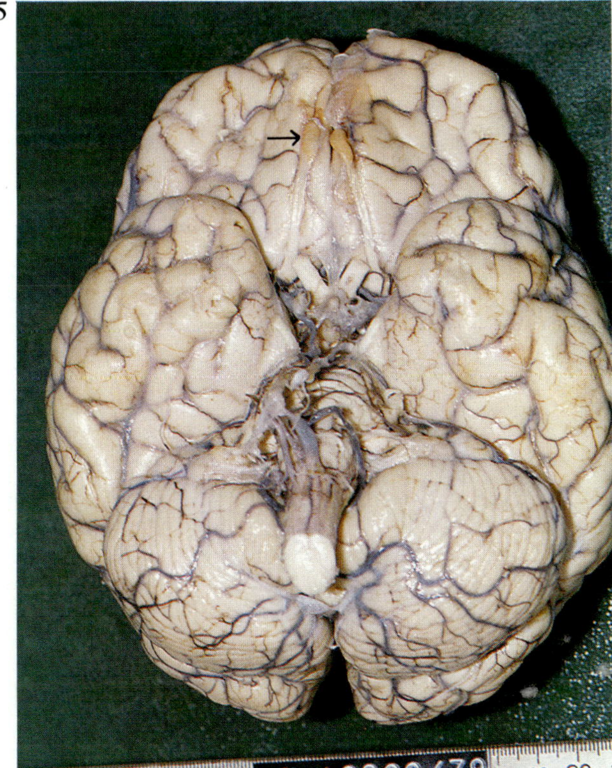

215   The base of the brain. Cortical contusion (arrow) around the olfactory bulbs. The xanthochromasia is in keeping with the age of the injury (many months previously). (*Formalin-fixed brain*)

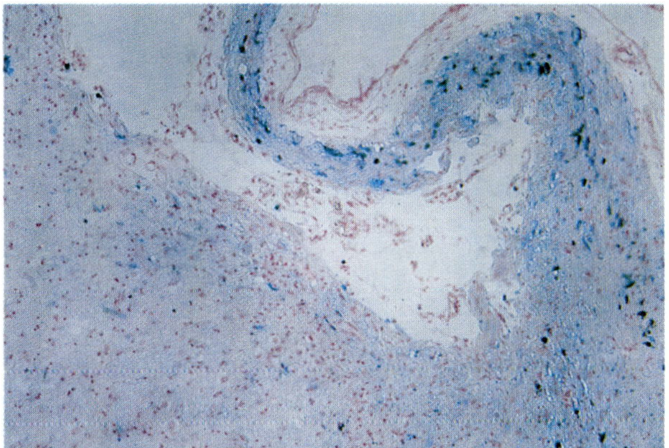

216   Cerebrum. An old focus of cerebral cortical contusion (8 months after injury), showing cystic change. Note the thickening of the leptomeninges with large amounts of haemosiderin (blue) here and in the cerebral cortex. (*Prussian blue ×25*)

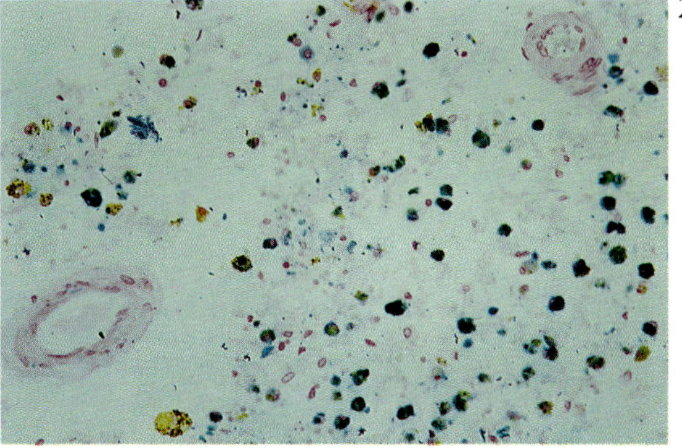

217   Cerebrum. An old focus of cystic change, exhibiting deposition of haemosiderin (blue) and haematoidin (yellow). (*Prussian blue ×60*)

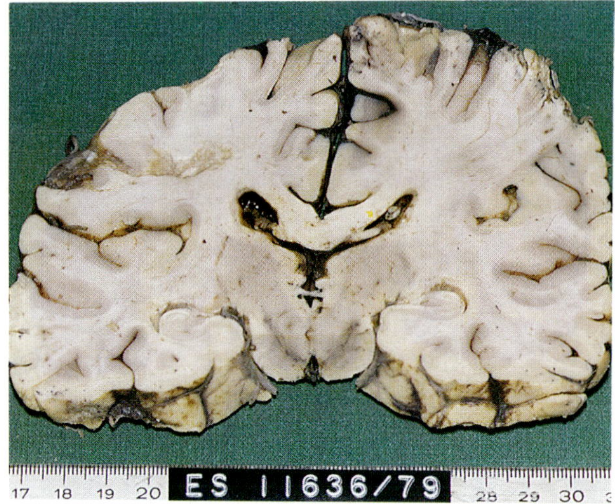

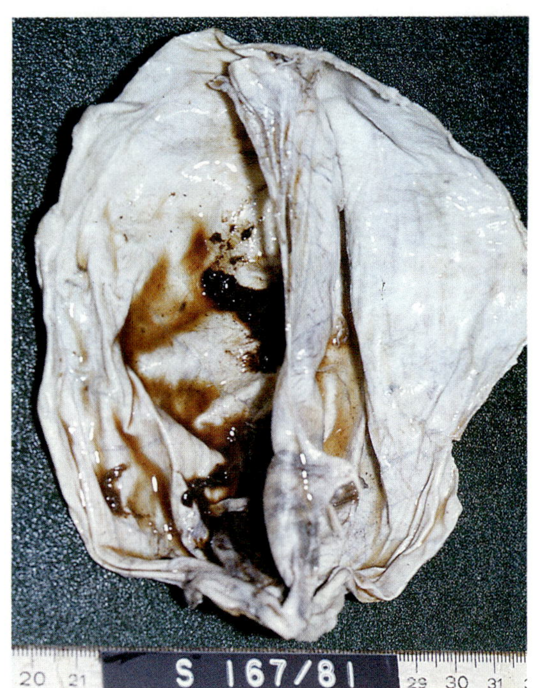

218 Compression of the left cerebral hemisphere by an epidural haematoma. In addition, areas of contusion and loss of parenchyma in the right parietal lobe.

219 Dura mater with subdural haemorrhage (4 days old) following a blunt head injury. (*Formalin-fixed specimen*)

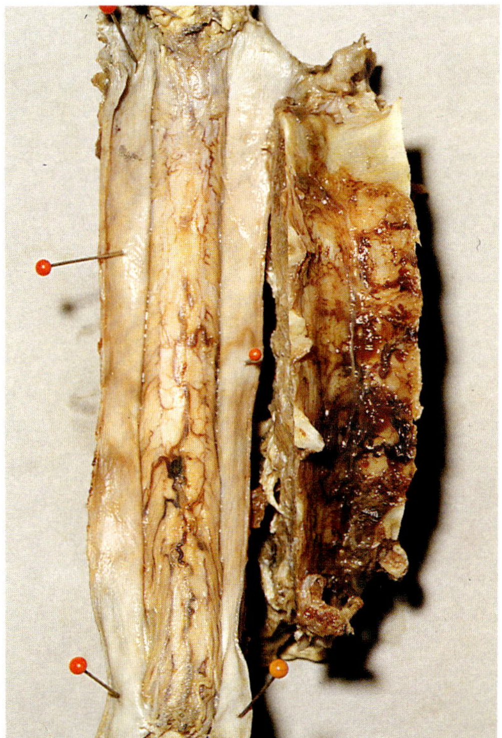

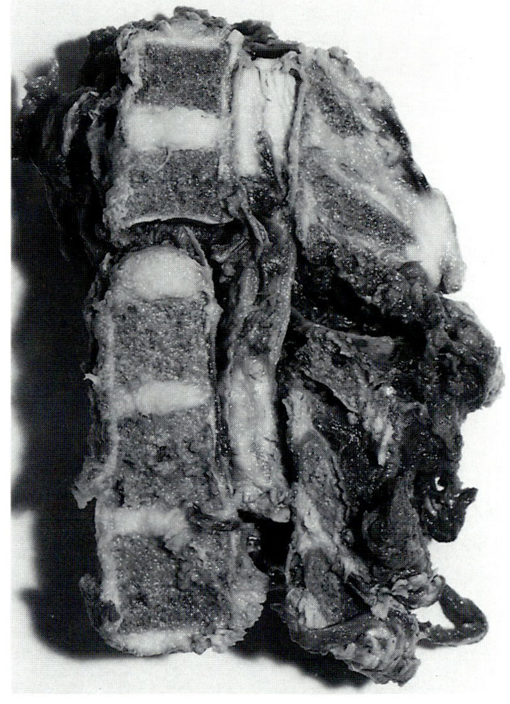

221 Fracture-dislocation in the cervical region of the vertebral column with tearing of the intervertebral disc, haemorrhage and crushing of the spinal cord. From a 22 year-old pedestrian who was run over by a car. (*Formalin-fixed specimen*)

220 Severe contusion of the spinal cord with hyperaemia and oedema. The corresponding segment of the vertebral canal shows areas of haemorrhage. Material from a 23 year-old man who died following a fall from a roof.

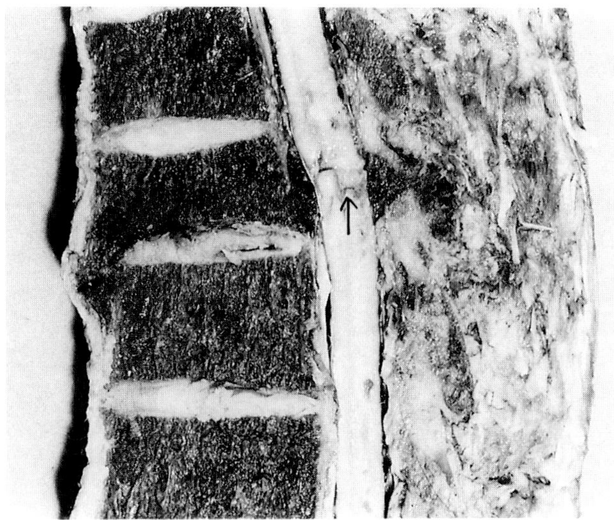

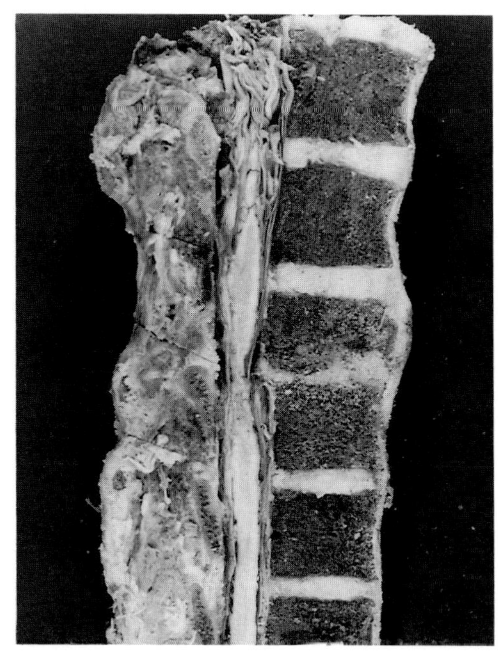

222 Blunt injury to the thoracic vertebral column with peripheral fractures in two adjacent vertebral bodies. In addition, crushing of the intervertebral disc, rupture of the anterior longitudinal ligament and an irregular transverse severing of the spinal cord. Material from a 25 year-old man who died 3 days after a motorcycle accident. (*Formalin-fixed specimen*)

223 Fractures in the lower thoracic vertebral bodies with subsequent crushing of the spinal cord.

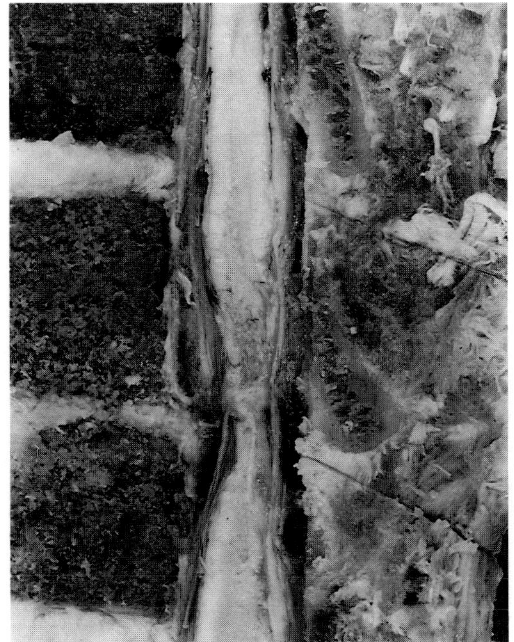

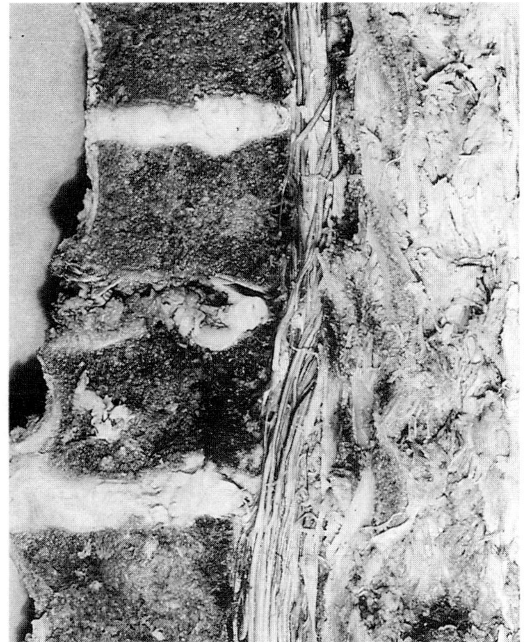

224 As in **223**. Close-up view of the spinal cord lesion.

225 Fracture of a lumbar vertebral body with traumatic disruption of an intervertebral disc and partial transection of the cauda equina. The 46 year-old victim was run over by a car and died 4 weeks later. (*Formalin-fixed specimen*)

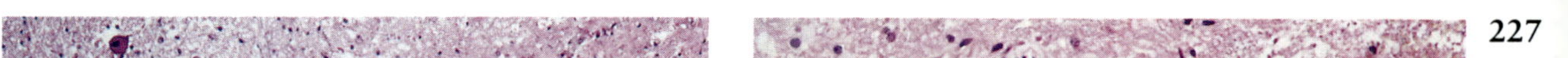

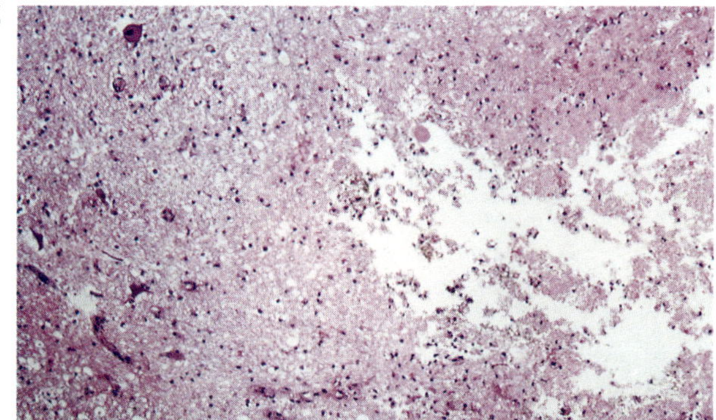

226 Cervical spinal cord. Compression as a result of a fracture of the seventh cervical vertebral body. Note the focal malacia (right) and marked oedema. Post-traumatic survival time: 5 days. (*H&E ×25*)

227 Cervical spinal cord. Compression injury to the spinal cord as in **226**. Important features are haemorrhage (right), oedema and progressive alterations in the glial cells. Post-traumatic survival time: 5 days. (*H&E ×600*)

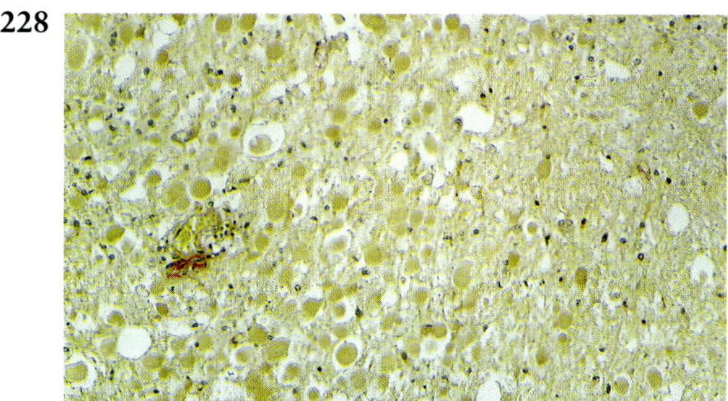

228 Cervical spinal cord showing an area of necrosis with numerous corpora amylacea. Post-traumatic survival time: 5 days. (*van Gieson ×40*)

229 Upper thoracic spinal cord. Compression injury caused by a fracture of the fifth thoracic vertebral body. As well as necrosis of neurons, a mobilisation of the glial cells can be seen. Post-traumatic survival time: 14 days. (*H&E ×60*)

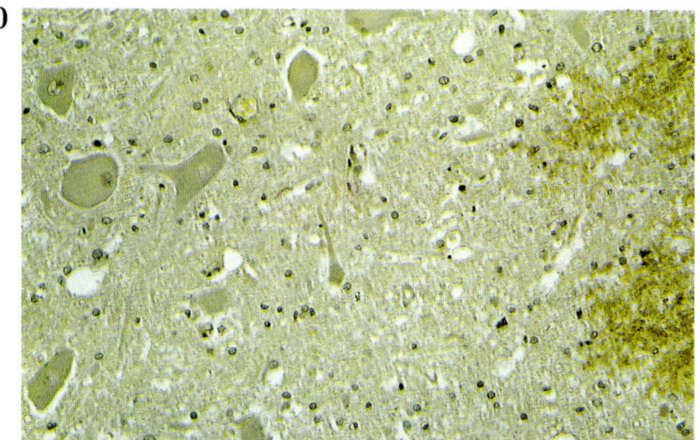

230 Cervical spinal cord showing haemorrhage (right) oedema and degenerative change in the anterior horn cells. Post-traumatic survival time: 1 week. (*van Gieson ×50*)

231 Cervical spinal cord. Marked degeneration of the anterior horn cells as a result of spinal cord compression. (*H&E ×60*)

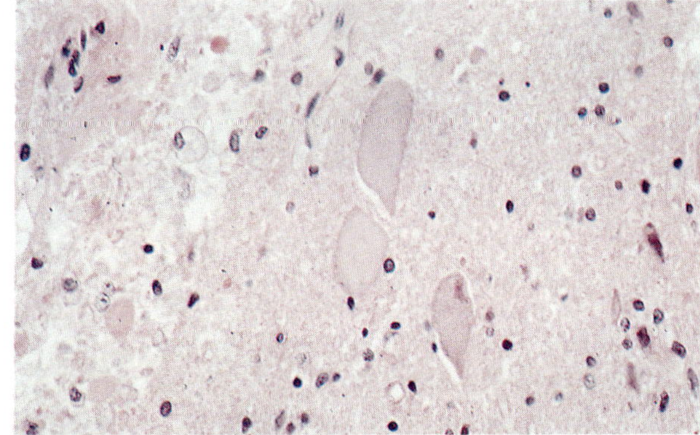

232   Cervical spinal cord. Compression injury to the spinal cord, demonstrating cloudy swelling of the anterior horn cells (middle) and single phagocytosing macrophage (left). Post-traumatic survival time: 8 days. (*H&E ×100*)

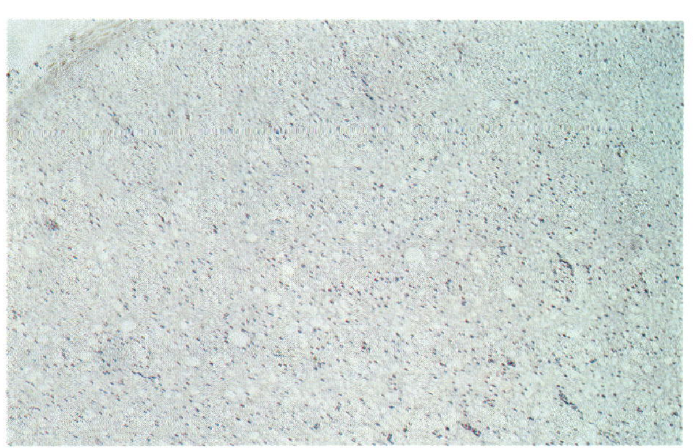

233   Cervical spinal cord. Compression injury of the seventh cervical vertebral body. Note the vacuolisation and oedema of the spinal cord. Post-traumatic survival time: 4 months. (*H&E ×16*)

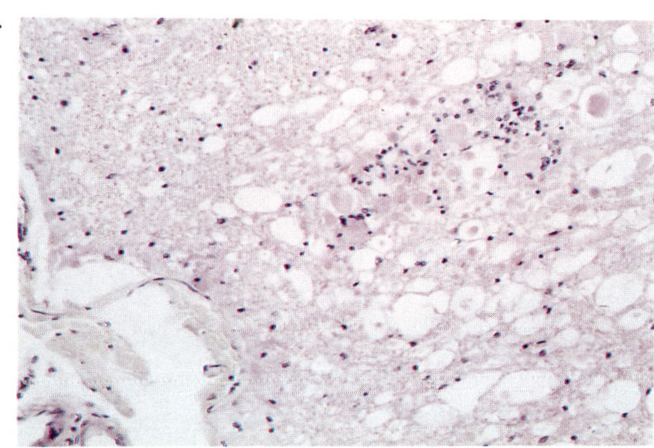

234   Cervical spinal cord. Compression injury as in **233**. Enlargement of an area of vacuolisation, showing corpora amylacea. Post-traumatic survival time: 4 months. (*H&E ×50*)

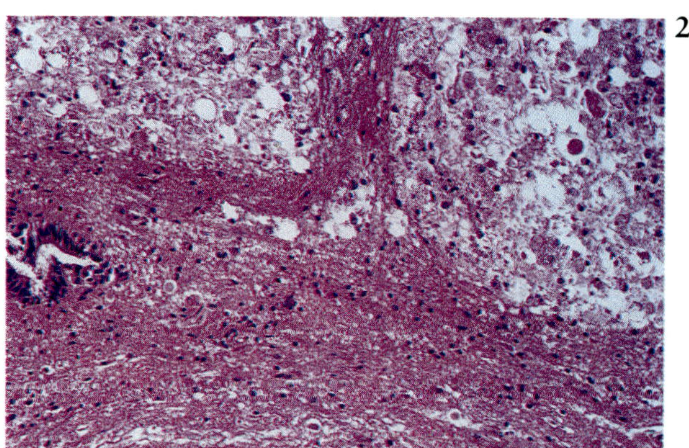

235   Spinal cord. Fracture of the vertebral body with compression of the spinal cord. Secondary degeneration of the spinal cord tracts can be seen in the upper half of the picture. (*H&E ×25*)

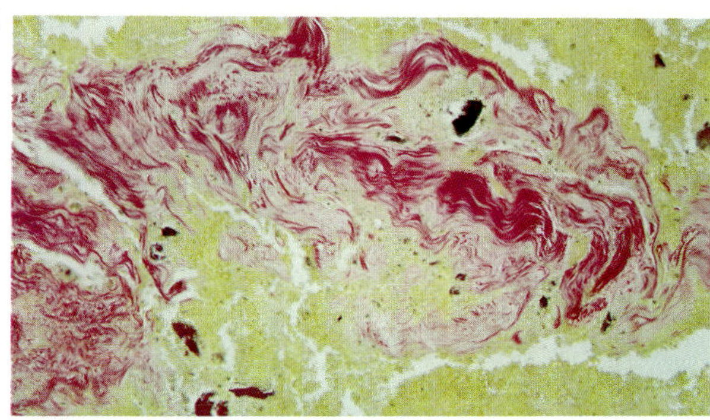

236   Dura mater. Severe closed head injury. Note the massive haemorrhage (stained green with van Gieson) with interspersion of bone spicules. Material from a patient who died 25 days after a road traffic accident. The autopsy was performed 3 days after death, so there are signs of decomposition and a decreased staining reaction of the cell nuclei. (*van Gieson ×25*)

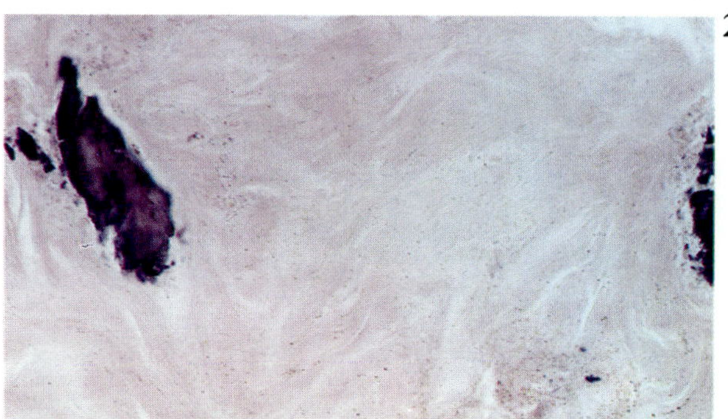

237   As in 236. (*H&E ×100*)

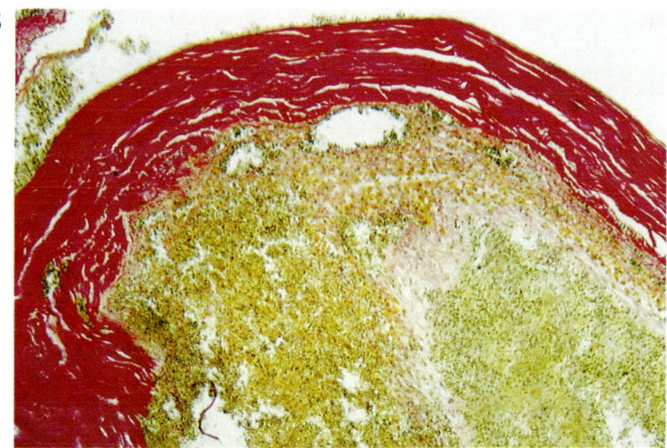

238 Dura mater. Subdural haematoma showing marked deposition of haemosiderin. Post-traumatic survival time: 5 weeks. (*van Gieson ×25*)

239 As in **238**. (*Prussian blue ×25*)

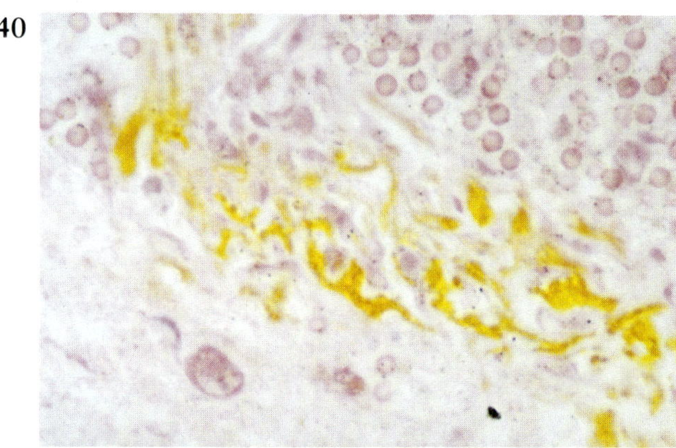

240 Dura mater. Severe closed head injury. Extensive tissue alteration as a result of decomposition. Note the haematoidin pigment (yellow), a bilirubin-like pigment formed from haemoglobin under conditions of reduced oxygen tension. (*H&E ×250*)

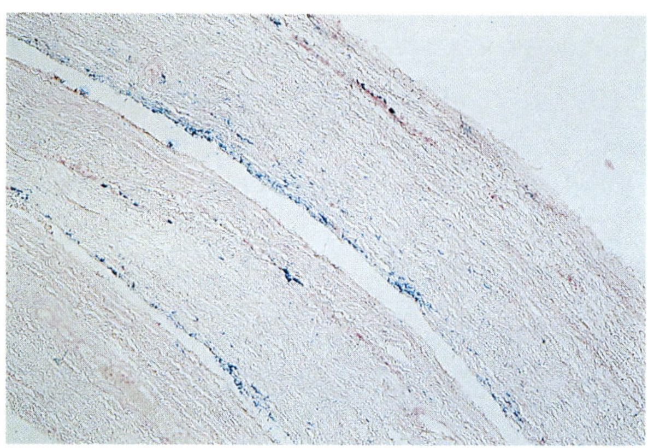

241 Dura mater from the cervical region, 4 months after a fracture of the seventh cervical vertebral body. Haemosiderin pigment (blue) of varying density is shown in the region of the internal aspect of the dura. The dura mater was rolled up before sectioning and the picture therefore shows three different regions. (*Prussian blue ×16*)

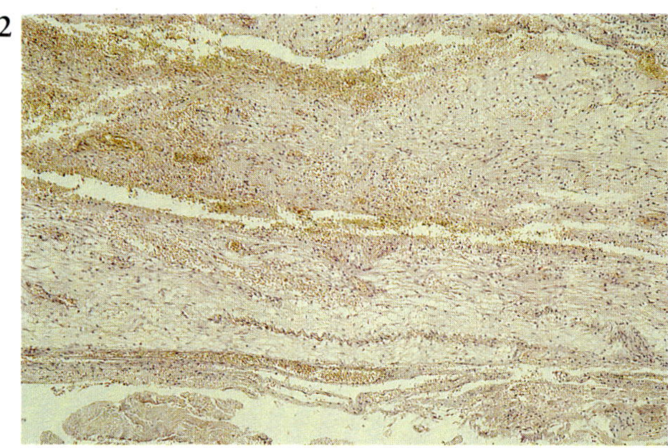

242 Hypophysis. Oedema and haemorrhage in the stalk of the pituitary following severe closed head injury. (*H&E ×20*)

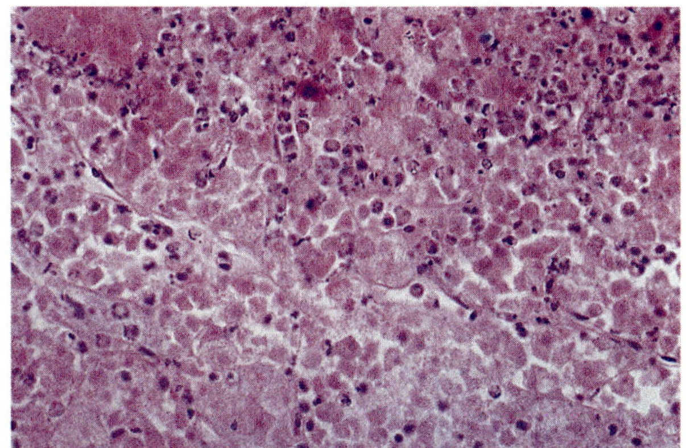
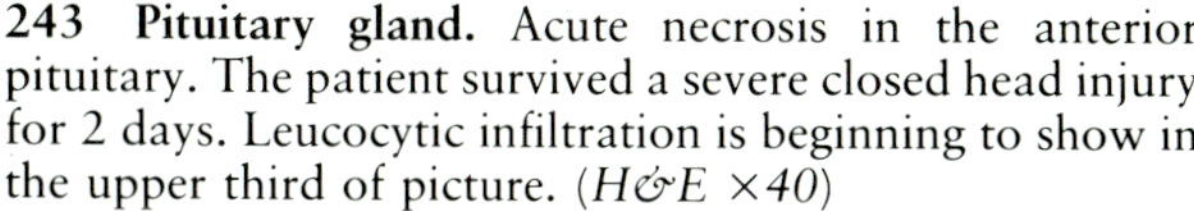

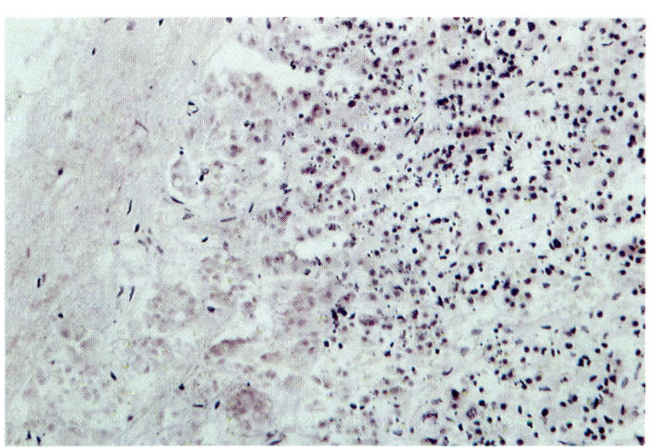

243 Pituitary gland. Acute necrosis in the anterior pituitary. The patient survived a severe closed head injury for 2 days. Leucocytic infiltration is beginning to show in the upper third of picture. (*H&E ×40*)

244 Pituitary gland. Area of necrosis (left) with a cellular inflammatory reaction in the anterior pituitary. Material from a patient who suffered a severe closed head injury in a road traffic accident. Post-traumatic survival time: 3 days. (*H&E ×63*)

5 Burns and Hyperthermia

The depth and extent of burns are clinically estimated using the 'rule of nines'. More severe forms of burns lead to a state of shock and later on to 'burn disease'. The local effects of burns are also important. Thus, for example, the inhalation of flames may cause severe damage to the respiratory tract. Carbon monoxide intoxication has long been recognised as an important factor to be treated in the acute management of casualties due to fire. In recent years, cyanide intoxication has been recognised as important, especially where plastics and paints are burning.

The pathologic morphologic changes that are associated with the four degrees of burn severity are as follows:

First degree burns (reddening):
Marked dilatation of capillaries; condensation of nuclear chromatin; hydrophilic swelling of the epidermal cell nuclei; occasional necrotic epidermal cells; oedema of the subepidermal connective tissue.

Second degree burns (blister formation):
Subepidermal oedema with blister formation; varying degrees of epidermal cell necrosis; reduced staining reaction of epidermal cell nuclei; in the upper part of the dermis, hyperaemia, oedema and a minimal perivascular accumulation of granulocytes, macrophages and occasional lymphocytes. According to Raasch *et al.* (1974) polymorphonuclear neutrophils have usually migrated into the dermis after 16 hours.

Third degree burns (complete destruction of skin):
Loss of epidermis and necrosis of the dermis (including the deeper layers); coagulation of collagenous fibres; necrosis of skin appendages; hyperaemia of neighbouring capillaries; along the edge of adjacent intact epidermis an elongation of cells and cell nuclei can be seen (palisade formation); neighbouring epidermal cells may contain cytoplasmic vacuoles; the necrotic areas become demarcated by polymorphonuclear leucocytes after 6–24 hours; dermal inflammation tends to lag by several days, although the subcutaneous tissue shows inflammatory cell infiltration by the second day. Metal traces may be found in cases of burns caused by metal objects (thermal metallisation).

Fourth degree burns (charring):
Complete destruction of skin and subcutaneous tissue, sometimes with exposure of bone.

Histochemical or scanning electron microscopic detection of superficial traces of metal allows a clear demarcation between thermal metallisation burns and lesions caused by an electric current. The morphological appearance of nuclear elongation is a non-specific change, which, according to Janssen (1977), can be found in the periphery of burns, lesions caused by blunt injury, alkali lesions and blisters caused by barbiturate poisoning and cold injury.

According to Janssen's studies (1977) of the respiratory tract (trachea, bronchi and lung tissue) following inhalation of flames, a variety of pathological changes are seen:

- Swelling and superficial coagulation necrosis of the cylindrical epithelium.
- Marked elongation of the epithelial cell nuclei with palisade formation
- Evagination of the superficial glands of the epithelium.
- Fragmentation and clumping of erythrocytes in the mucosal blood vessels.
- Oedema of the submucosa.
- Generalised epithelial hyperaemia.

In fatal cases of **acute** hyperthermia no specific macroscopic or microscopic alterations are to be found.

In heat stroke the homeostatic heat regulatory mechanism is overwhelmed by the amount of heat energy to which the body is exposed. A decompensation is inevitable. This disease complex is classified thus:

- Heat stroke.
- Hyperpyrexia.
- Anhidrotic heat exhaustion.

In cases of hyperthermia (heat stroke), distinct changes can be found in a variety of organs. Malamud *et al.* (1946) have detailed the effects of severe heat stroke on parenchymatous organs, especially the liver, heart, adrenal glands and kidneys. Of pathophysiological importance is dehydration with subsequent haemoconcentration resulting from the heat. Haemoconcentration leads to increased blood viscosity and hence to disturbances in blood flow and to electrolyte imbalance. In the brain, for example, these processes lead to perivascular oedema, with widening of Virchow–Robin spaces, and to focal areas of haemorrhage. In the lung, haemorrhagic pulmonary oedema is often found in fatal cases.

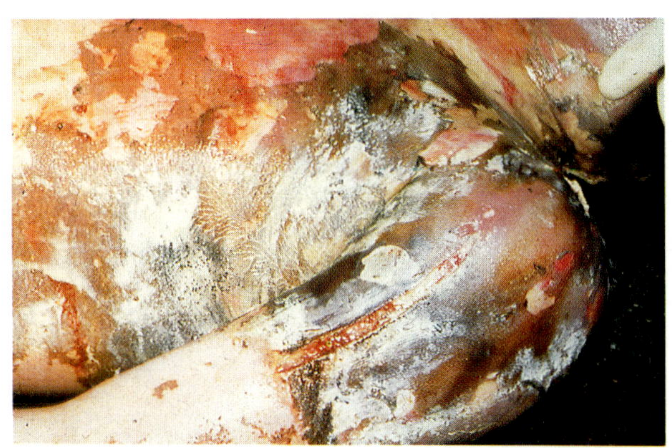

245 **Extensive third degree burns on the left side of the neck** and the thorax as well as on the upper arm.

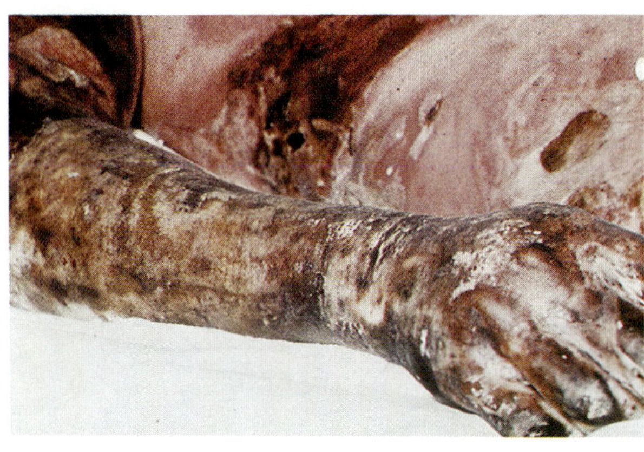

246 **Third to fourth degree gasoline burns** on the arm, hip and thigh of a 28 year-old man.

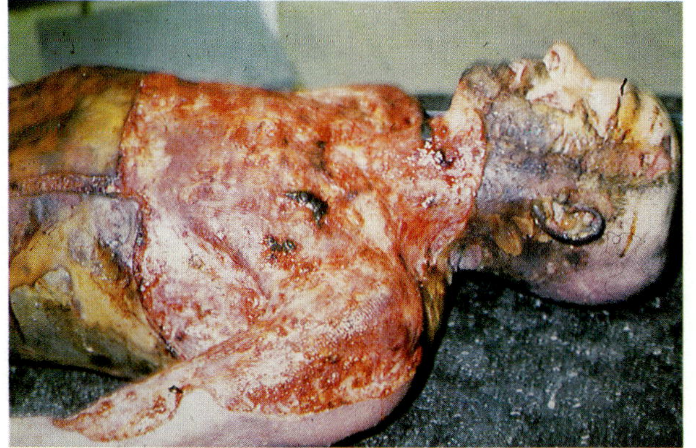

247 **Extensive third degree scalding.**

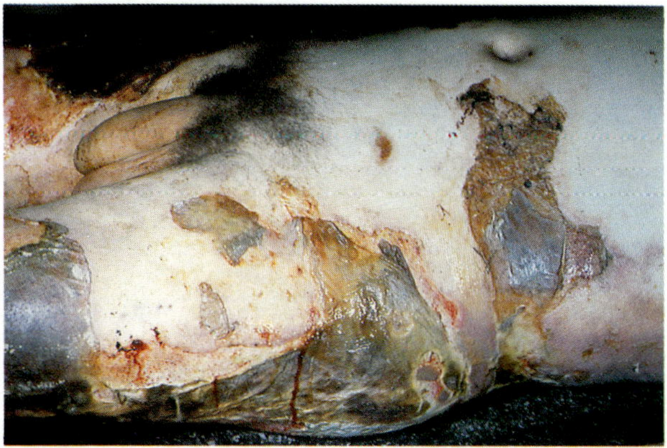

248 **Second and third degree scalds on the left flank, buttock and thigh.** Peripheral areas show extensive blisters.

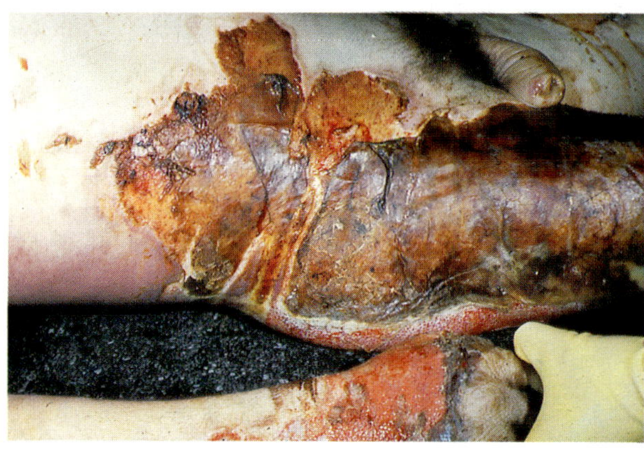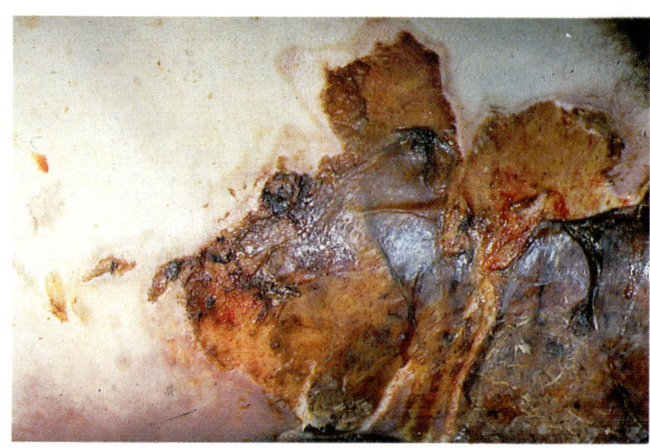

249 and **250** **Extensive scalding** to the right side of the abdomen, thigh, forearm and hand with superficial desiccation giving the appearance of leather. Marked hyperaemia of the skin in peripheral areas is shown.

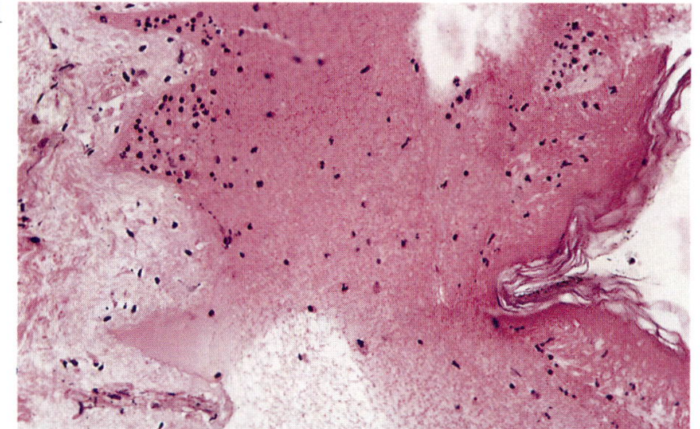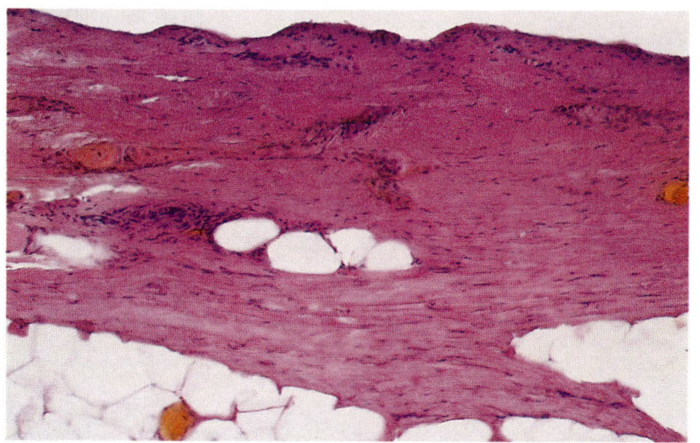

251 **Skin.** The important features are necrosis of the epidermis (extreme right), marked oedema of the dermis and dermal infiltration by leucocytes. Post-traumatic survival: 2 days. (*H&E ×250*)

252 **Skin** from a 5 year-old child exposed to convection heat (the child lay some metres from the flames from a house fire: the cause of death was carbon monoxide poisoning). Complete loss of the epidermis, heat coagulation of the dermis with nuclear pyknosis and capillary dilatation. (*H&E ×100*)

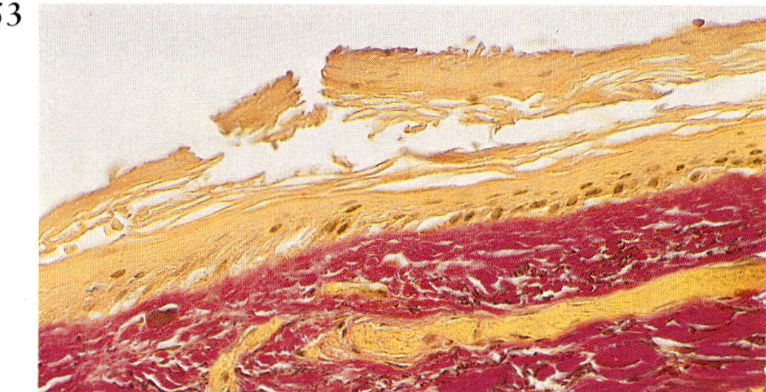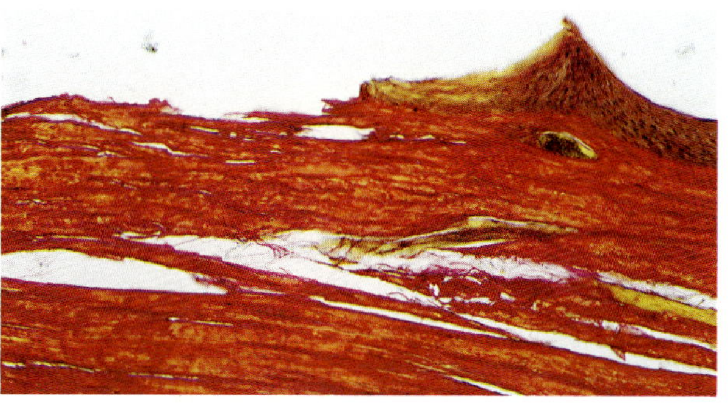

253 Same as **252**. Skin, showing oedema (and therefore friability) of the epidermis (upper, yellow), as well as decreased nuclear staining reaction and vacuolation of the stratum basale. (*van Gieson ×250*)

254 **Skin.** Third degree burn, showing complete loss of the epidermis with exposure of the dermis. In the latter, note the heat coagulation of the collagen fibres, which demonstrate variable staining intensity, and loss of nuclear staining reaction. Post-traumatic survival time: 3 days. A thick section was cut to preserve the structure of the friable material. (*van Gieson ×160*)

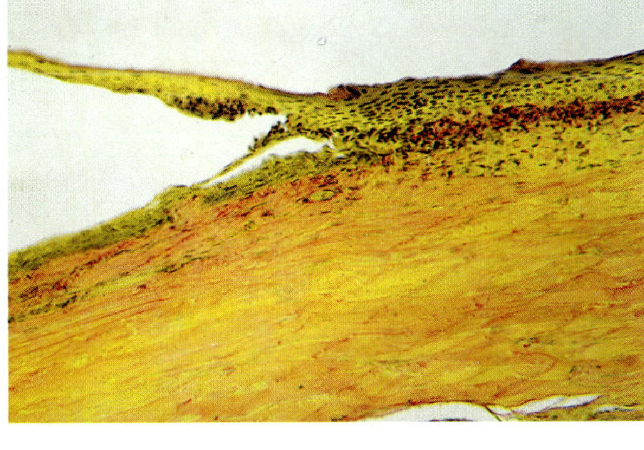

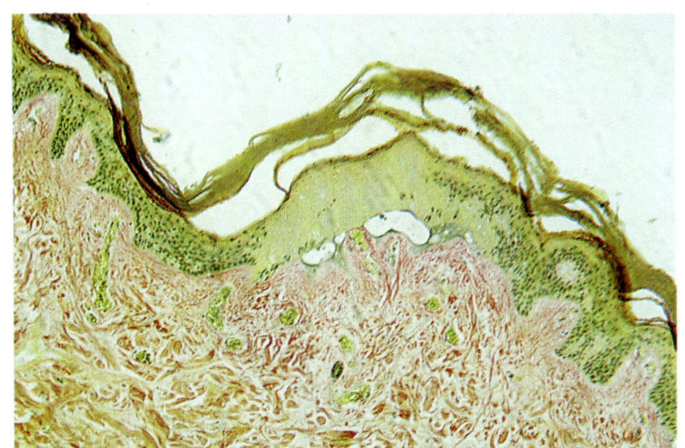

255   Skin. Peripheral part of a second degree skin burn, showing intraepidermal blister formation and partial necrosis of the epidermis (upper left). The dermis shows heat coagulation changes. (*van Gieson ×100*)

256   Skin. Localised burn with necrosis of part of the epidermis and formation of subepidermal blisters. (*van Gieson ×100*)

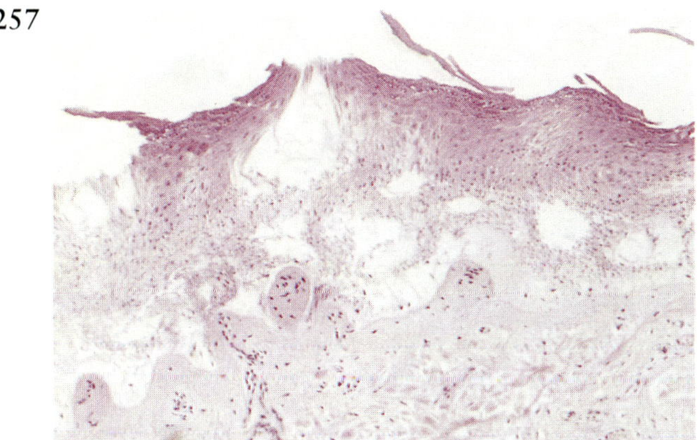

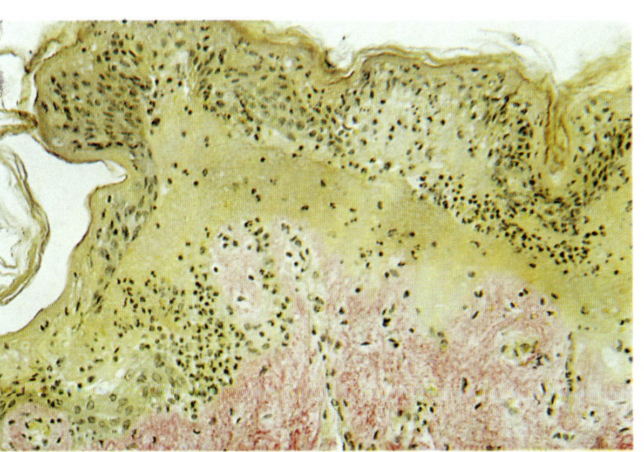

257 Skin from the hand. Autopsy material from a patient who died of carbon monoxide poisoning. The picture shows a pre-terminal skin lesion caused by a burning cigarette. Note the subepidermal blister formation. (*H&E ×160*)

258 Skin. First/second degree burn. Important features are the oedema of the epidermis, haemorrhage and a leucocytic reaction in the dermis. Post-traumatic survival: 5 days. (*van Gieson ×250*)

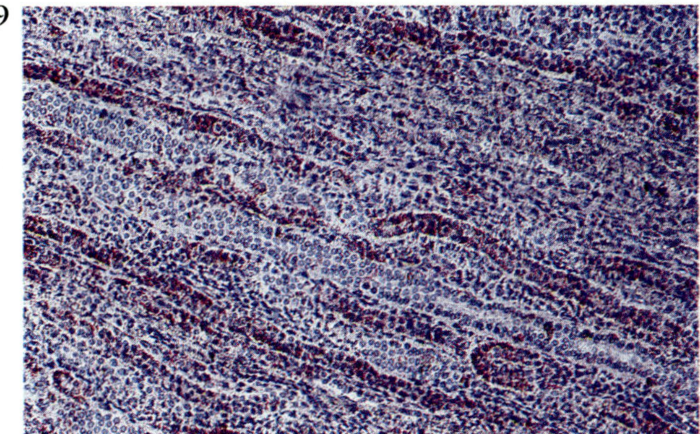

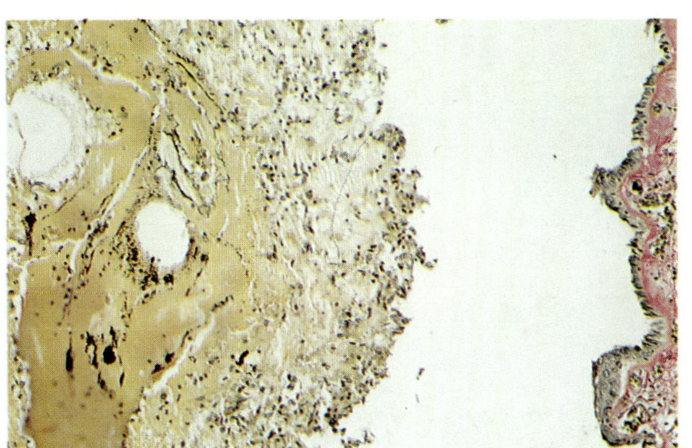

259   Kidney. Toxic fatty change of the epithelium of the collecting tubules caused by burns to 15 per cent of the body surface. Material from a one year-old male. Post-traumatic survival: 2 days. (*Sudan stain ×100*)

260   Lung. Soot inhalation. The soot particles (black) are seen in the bronchial secretions (yellow–brown, left), evidence of spontaneous breathing before death by burning. (*van Gieson ×160*)

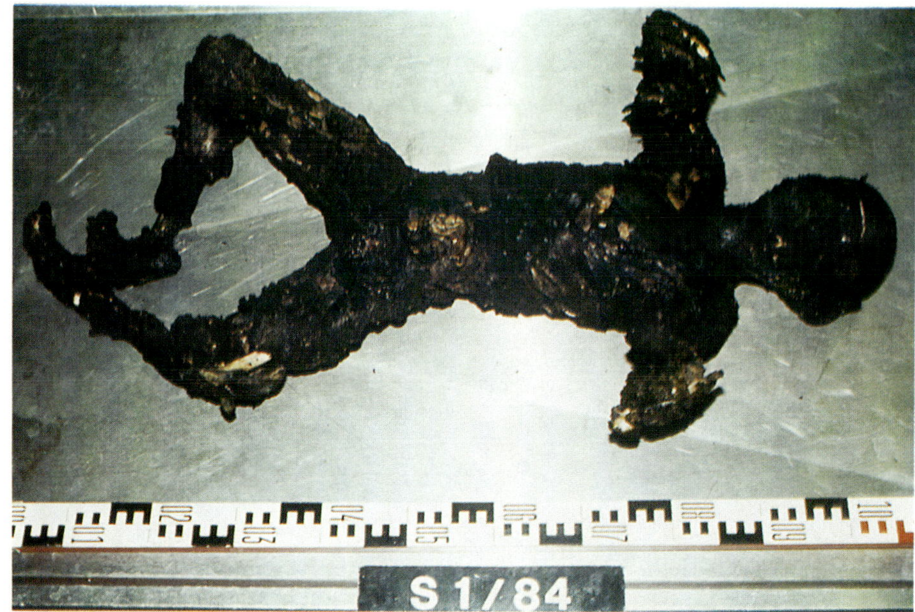

261 **Burnt corpse** in typical 'fencer' position (pugilistic attitude). 12 year-old boy.

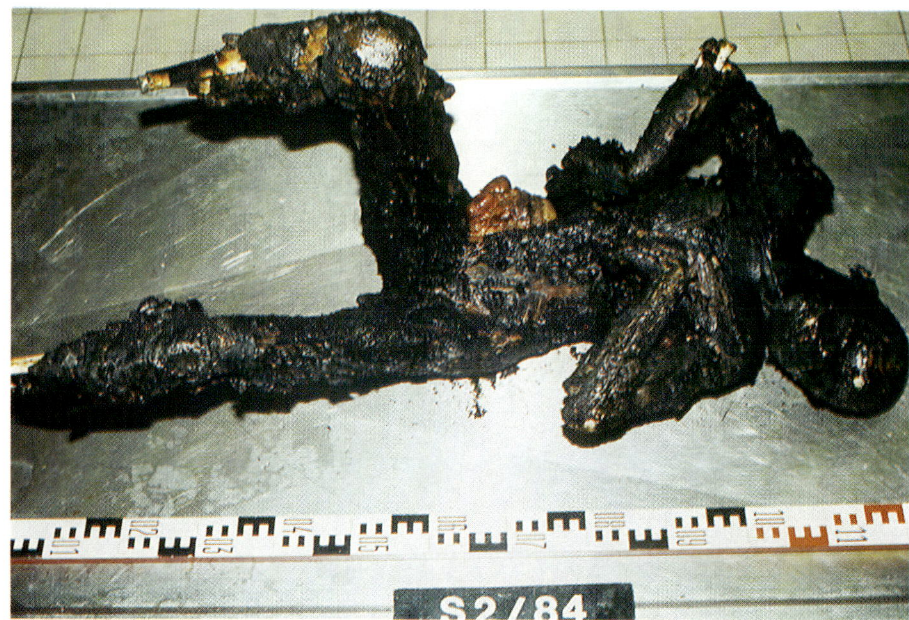

262 **Burnt corpse** with marked superficial charring and loss of both feet and parts of the leg. 14 year-old boy.

Note that the unusual postures of burnt bodies are due to post-mortem contraction of the muscles caused by heat. They have NO correlation whatever with pre-mortem activity. Lay investigators must be warned against interpreting the position of the corpse as indicative of some specific activity prior to the fire.

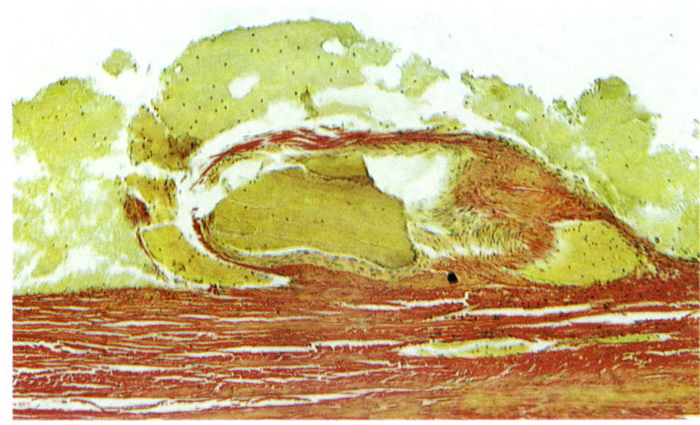

263 Dura mater. Epidural burn haematoma (green) following severe burns to the head. The haematoma arises from post-mortem extravasation of blood into the epidural space. It results from the heating of the brain, which expands, and contraction of the dura. It is **not** related to pre-mortem trauma. (*van Gieson ×100*)

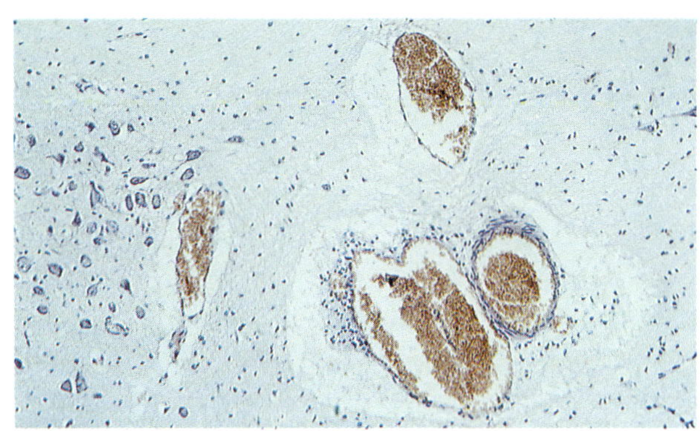

264 Cerebrum. Hyperthermia in a 3 month-old boy. Note the marked perivascular oedema, as well as hyperaemia. (*H&E ×250*)

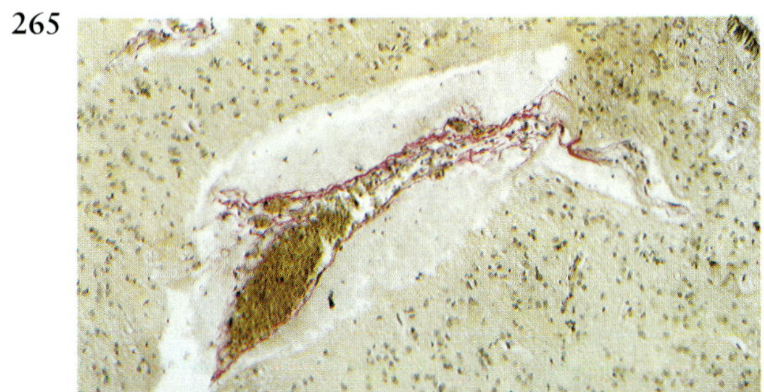

265 Cerebrum. Same case as **264**. Subependymal region, showing perivascular (Virchow–Robin space), protein-rich oedema (dysoria). (*van Gieson ×160*)

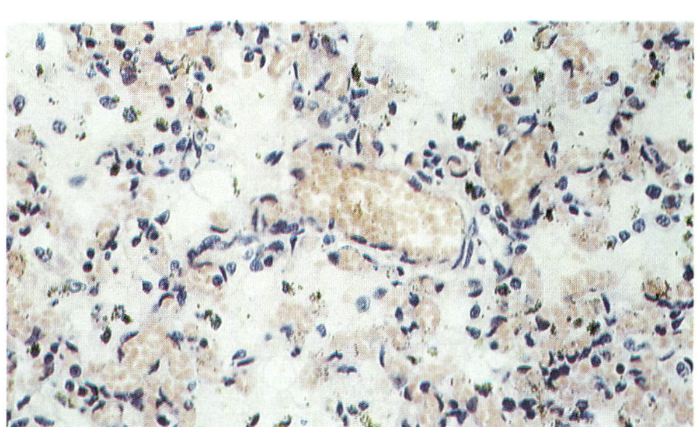

266 Lung. Hyperthermia. Same case as in **264**. The capillaries display a marked dilatation. Moreover, there are signs of beginning haemorrhagic pulmonary oedema. The black particles are formalin pigment precipitates. (*H&E ×400*)

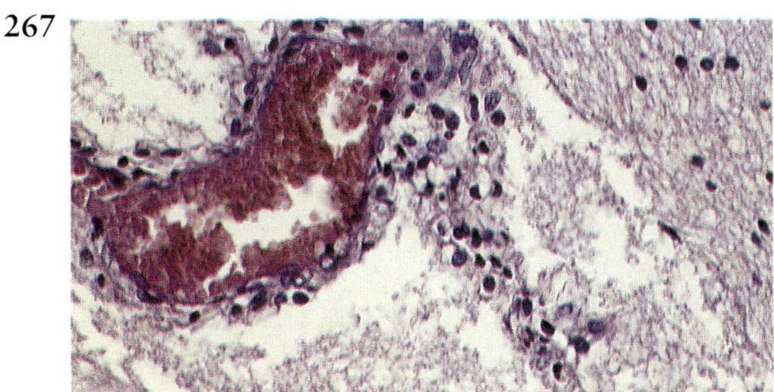

267 Cerebrum. Hyperthermia caused by an acute respiratory tract infection in an 18 months-old boy. Death occurred suddenly. Note the hyperaemia of the blood vessels and the presence of protein-rich perivascular oedema. (*H&E ×100*)

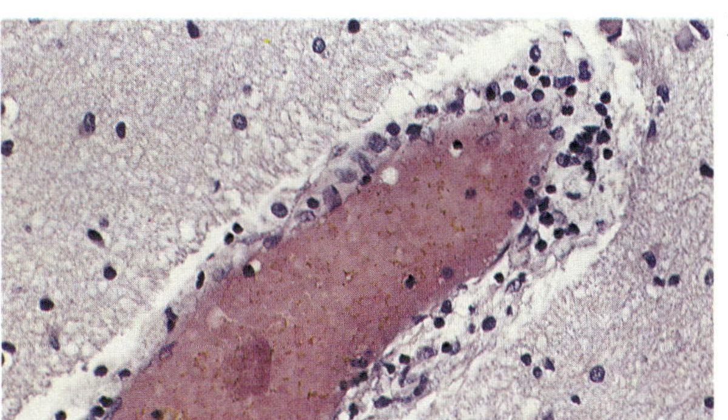

268 Cerebrum. Perivascular cellular accumulation consisting principally of lymphocytes. Such a picture may be found in cases of heat stroke, where the patient survives for a few days. If heat stroke can be excluded from the case history, such a finding is most likely a residual infiltration from a previous viral meningitis. (*H&E ×100*)

6 Effects of electric current

The morphological hallmarks of the injury caused by electric current are the 'current mark' and the electrothermal burn. The severity of these changes depends on a variety of factors, including the resistance of the skin, the size of the contact surface, and the voltage applied. Thus, with a large contact surface or in cases in which the skin is wet, current marks may be absent. In the latter case, the wet skin offers minimal resistance and minimum Joule effect.

In high voltage electrocutions severe and extensive entrance and exit burns may be produced. Current marks caused by low voltage injury are particularly obvious in areas of the body with a well developed horny layer, as on the fingers and palms of the hand or on the soles of the feet. The heat generated causes the formation of spherical vacuoles in the horny layer (stratum corneum) of the skin with splitting of the layers of the epidermis.

More marked histological changes can be seen if more heat has been generated. Thus, a honeycomb (or Swiss cheese) appearance may be produced by blister formation in the epidermis. Cell necrosis may also be observed with pyknosis of the nuclei and loss of a clear demarcation between the epidermal cells. The ducts of sweat or sebaceous glands may also show areas of necrosis.

Further features of electric current injury are the elongation of cell nuclei and cells in the epidermis, and the formation of approximately parallel cellular sheets (palisading), particularly in the basal and spindle cell layers. This cellular arrangement often produces a whorled appearance, which can also be seen in the sweat and sebaceous glands of the dermis, or, more rarely, in the walls of dermal blood vessels.

A denaturation of dermal connective tissue and subcutaneous muscle cells may occur and manifests itself as indistinct outlines of individual cells with altered staining reaction (increased basophilia).

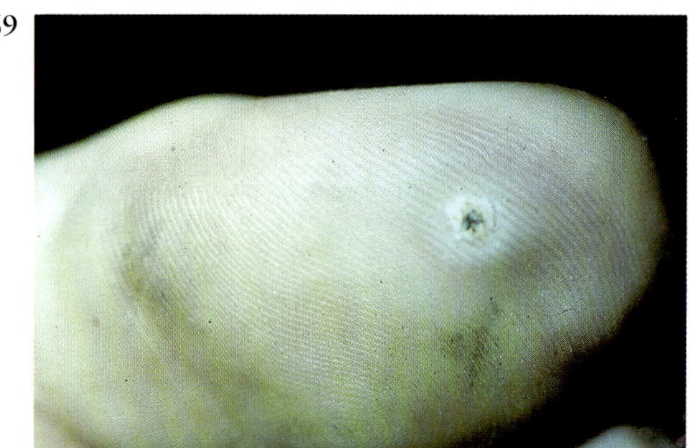

269 Lesion on the tip of the finger caused by electrocution.

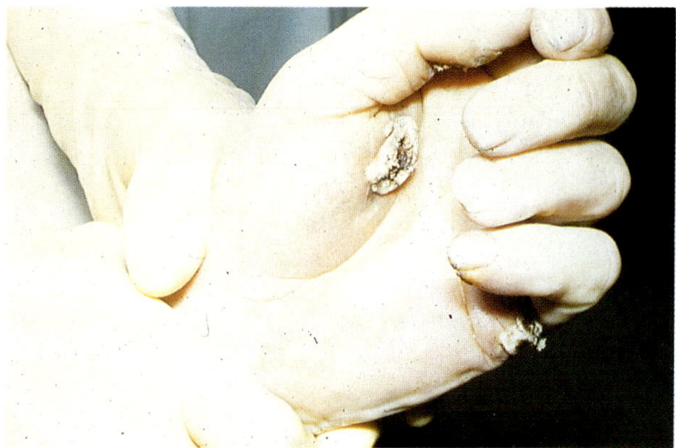

270 Electric burn on the palm of the hand.

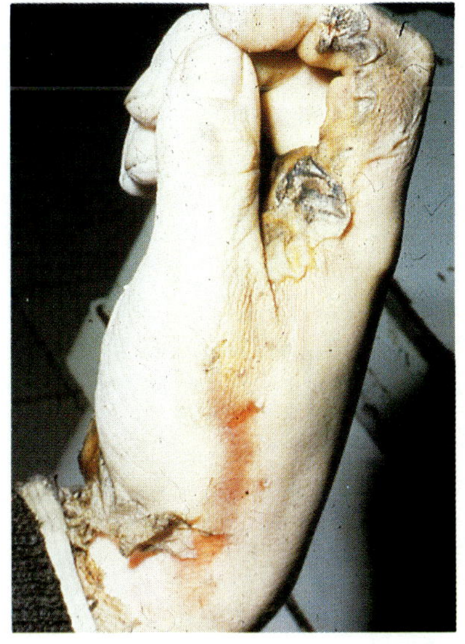 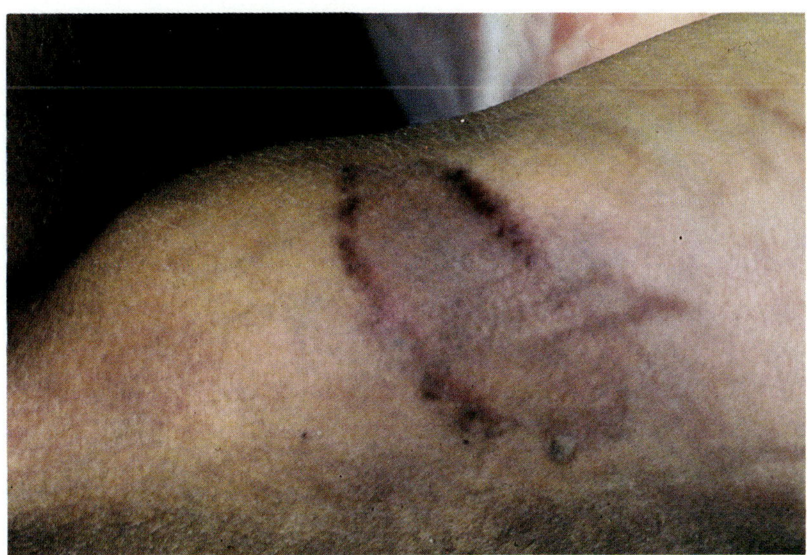

271   **High voltage electric burn** to the right hand.

272   **Extensive skin lesion** caused by electric current.

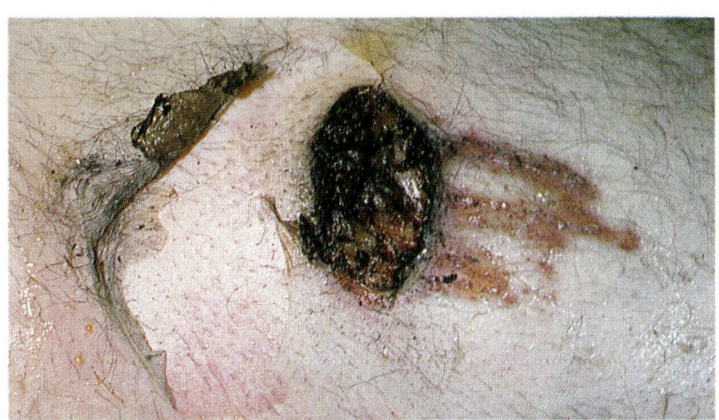 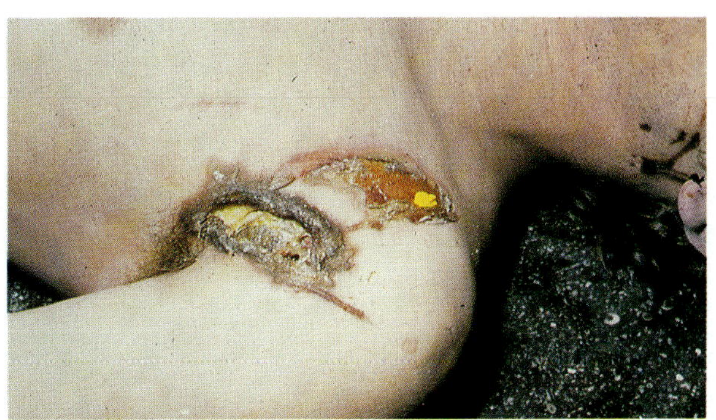

273   **High voltage lesion** on the thigh with third degree burns. The epidermis is separated from the dermis due to heat, and has been pushed into a roll to the left.

274   **High voltage lesion** on the left shoulder. Same case as in **273**.

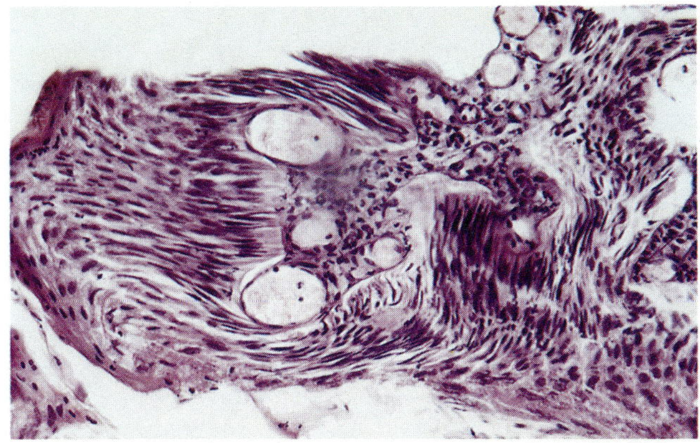 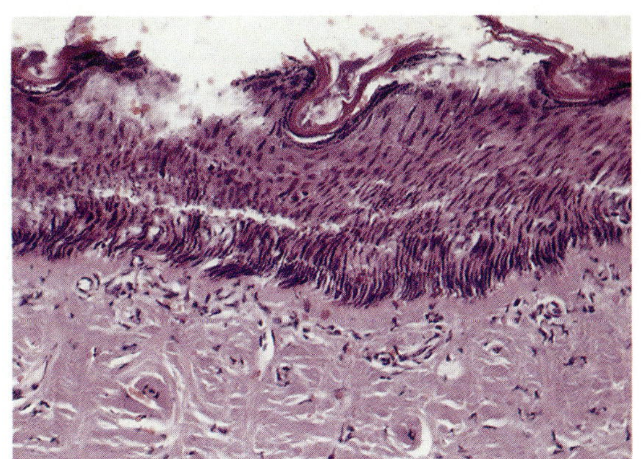

275   **Penile condyloma** following removal by cauterisation. The tissue shows evidence of the action of electric current — the cells are elongated, spindle-shaped and are arranged in parallel sheets. (*H&E ×250*)

276   **Foreskin.** Effects of cauterisation. The electric current has caused an elongation of the cell nuclei in all epidermal strata, especially in the basal layer. (*H&E ×100*)

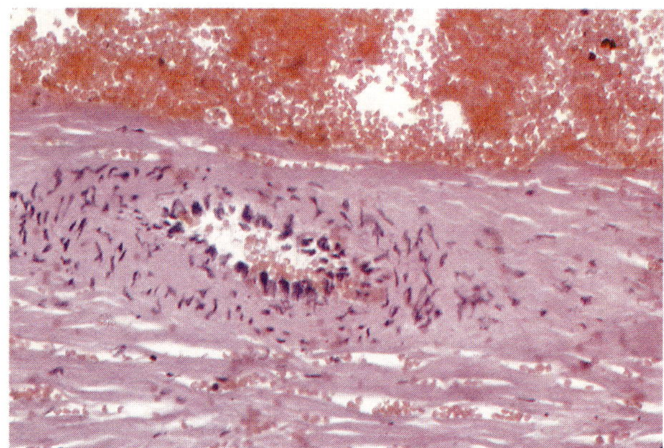

277 Subcutaneous tissue. Alterations caused by electric current in a blood vessel wall in the dermis. The nuclei are markedly elongated. (*H&E ×250*)

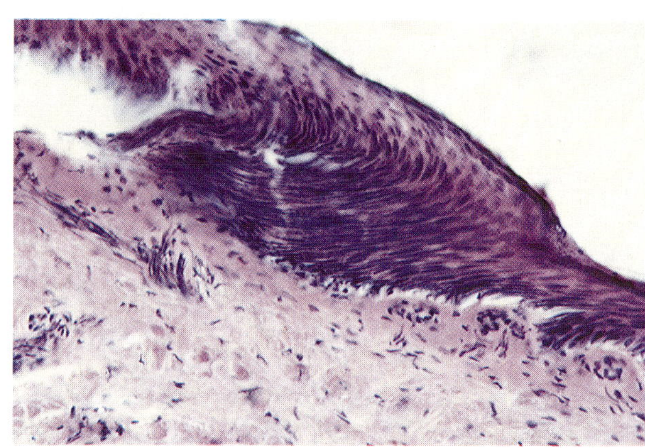

278 Skin (finger). Death from electrocution. The epidermis has been partially elevated by vaporisation of water at the dermoepidermal junction (upper left). The typical elongation of the cell nuclei is also evident in the dermis as well as in the epidermis. (*H&E ×250*)

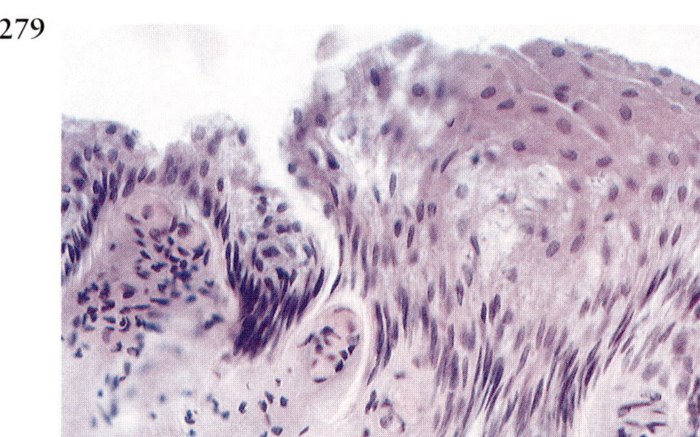

279 Skin (finger). Material from a male who died following electrocution. The cells of the basal layer show marked nuclear elongation, while vacuolisation is seen in the cells of the spindle cell layer. (*H&E ×400*)

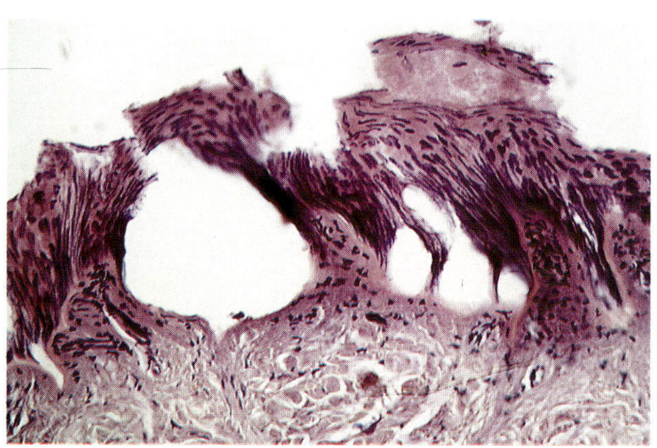

280 Skin (finger). Death from electrocution (220 volt AC) in a 19 year-old male. Blister formation and elongation of cell nuclei can be seen in the epidermis. (*H&E ×250*)

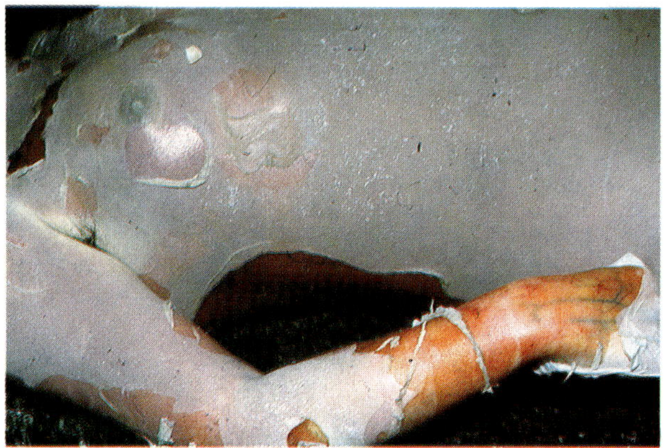

281 Death by electrocution in the bath.

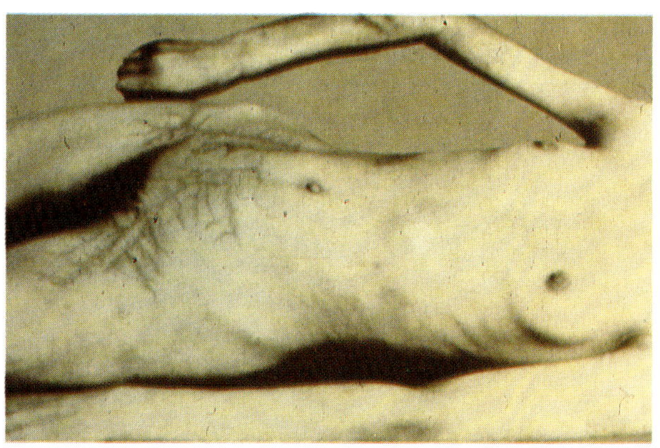

282 Lesions caused by lightning which struck the lower abdomen and thigh. The arboral pattern is characteristic of lightning strikes, and is caused by passage along the skin.

7 Poisoning

Toxicology is a vast field, embracing the entire spectrum of poisons, including gases, organic solvents, corrosive poisons, pesticides, metals and therapeutic agents. This chapter outlines the main pathological changes associated with various forms of poisoning.

Poisons can act on the body in two principal ways:

- **Locally,** at the site of administration — corrosive destruction of skin caused by concentrated acid.
- **Systemically,** for example, following absorption, the poison is carried by the circulation to different organs where it, or a metabolite, exerts its effect.

Poisons may be absorbed in various ways:

(a) **Via the gastrointestinal tract:**
Oesophagus and stomach. Under the action of corrosive agents, superficial epithelial defects arise with marked dilatation and hyperaemia of blood vessels and morphological evidence of toxic circulatory damage.
Liver. Marked capillary hyperaemia is seen, evidence of acute congestion as a result of circulatory failure.
Kidney. If the victim lives for some hours following poisoning, a toxic nephrosis with swelling of the renal tubular epithelium in the presence or absence of cytoplasmic vacuolation may be seen.
Brain. In, for example, cases of barbiturate poisoning, perivascular oedema (filling of the Virchow–Robin space with weakly staining eosinophilic transudate) can be found, sometimes with extravasation of erythrocytes.

(b) **Via the respiratory tract:**
Lungs: Nitrogenous gases and various smoke gases cause a proteinaceous pulmonary oedema, which is eosinophilic on routine H&E staining. This is followed a few days later by a fibroblastic reaction. Haemorrhagic pulmonary oedema is often seen in cases of severe poisoning. Chemical damage to the bronchial epithelium manifests itself as superficial necrosis or degenerative change in the epithelial cells.

The effects of inhaled CS gases have been described by Chapman and White (1978). After 48 hours there is extensive necrosis and ulceration of the mucosal epithelium of larynx, trachea, and bronchi, and its replacement by a pseudomembrane of fibrin-rich exudate containing polymorphonuclear leucocytes and their degenerating forms. Scattered areas of bronchopneumonia are present, all clustered about exudate-filled bronchioles. Oedema and minimal intra-alveolar haemorrhage are observed.

Tear gas can also produce pulmonary changes. Thus, 14 days after inhalation, intra-alveolar haemorrhage with loss of epithelium lining the respiratory bronchioles and alveoli may be observed. In many places the respiratory bronchioles are lined by a proteinaceous exudate resembling hyaline membrane disease. The alveolar septa are widened and show proliferation of young fibroblasts.

(c) **Via the skin:**
An example of percutaneous poisoning is the absorption of solvents such as benzene. This causes damage to parenchymatous organs, especially liver, kidney and bone marrow. The highly toxic esters of phosphoric acid are enzyme poisons and inhibit acetylcholinesterase. Death occurs so rapidly that morphological changes in the various organs do not have time to develop.

Corrosive agents

Whereas acids cause a tissue hardening and brittleness when applied, for example, to skin or mucous membranes, alkalis cause a liquefaction of tissue by denaturation of protein and saponification of fats. In the latter case the affected tissue swells, becomes soft and assumes a slimy consistency. The formation of haematin pigment results in a brown colouration of the tissue.

Corrosive agents are often ingested orally and may cause severe local and systemic changes. Lesoine (1965) classified corrosive trauma to the oesophagus into five stages:

- Primary local damage. This takes the form of tissue necrosis, mucosal ulceration and oedema.
- General intoxication.
- Oesophagitis, with acute, subacute and chronic forms.
- Healing, with fibrous tissue formation and the possibility of oesophageal stricture.
- Late complications.

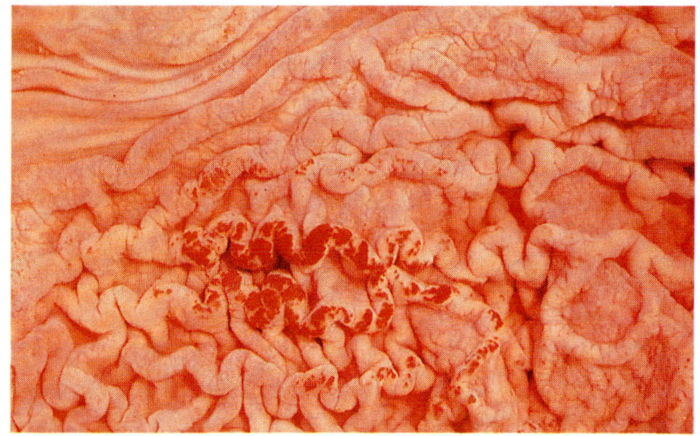

283 Toxic gastric mucosal haemorrhage. Suicide using turpentine-containing solution.

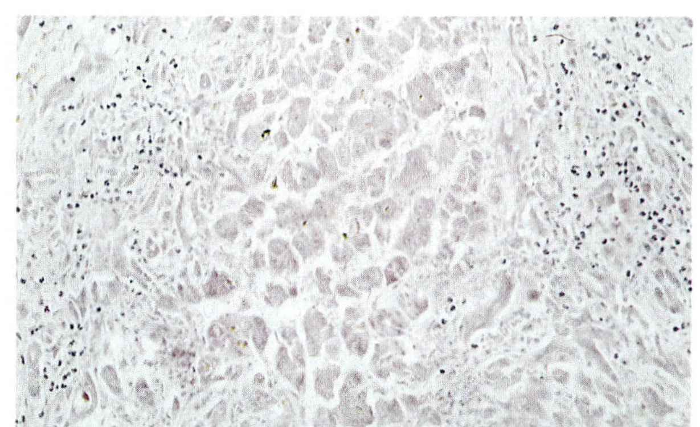

284 Liver. Mushroom poisoning (*Amanita phalloides*), showing areas of hepatocyte necrosis (centre) surrounded by a leucocytic infiltration. Blue pigment (yellow, below) is also visible. Material from a 35 year-old male who survived for 2 days. (*H&E ×200*)

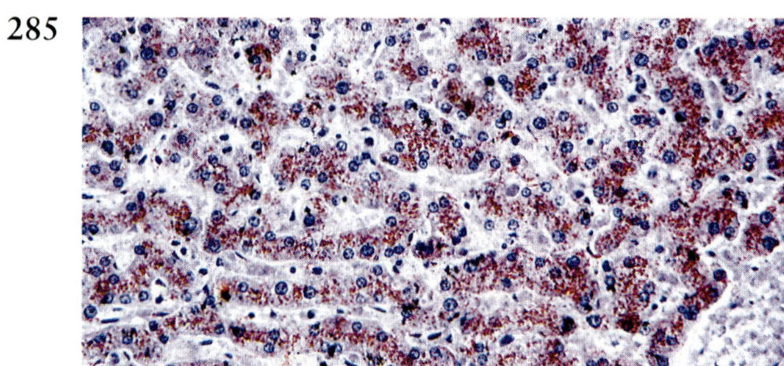

285 Liver. Barbiturate poisoning. Note the extensive fatty change in the hepatocytes (as a result of hypoxia) which contain small droplets of fat (red). The changes are non-specific but are observed in such cases of poisoning. The patient died 3 days after the overdose. (*Sudan stain ×250*)

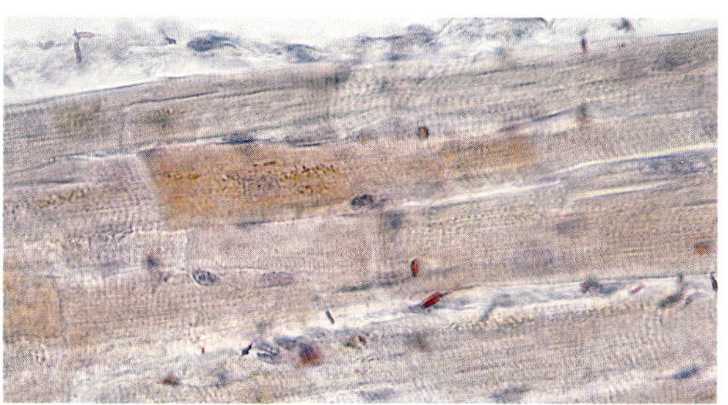

286 Heart. Mushroom poisoning. The cardiac muscle cells contain very fine lipid droplets (red), the result of toxic and/or hypoxic changes. Material from a 35 year-old male, who lived for 2 days after ingestion. (*Sudan stain ×640*)

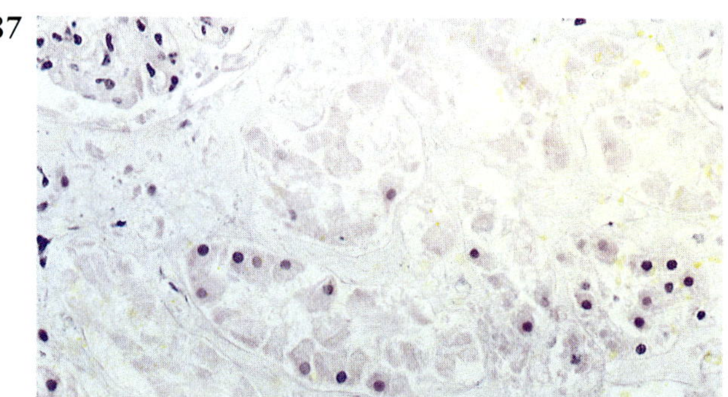

287 Kidney. Mushroom poisoning (*Amanita phalloides*) in a 35 year-old male who died 2 days later. A renal tubulonecrosis is seen with selective necrosis of epithelial cells of numerous renal tubuli. In some cells, the nucleus is no longer demonstrable; in others, the nuclei are pyknotic, whilst a few cells are still intact. (*H&E ×400*)

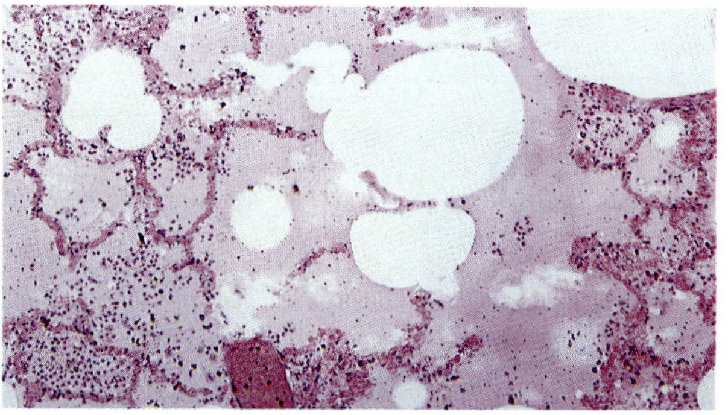

288 Lung from suicide by E 605 ingestion (organic phosphate parathion). The lung shows a marked hyperaemia and intra-alveolar oedema with disruption of alveolar lining cells. Leucocytes are visible in some alveoli, evidence that bronchopneumonia has begun to appear. Putrefied blisters are present. The patient survived for a few hours. (*H&E ×100*)

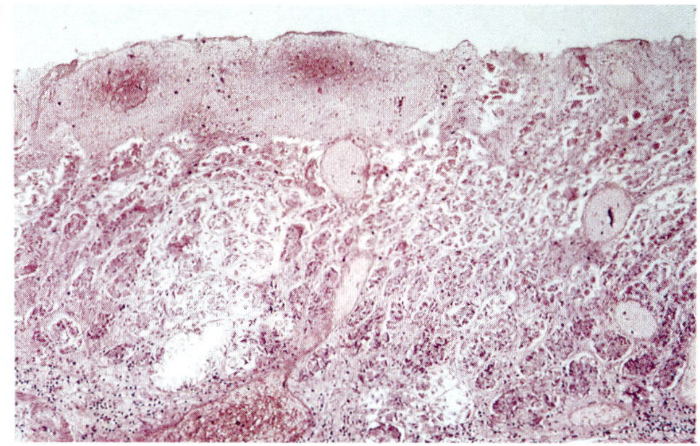

289 Stomach. Suicide by E 605 (parathion) ingestion. The blood vessels of the mucosa are markedly dilated and hyperaemic. Haemorrhage is also a feature seen in the autolytic mucosa. The patient died a few hours after ingestion. (*H&E ×100*)

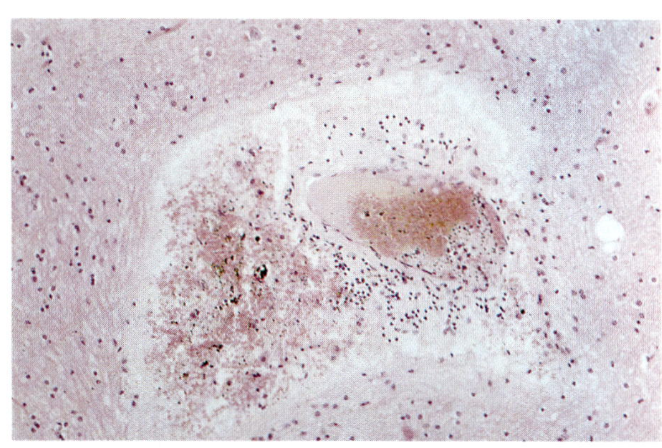

290 Cerebrum. Barbiturate poisoning in a 15 year-old girl, who died one day later. Note the changes caused by hypoxia: perivascular oedema and haemorrhage (Virchow–Robin space) and a perivascular leucocytic infiltrate. The brown–black pigment in the area of haemorrhage is formalin pigment. (*H&E ×160*)

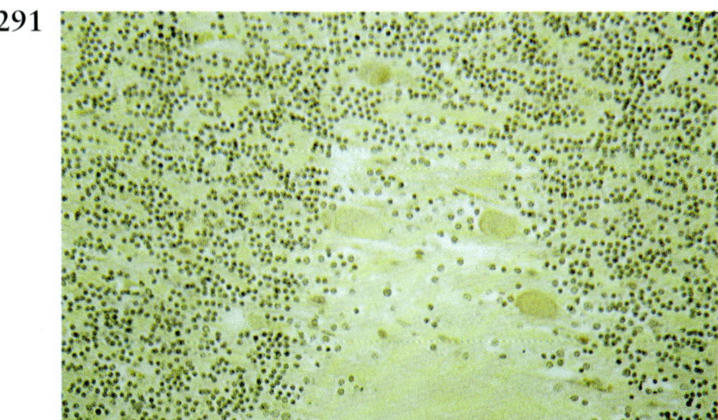

291 Cerebellum. Barbiturate poisoning (same case as **290**). The Purkinje cells (large cells) show degenerative changes with cytoplasmic swelling, loss of clear demarcation of the nuclear membrane and decreased nuclear staining reaction. (*van Gieson ×250*)

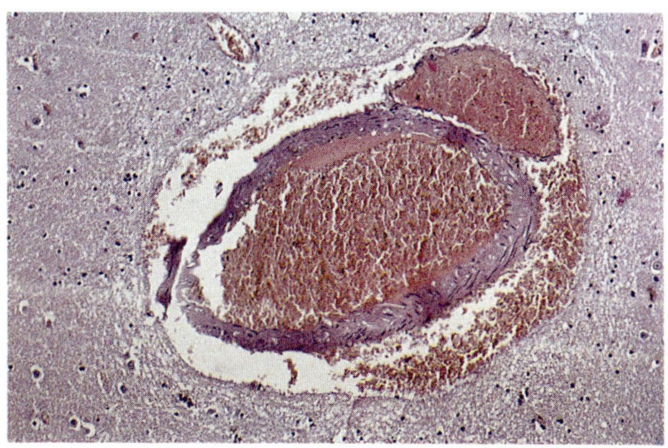

292 Suicidal intoxication with alcohol and chloromethiazole. Brain, showing hyperaemia and perivascular haemorrhage. (*H&E ×100*)

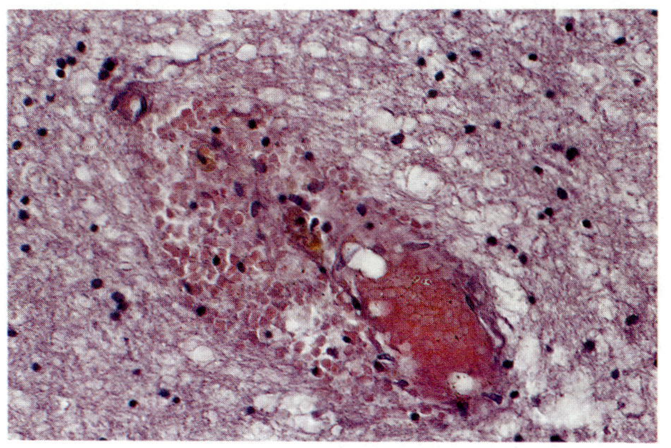

293 Same case as in **292**. Hyperaemia, perivascular haemorrhage and marked oedema in the neighbouring parenchyma. (*H&E ×100*)

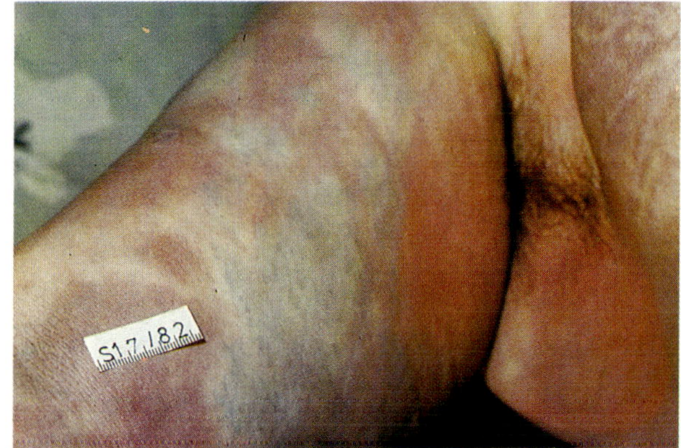

294 **Cherry red post-mortem lividity** in a case of carbon monoxide poisoning, best seen in the axilla in this photograph.

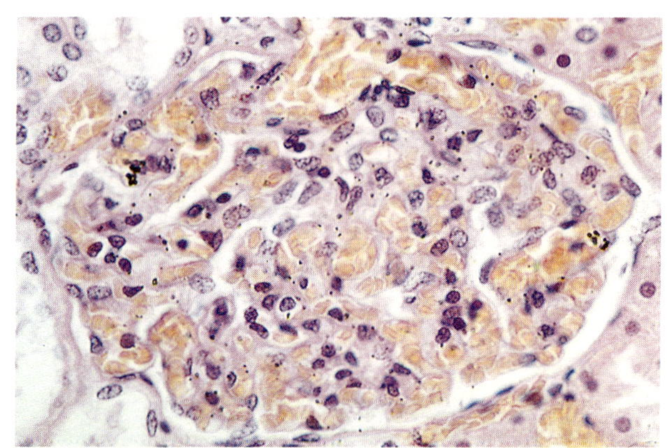

295 **Kidney.** Carbon monoxide poisoning in a 30 year-old male who died approximately 10 hours after being poisoned. The glomerulus shows very marked congestion in the capillaries. (*H&E ×640*)

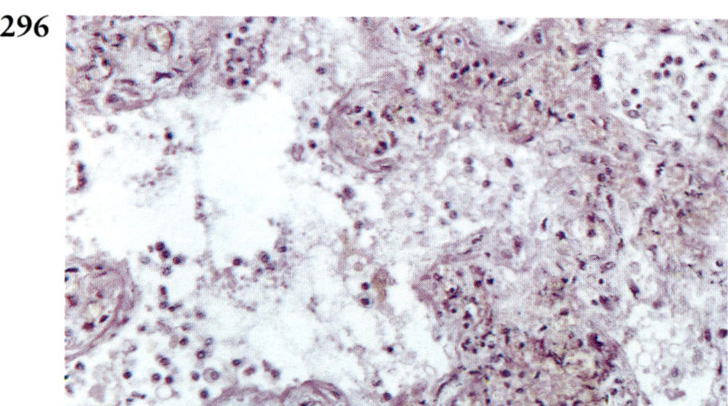

296 **Lung.** Zinc chloride poisoning (from a smoke bomb). The small pulmonary blood vessels are markedly dilated, the alveolar lining cells are swollen, and in some cases desquamated. Intra-alveolar leucocytes are also visible, as well as the formation of hyaline membranes lining the alveoli. From a 24 year-old male who died 6 days later. (*H&E ×250*)

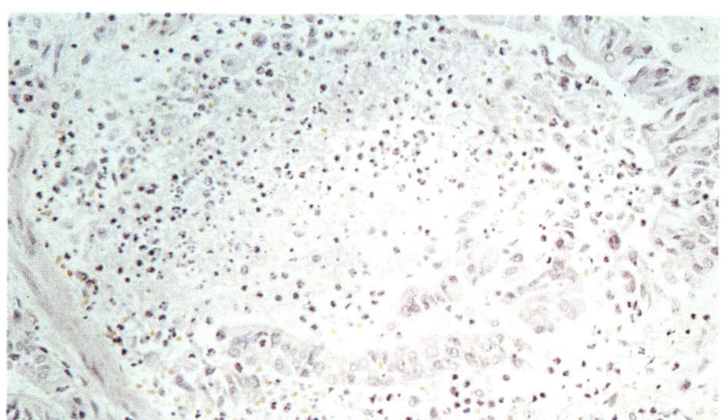

297 **Lung.** Same case as in **296**. The bronchial epithelium is partially necrotic (upper left). A purulent bronchitis is also evident from the numerous leucocytes in the bronchial lumen. (*H&E ×250*)

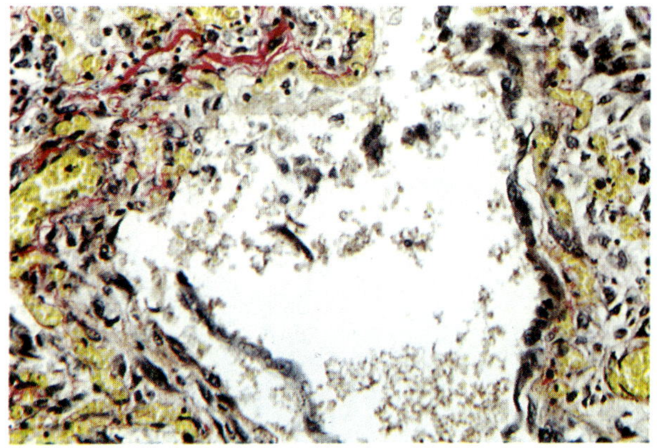

298 **Lung.** Same case as in **296**. The disruption of the partially necrotic bronchial epithelium is depicted. (*van Gieson ×250*)

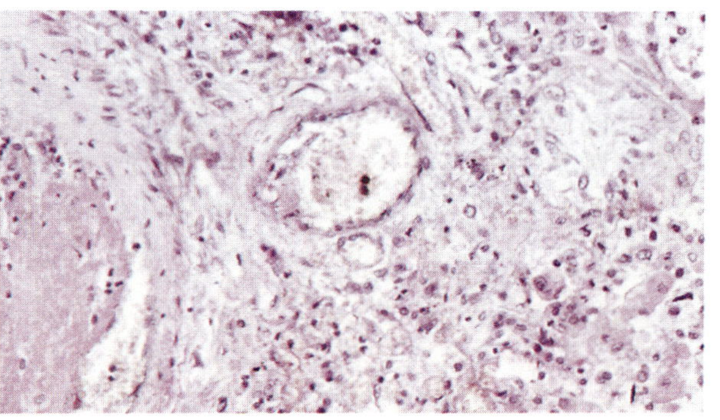

299 **Lung.** Zinc chloride poisoning. Same case as in **296**. A partially organised thrombus is visible in a branch of the pulmonary artery (left). (*H&E ×250*)

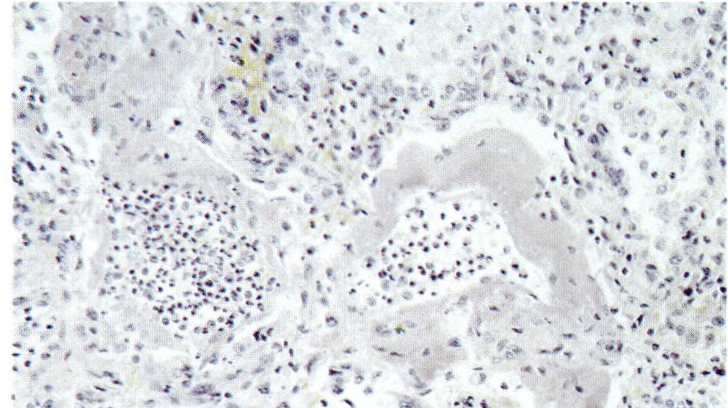

300 **Lung.** Zinc chloride poisoning (smoke bomb) in a 20 year-old male who died 11 days later. A marked swelling and desquamation of the alveolar lining cells is seen, as well as large hyaline membranes and a purulent bronchiolitis (leucocytes in the bronchiolar lumen). (*H&E ×250*)

301 **Lung.** Same case as in 300. The lung shows an extensive connective tissue proliferation as in carnification of a pneumonia. (*van Gieson ×160*)

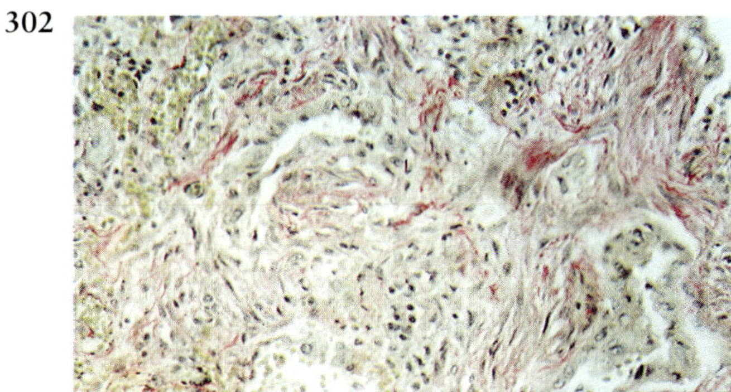

302 **Lung.** Same case as in 300, demonstrating the connective tissue proliferation (collagen fibres red) with formation of bronchiolitis obliterans (obliteration of the bronchiolar lumen). (*van Gieson ×250*)

303 **Lung.** Bronchiolitis obliterans caused by zinc chloride poisoning. The bronchiolar lumen contains immature collagen fibres (yellow–orange, centre). (*van Gieson ×200*)

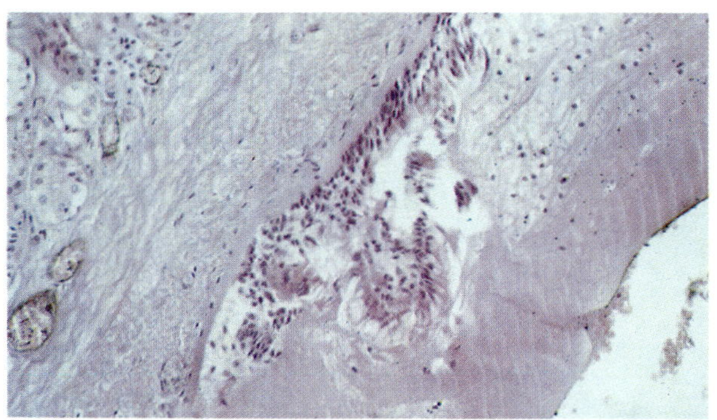

304 **Lung.** Paraquat poisoning in a 39 year-old man who inhaled paraquat vapour. Death occurred 6 hours later. The mucosa of the distal trachea shows partial disruption of the superficial epithelium and deposition of large amounts of fibrinous material. (*H&E ×250*)

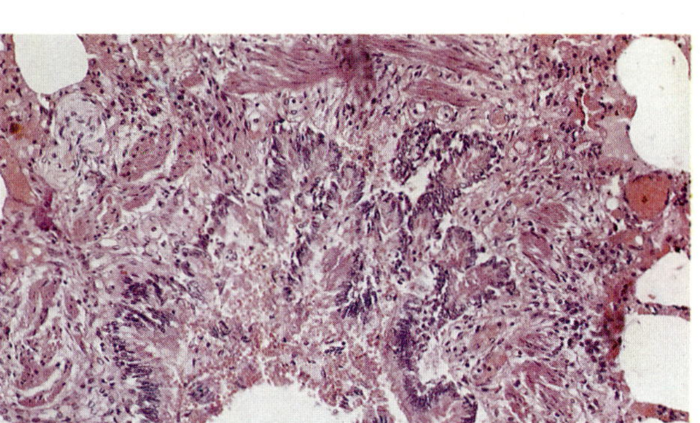

305 **Lung.** Inhalation of concentrated sulphuric acid vapour in a 58 year-old male. Part of a bronchus, in which haemorrhagic secretions can be seen in the lumen. The structure of the bronchial epithelium is for the most part well preserved, although signs of epithelial disruption are visible. Peribronchial haemorrhage is also present (left). The patient died 3 hours after inhalation. (*H&E ×250*)

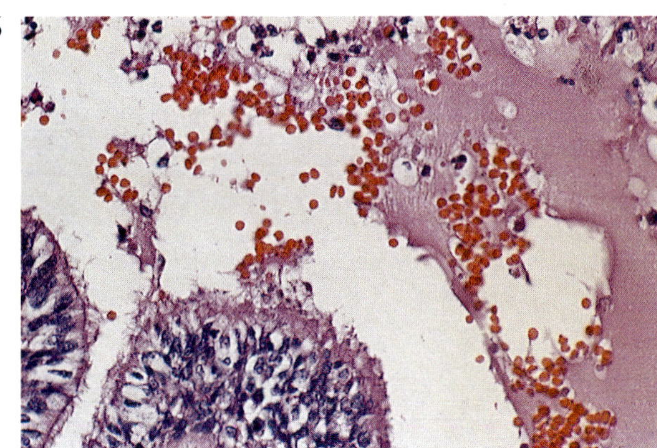

306 Lung. Same case as in 305. Part of a bronchus showing relatively normal epithelium (extreme lower left) and epithelium with superficial damage from the corrosive action of the sulphuric acid. The bronchial lumen contains oedematous fluid with erythrocytes (upper right). (*H&E ×200*)

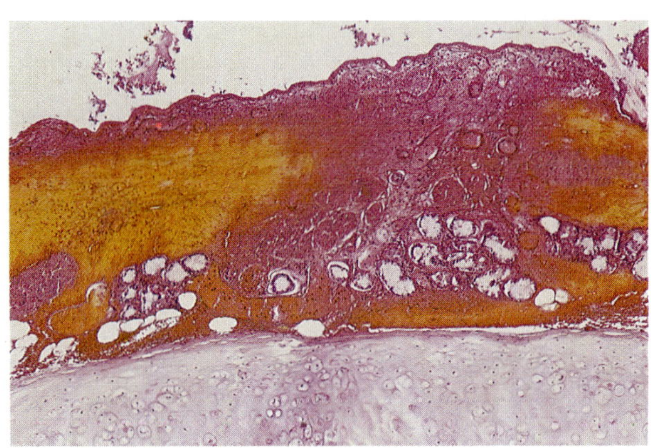

307 Lung. Same case as in 305. Part of a bronchus is illustrated, in which the epithelium has been destroyed by the sulphuric acid vapour. Epithelial remains can be seen in the upper right of the picture. The submucosa is markedly altered by haemorrhage. Bronchial cartilage can also be seen (below). (*H&E ×160*)

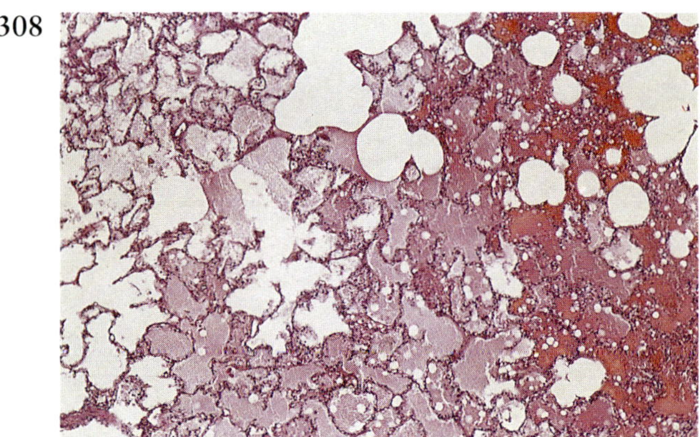

308 Lung. Same case as in 305. Areas of intra-alveolar haemorrhage (right) and intra-alveolar oedema (left) can be seen. (*H&E ×100*)

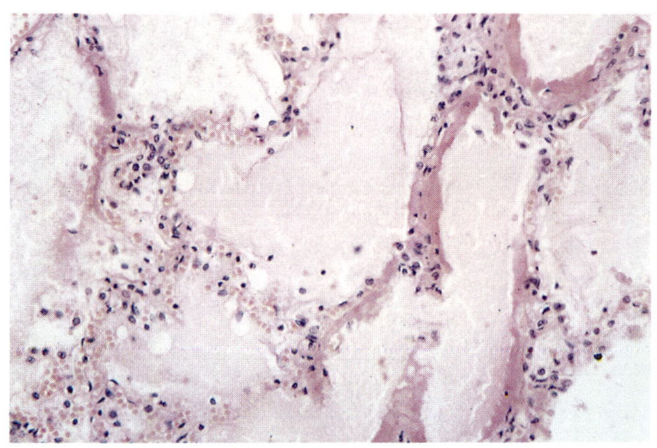

309 Lung. Poisoning with a mixture of nitrous and nitric oxides caused by an accident with a bottle of concentrated nitric acid. The 30 year-old victim died one day later. Note the filling of the alveoli with protein-rich oedema fluid and the eosinophilic hyaline membranes lining the alveoli. The latter is most probably the result of intensive artificial respiration. There is no inflammatory cell infiltration. (*H&E ×63*)

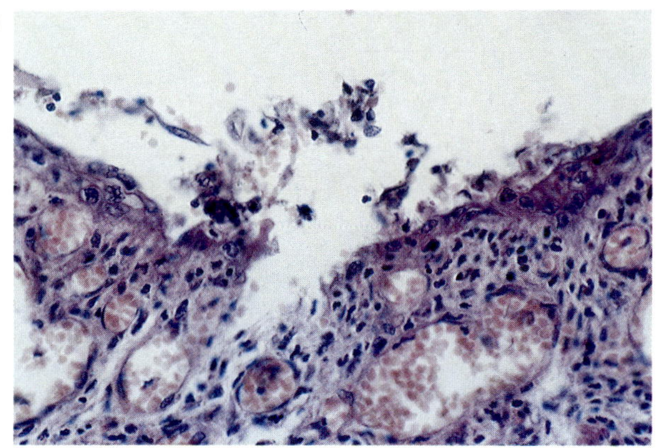

310 Oesophagus. Material from a 4 day-old baby who was given a household cleaning agent (the exact composition could not be established). Death occurred within half an hour of ingestion. The picture shows partial destruction of the oesophageal epithelium (middle). (*H&E ×400*)

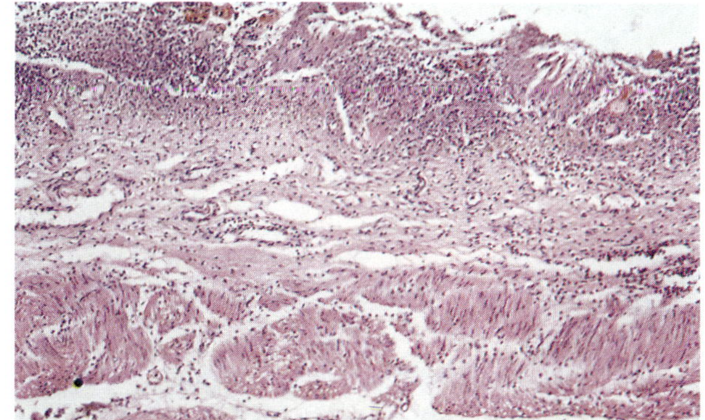

311 Oesophagus. Corrosion by concentrated alkali. Material from a 33 year-old male who died 36 hours after ingestion. The oesophageal muscle is depicted (bottom). An important feature is the loss of the oesophageal epithelium, which ·has been replaced by fibrin and numerous polymorphonuclear leucocytes. (*H&E ×100*)

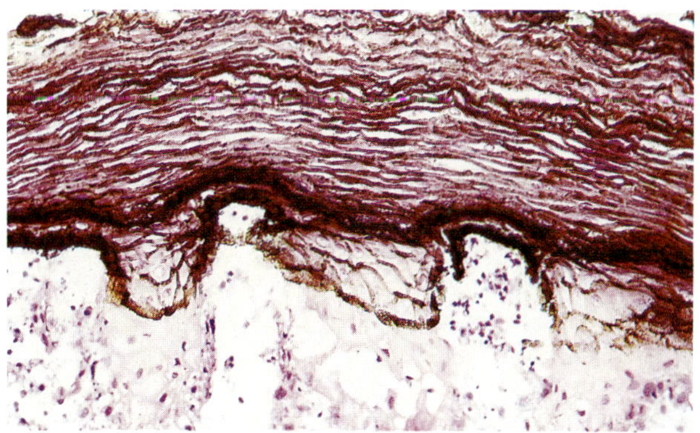

312 Oesophagus. Same case as in **311.** Here some remaining oesophageal epithelium is seen (below), as well as sheets of proteinaceous material containing alkaline haematin (red, above) deposited on the luminal side of the epithelium. (*H&E ×250*)

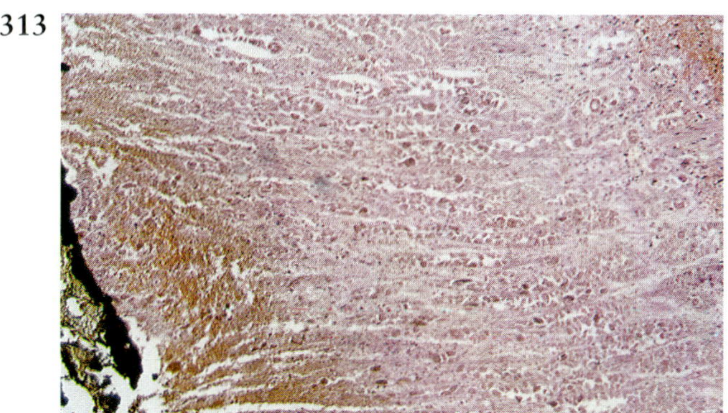

313 Stomach. Same case as in **311.** The corpus epithelium shows haemorrhage in the deepest part of the mucosa (right), as well as superficial necrosis and formation of a darkly staining eschar (left). (*H&E ×100*)

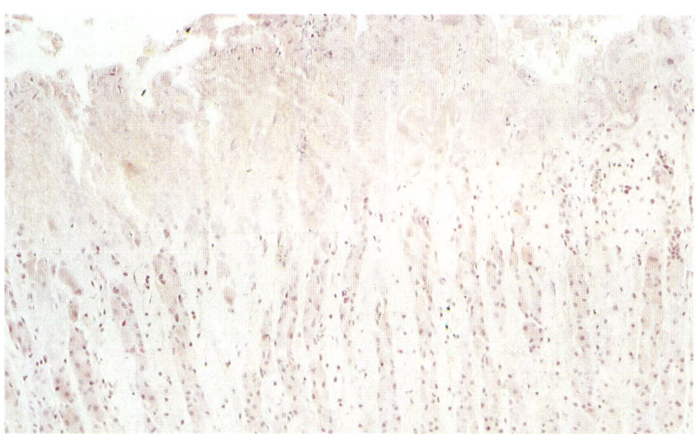

314 Stomach. Corrosion of the stomach mucosal lining following ingestion of fluid from a galvanising bath. Death resulted from cyanide poisoning. The superficial necrosis of the lining epithelium is shown, but because of this necrosis the tissue is faintly stained. (*H&E ×160*)

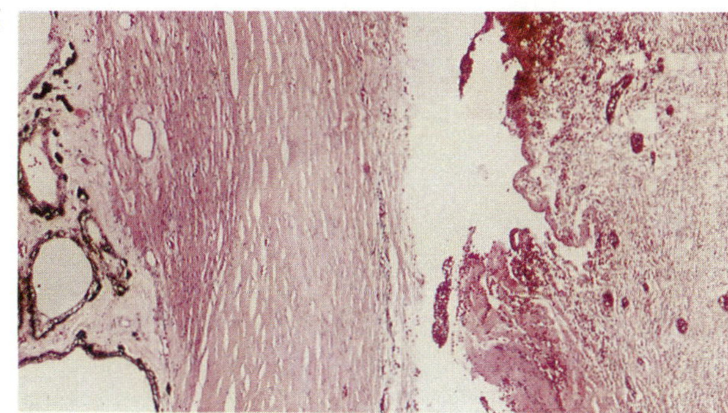

315 Eye. Enucleation after tear gas corrosive injury 2 years previously. Material from a 31 year-old man. Note the broad fibrous tissue layer (right) in place of the sclera. Part of the ciliary body is also depicted (left). (*H&E ×40*)

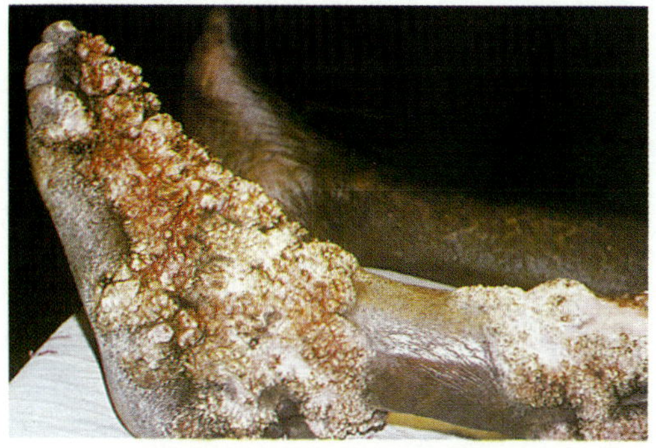

316 A week-old bite from an otter (*Bitis arietans, Clotho arietans,* grey) on the foot of a 12 year-old boy, with marked secondary infection by various organisms.

8 Post-traumatic complications

Embolism

Fat embolism

On the whole, fat embolism is usually related to trauma, especially bone, and can be seen in the pulmonary blood vessels. It is also present in the organs supplied by the systemic circulation, though they are affected to a variable degree.

Fat embolism is assessed at a magnification of $\times 25$ using the following classification scheme:

> 0 No fat embolism or occasional embolic fat droplets.
>
> I Low grade fat embolism: single or multiple embolic fat droplets in every microscopic field.
>
> II Marked fat embolism: numerous fat droplets in every microscopic field.
>
> III Massive fat embolism: more than 50 per cent of the pulmonary capillaries contain fat droplets.

Fat droplets in blood vessels can also be demonstrated in:

- Cases of burns with emulsification of blood lipids.
- Decomposition.

Fat embolism, in the form of sausage-shaped neutral fat droplets, can be demonstrated many months after death. As well as Sudan III, Sudan black, Nile blue sulphate and Oil red O can be recommended as staining reagents.

In *tissue embolism*, particles of bone marrow, or rarely of liver or brain, can be seen.

Air embolism is seen in cases of severe trauma to major veins, especially in the neck, occasionally during intravenous infusion under pressure, and in cases of criminal abortion. The demonstration of air embolism is **macroscopic** — for example, by opening the heart under water and by the presence of foamy blood in the veins. The latter is to be interpreted with care in cases of decomposition.

The *laminated thrombus* cannot always be easily distinguished from the so-called *red thrombus*. The former, however, demonstrates a definite stratification of fibrin and blood cells, especially leucocytes. At its site of formation, the thrombus adheres to the intima of the blood vessel. The mixed thrombus contains a laminated portion and a red thrombus portion at one end.

The following guidelines can be used to determine the age of a thrombus:

- Recent   Unaltered polymorphonuclear leucocytes and monocytes.
- After 24 hours   Disintegration of polymorphonuclear cells and swelling of monocytes.
- After 7 days   Fibroblastic proliferation beginning in the region of the thrombus adherent to the intima.
- After 14 days   Formation of collagen fibres.

A more detailed account of the chronological course of the process of thrombus organisation is given by Janssen (1977):

- 1–3 days: Absence of a reaction between endothelium and thrombus. Leucocytes, as well as fibrin strands and thrombocytes, are structurally unchanged. In the central portions of the thrombus, the erythrocytes tend to be closely packed, and at the periphery more loosely arranged.
- 3–8 days: Infiltration of endothelial sprouts. The free (nonadherent) surface of the thrombus may be invested in an endothelial cell layer. Hyalinisation usually begins centrally. The entrapped leucocytes are pyknotic. Monocyte nuclei are enlarged and stain more lightly. As a result of thrombus contraction, peripheral clefts and sinuslike cavities may arise and contain loosely clumped erythrocytes.
- 4–20 days: The first capillaries, fibroblasts, mesenchymal cells and haemosiderin-laden histiocytes can be seen. The hyalinising process tends to divide the thrombus into a few large compartments. Evidence of nuclear debris from leucocytes can be seen. The swelling of the monocytes is also a feature.
- 8 days–2 months: Fibroplasia (formation of argyrophilic and collagen fibres). Numerous capillaries. In hyalinised thrombi, the nuclear debris from polymorphonuclear cells is seen only as indistinct shadows. After between 8 and 17 days, monocyte swelling is not observed.
- 2–8 months: Few cell elements are visible. Occasional capillaries, argyrophilic and collagen

fibres, as well as a few elastic fibres, are seen. In the completely hyalinised thrombus, groups of spindle-shaped cholesterol crystal spaces may be present. Rarely, small blood vessels may be seen sprouting from the adventitia. In the central regions, unaltered blood from the vessel lumen or fragments of the thrombus may be observed in the sinus-like cavities.

- After 6–12 months: Complete recanalisation of the thrombus in larger vessels. The remains of the thrombus consist of a connective tissue rich in fibres, but with few cells.

Aspiration

Aspiration associated with trauma is usually found in unconscious patients, particularly if the injured person is lying supine. Aspiration can become a serious problem when positive pressure breathing or resuscitation apparatus is used by unskilled persons. If the flow of gas enters the stomach, gas pressure will force the stomach contents into the trachea.

Brain tissue can also be aspirated in cases of severe head injury, in which the frontobasal regions of the base of the skull are extensively fractured.

Stress ulcer (acute peptic ulcer, Curling's ulcer, etc)

Severely injured patients are liable to develop gastric or duodenal ulcers, for example following an operation.

Characteristic features are:

- Development following trauma, in particular after head injury, operation, burns (Curling's ulcer).
- The clinical picture extends from upper abdominal pain to acute, often fatal haemorrhage.
- Usually no previous history of gastric ulceration.
- Aetiological factors include the overproduction of corticosteroids as a stress reaction, or the therapeutic administration of corticosteroids.
- Onset usually between the first and eighth days, up to 2 weeks following trauma. Cases arising after as long as 45 days have been reported.

The histological picture reveals a mucosal defect without increase in connective tissue or the presence of a marked chronic inflammatory reaction.

Post-traumatic pneumonia

Contusion pneumonia. This arises following blunt injury to the thorax and is caused by secondary infection of an intrapulmonary haematoma.

Aspiration pneumonia. This takes the form of a bronchopneumonia following aspiration into the distal airways of vomited gastric contents, inhaled food and mucous from the pharynx. The right lower lobe is particularly commonly affected because of the position and direction of the right main bronchus. The aspiration of chemically active substances, such as hydrochloric acid and pepsin, from the stomach provides the ideal conditions for growth of the simultaneously aspirated bacteria from the laryngeal and pharyngeal regions. The result is a rapidly developing suppurative and gangrenous inflammation.

Bronchopneumonia. Insufficient ventilation and the accumulation of secretions in patients with circulatory disturbances and who are confined to bed promote the development of a bacterial pneumonia. A bronchopneumonia can develop from a purulent bronchitis or bronchiolitis or develop in the basal regions of the pulmonary lower lobes. In the latter case failing cardiac function can cause a hypostatic oedema to develop a haemorrhagic component. The development of an infection here leads to a *hypostatic pneumonia.* The enlargement of bronchopneumonic foci can lead to the formation of a so-called *confluent bronchopneumonia.*

Infarction pneumonia. This pneumonia develops in an infarcted area of lung, caused by pulmonary embolism. Embolism in smaller branches of the pulmonary arterial tree result in wedge-shaped infarcts in the lung periphery.

Renal failure (traumatic uraemia)

Renal failure is a life-threatening complication of various forms of traumatic injury from severe crush injury to shock to septicaemia. The characteristic changes associated with renal failure following shock are discussed in Chapter 9.

Thrombosis

Thrombosis can be a severe complication of trauma. Among the many predisposing factors are obesity and long confinement to bed. The leg and pelvic veins are particularly vulnerable. The histology and age determination of thrombi have been discussed above.

Post-traumatic osteomyelitis

Post-traumatic or postoperative osteomyelitis, a complication not unusual in fractures of the long bones, serves as one of the arguments used by opponents of osteosynthesis. Open fractures are the main cause of osteomyelitis.

A main factor in the occurrence and continuation of a bone infection is an unstable osteosynthesis.

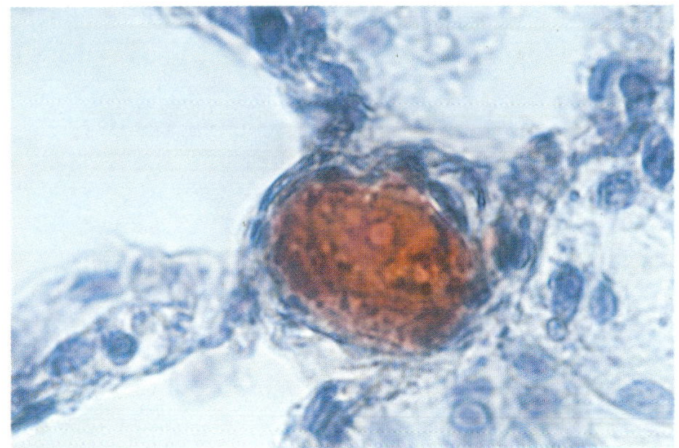

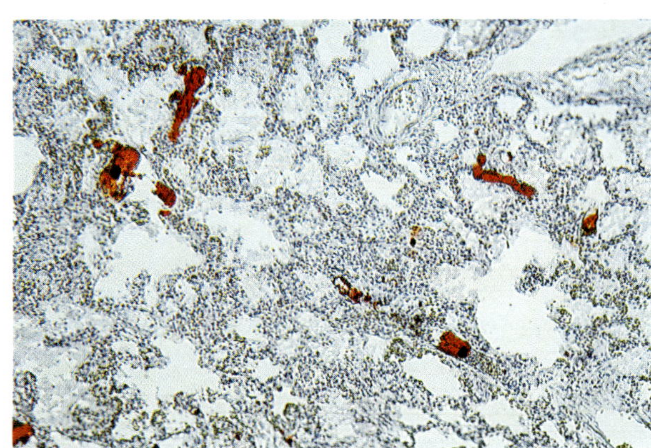

317 Lung. Recent fat embolism. A capillary containing a fat droplet (red) is shown. The patient died a few hours after sustaining multiple fractures in a road traffic accident. (*Sudan stain ×1000*)

318 Lung. Fat embolism in the lung of a battered child. Elongated fat droplets (red) can be seen in the pulmonary capillaries. (*Sudan stain ×100*)

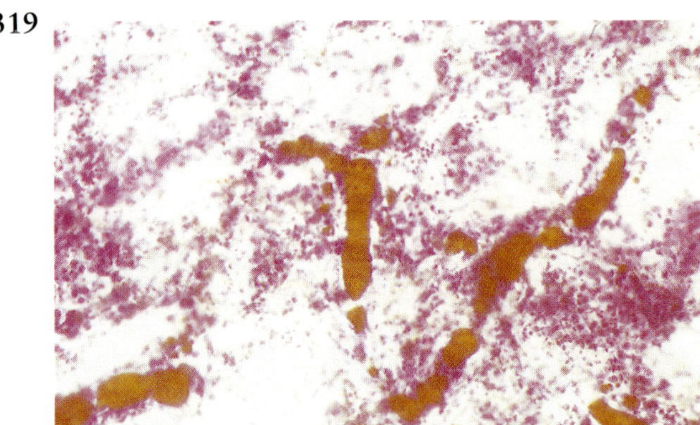

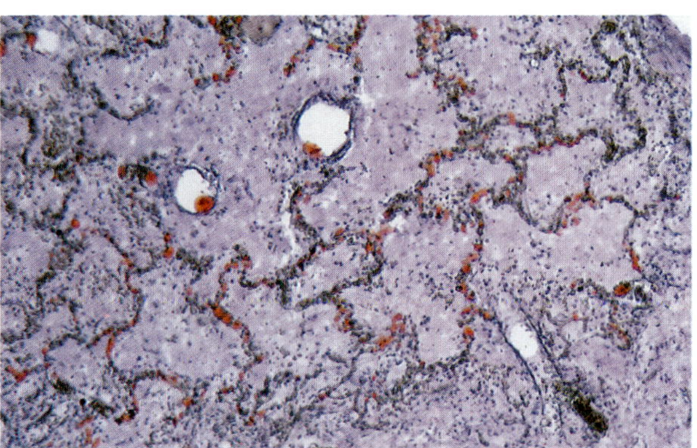

319 Lung. Massive fat embolism, showing numerous elongated and branching fat droplets in the pulmonary capillaries. (*Sudan stain ×250*)

320 Lung. Fat embolism with numerous intracapillary fat droplets (red). In addition, intra-alveolar oedema and disruption of the alveolar lining cells can be detected. The patient died 4 days after sustaining multiple fractures in a road traffic accident. (*Sudan stain ×100*)

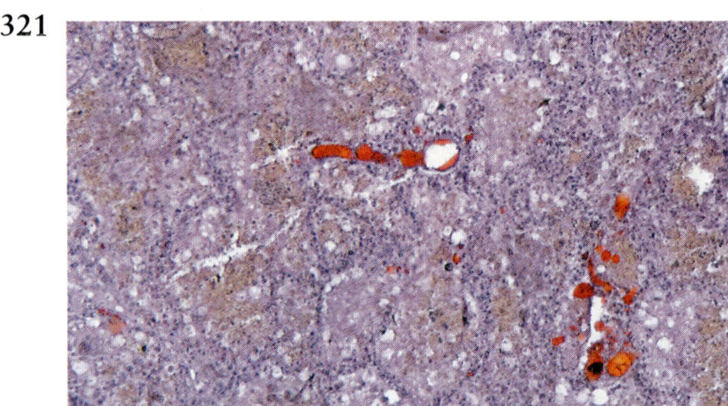

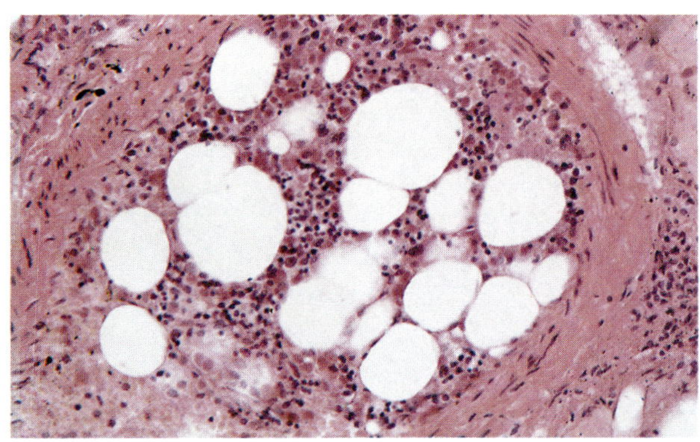

321 Lung. Fat embolism with accompanying intra-alveolar oedema and early bronchopneumonia in a 21 year-old male who died 5 days after severe crush injury to the thorax. (*Sudan stain ×100*)

322 Lung. Bone marrow embolus with numerous marrow cells and fat vacuoles in a branch of the pulmonary artery. Material from a 26 year-old pilot who died a few hours after an aeroplane crash. (*H&E ×250*)

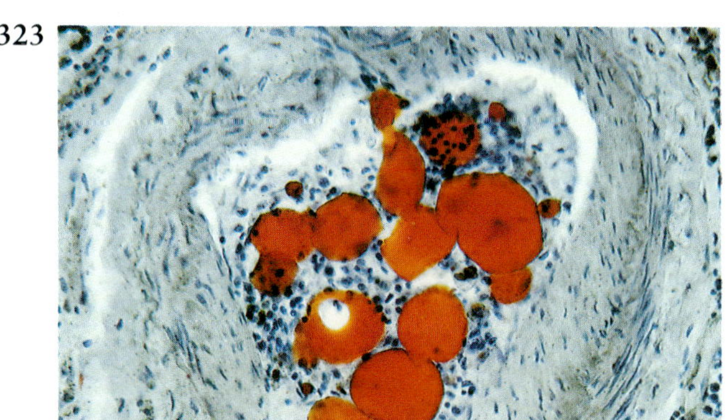
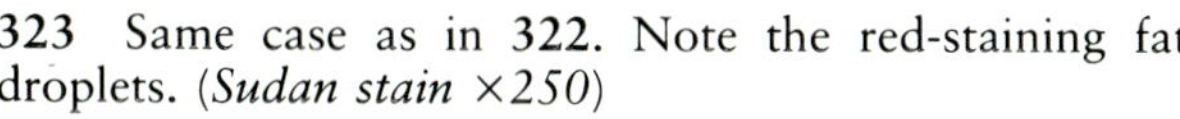

323 Same case as in **322**. Note the red-staining fat droplets. (*Sudan stain ×250*)

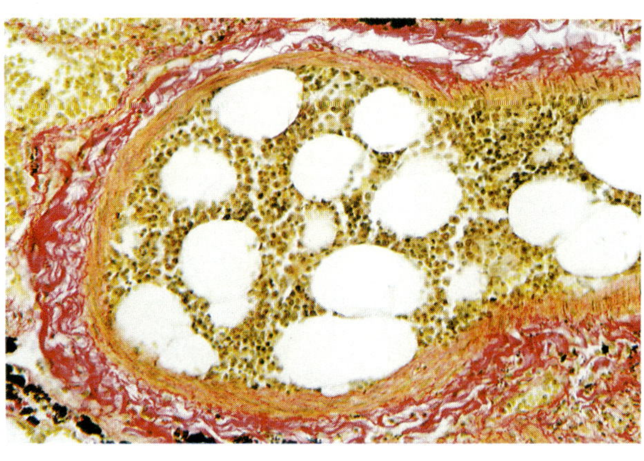

324 Same case as in **322**. Appearance of the bone marrow embolus with a connective tissue stain. (*van Gieson ×250*)

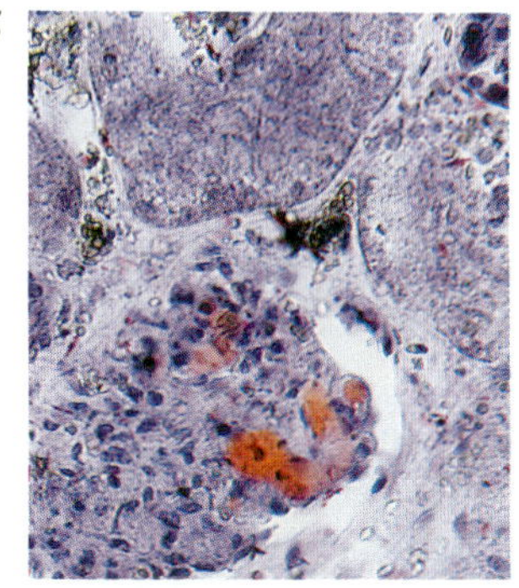

325 **Kidney.** Fat embolism with fat droplets (red) in a glomerulus. The adjacent tubular epithelial cells are markedly swollen. (*Sudan stain ×250*)

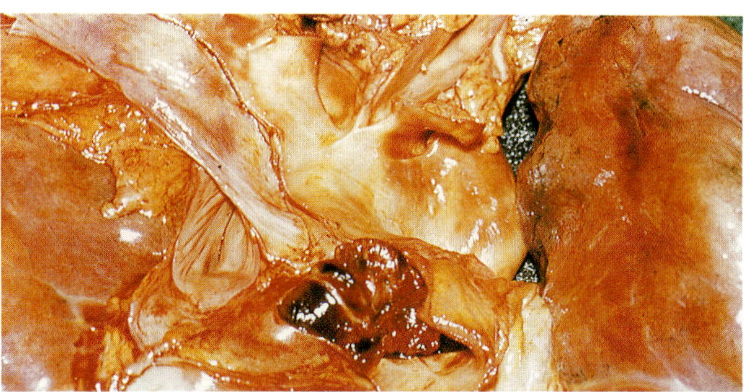

326 **Anterior view at autopsy** of the bifurcation of a fatal pulmonary embolism *in situ* in the main pulmonary artery extending into both right and left branches. This is sometimes called a 'saddle' embolus and is not consistent with survival.

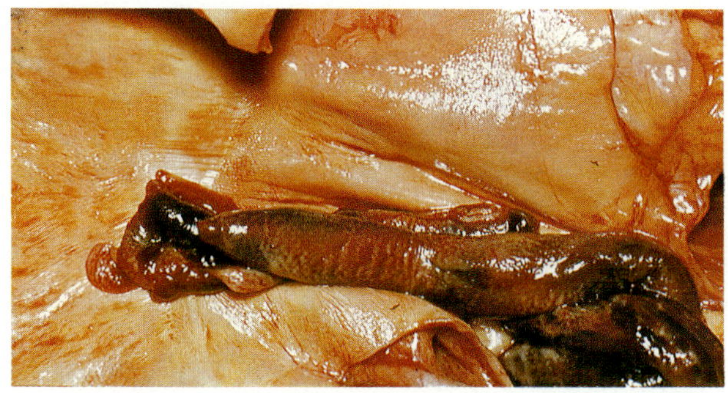

327 **A massive pulmonary embolism.** The embolus originated from thrombi in the large pelvic veins.

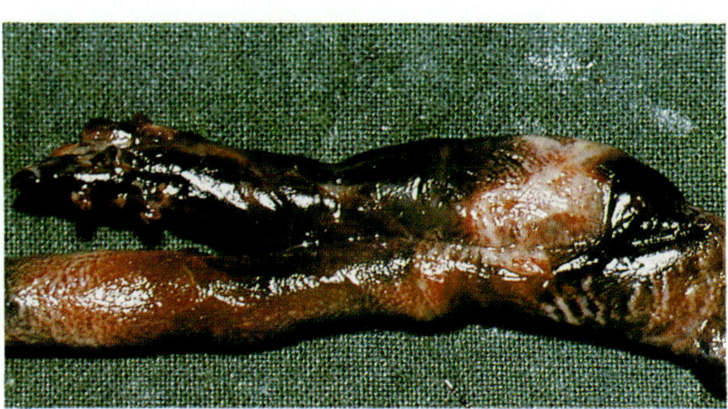

328 **Embolus** found in a branch of a pulmonary artery. Note the wavy structure of the embolus.

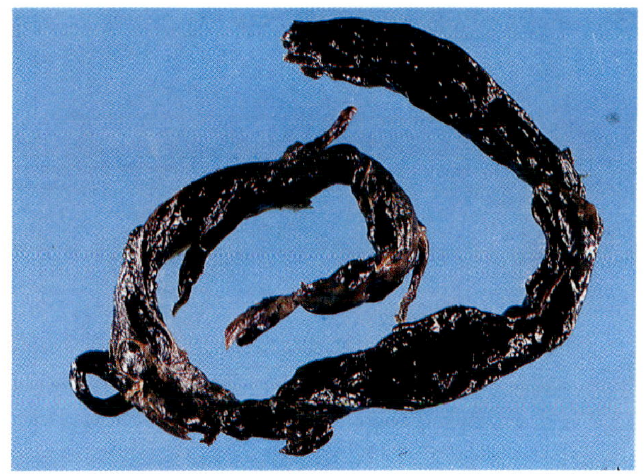

329 A long embolus found in the main pulmonary artery.

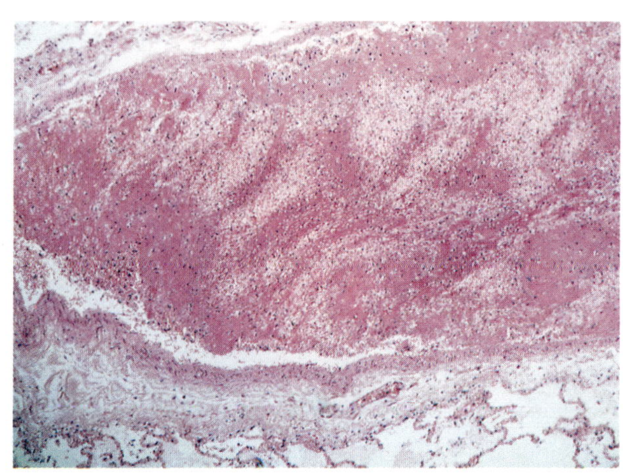

330 Lung. Recent thromboembolus, showing a layered structure. (*H&E ×100*)

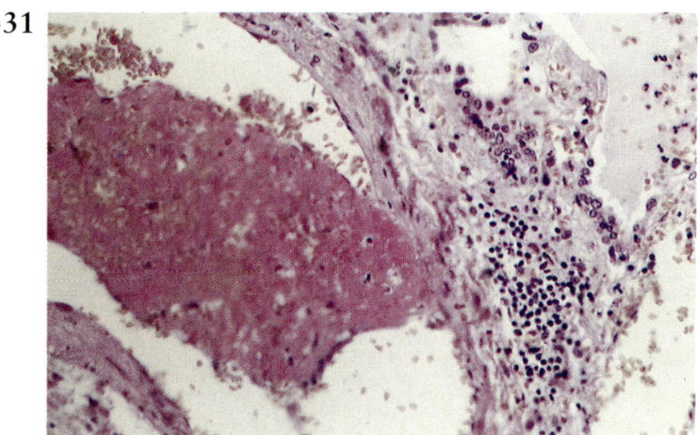

331 Lung. Branch of the pulmonary artery containing a partially adherent thromboembolus. (*H&E ×250*)

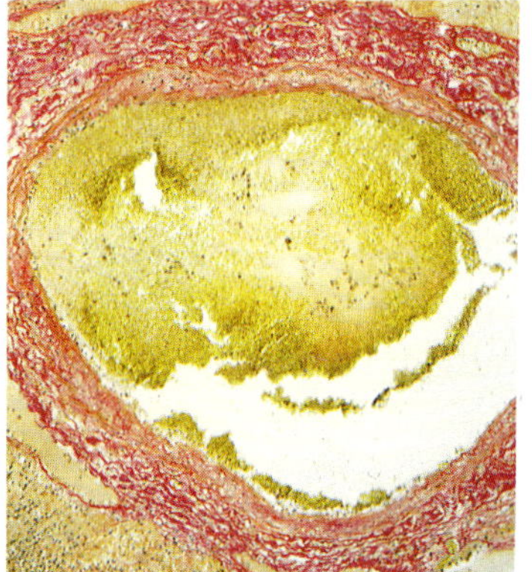

332 Lung. Branch of a pulmonary artery containing a thromboembolus which has become adherent to the vessel wall. (*van Gieson ×100*)

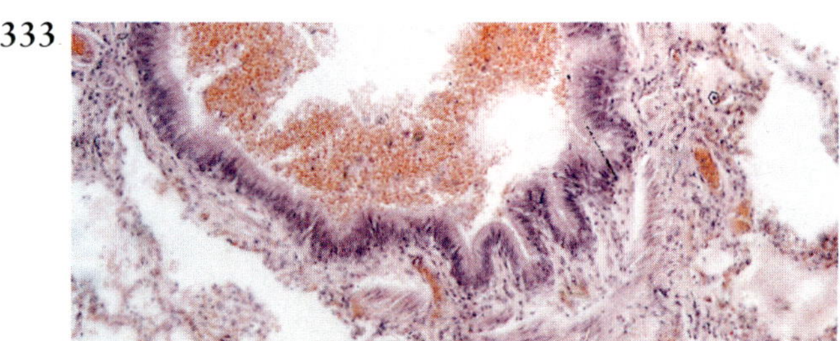

333 Lung. Following a road traffic accident with severe head injury and unconsciousness, blood has been aspirated into the lung. The picture shows part of the bronchial tree with blood in the bronchial lumen. Very short survival time, hence the absence of cellular reaction. (*H&E ×100*)

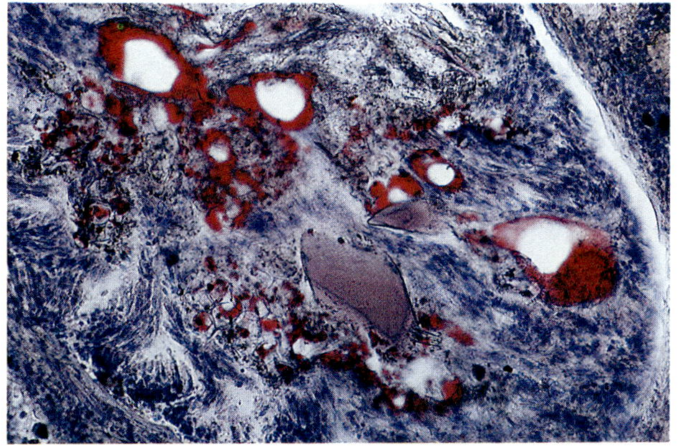

334 Bronchus. Aspirated food, seen as amorphous material and fat droplets (red) in the lumen of a bronchus, in which the epithelium has been partially disrupted. Material from a patient who died following a road traffic accident. (*Sudan stain ×160*)

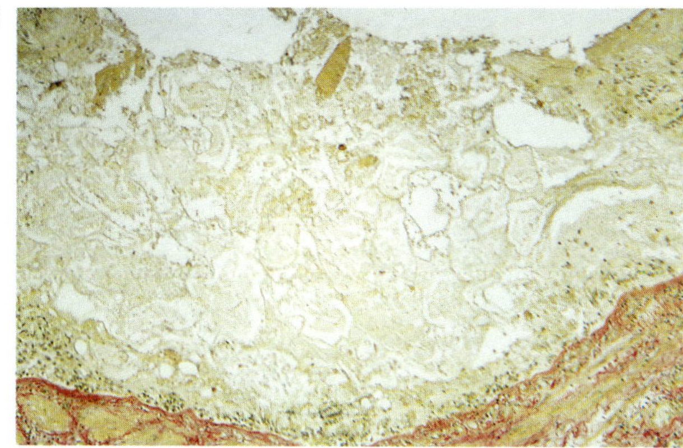

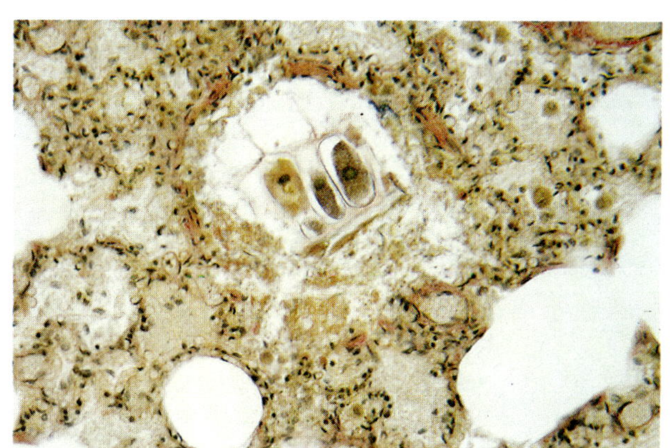

335 Bronchus. Aspirated stomach contents seen as ghost-like amorphous structures in the bronchial lumen. Material from a 25 year-old man who died in a road traffic accident. (*van Gieson ×160*)

336 Lung. Aspirated stomach contents showing the typical plant-cell structure of the food particles. Material from a 6 month-old child who died after falling downstairs. (*van Gieson ×250*)

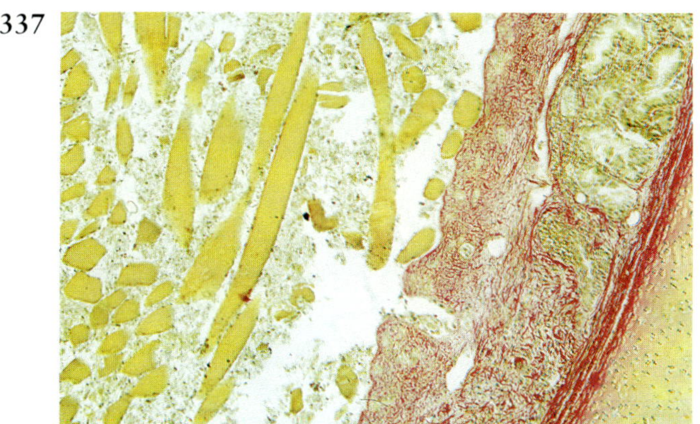

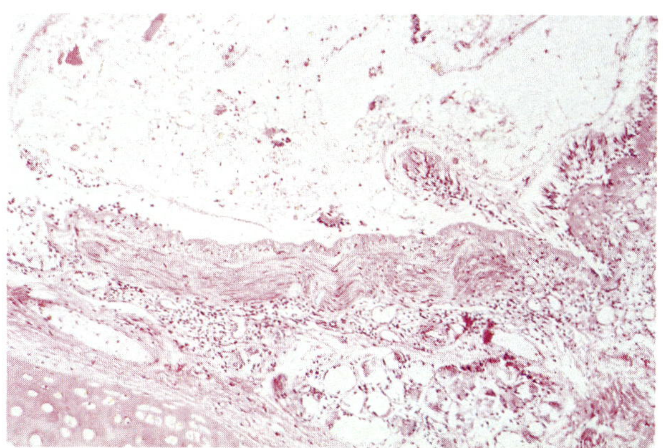

337 Bronchus. Massive aspiration of meat particles (muscle fibres) in the lumen. The bronchial epithelium has been totally disrupted. Material from a 2 year-old boy. (*van Gieson ×100*)

338 Bronchus. Massive aspiration of stomach contents. Food particles (amorphous, red) are seen in the lumen along with disrupted bronchial epithelial cells and bronchial secretions in the lumen. Material from a patient who died after receiving severe head injuries. (*H&E ×15*)

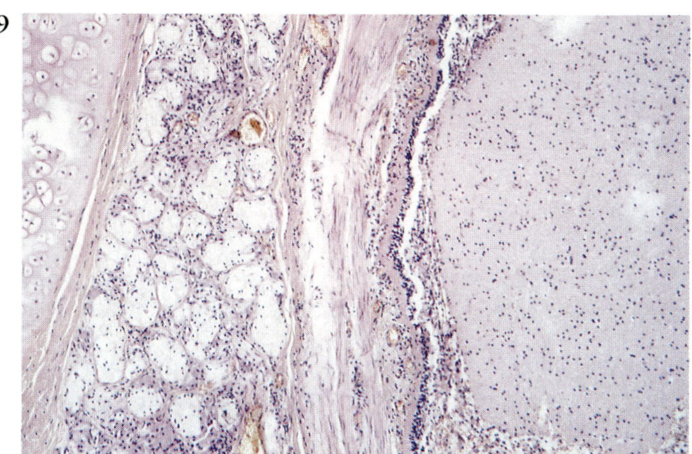

339 Lung. Aspirated brain tissue (right) in a branch of the bronchial tree. The bronchial cartilage, glands and lining epithelium can be clearly seen. The patient died almost instantaneously following severe head injuries with multiple fractures of the frontobasal parts of the base of the skull. (*H&E ×100*)

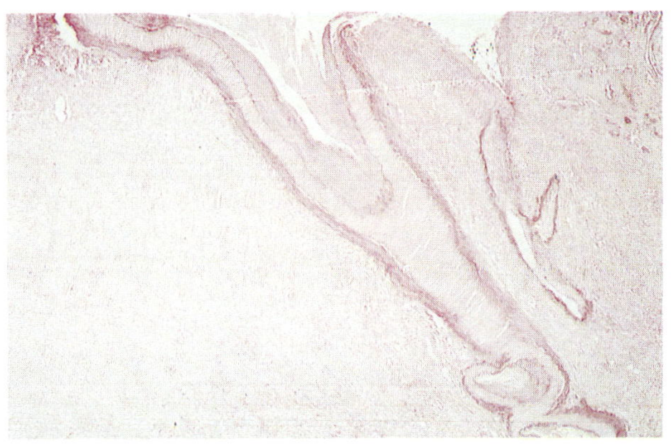

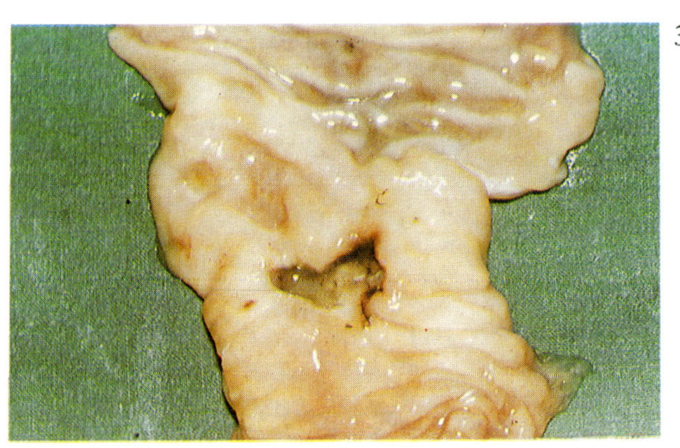

340   Stomach. Acute stress ulcer in the stomach epithelium with erosion of an artery. Material from a 50 year-old male injured in a road traffic accident. Cause of death was haemorrhage from the eroded vessel. (*H&E ×15*)

341   Duodenum. Stress ulceration. Note the well-defined ulcer edges.

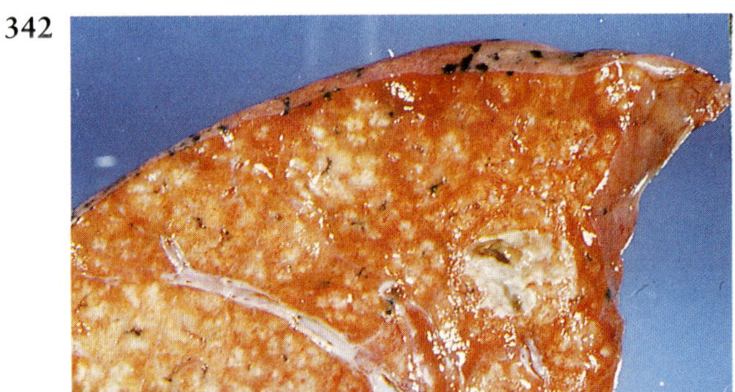

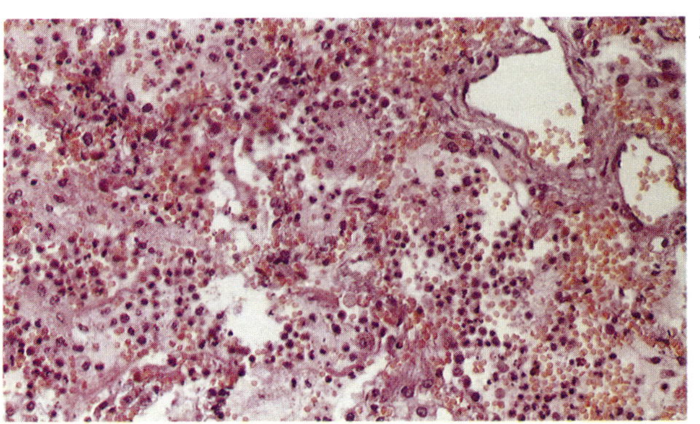

342   Confluent bronchopneumonia caused by aspiration in a patient who suffered a head injury. This complication often arises as a result of immobilisation, particularly in old people.

343   Lung. Post-traumatic bronchopneumonia, with numerous polymorphonuclear leucocytes in the pulmonary alveoli. (*H&E ×100*)

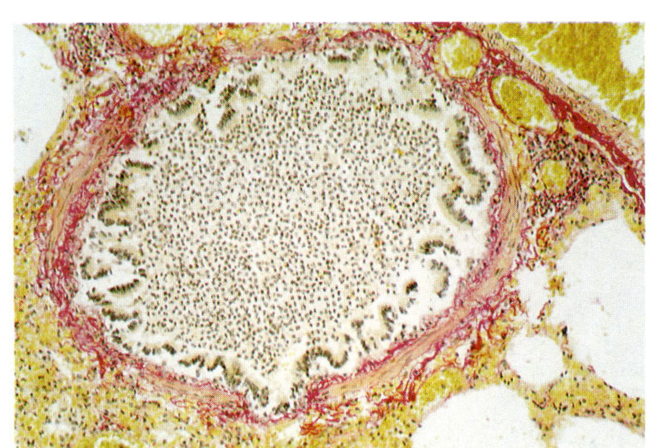

344   Bronchus. Purulent bronchitis, showing numerous polymorphonuclear leucocytes in the lumen of a branch of the bronchial tree. (*van Gieson ×160*)

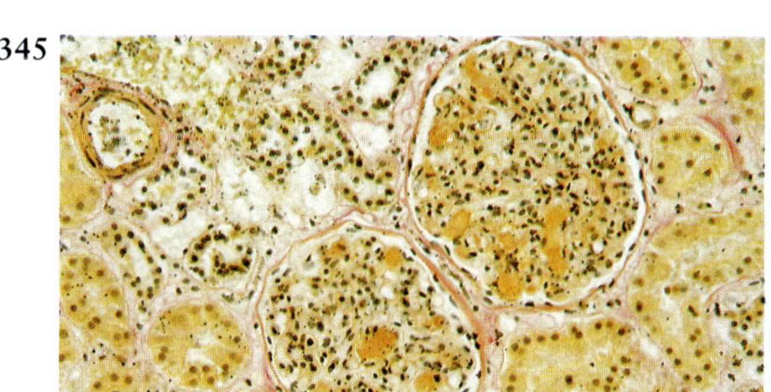

345 **Kidney.** Post-traumatic renal failure caused by septic shock. Fibrin thrombi can be seen in the glomeruli. Fairly well preserved cells of the proximal and distal convoluted tubules. (*van Gieson ×250*)

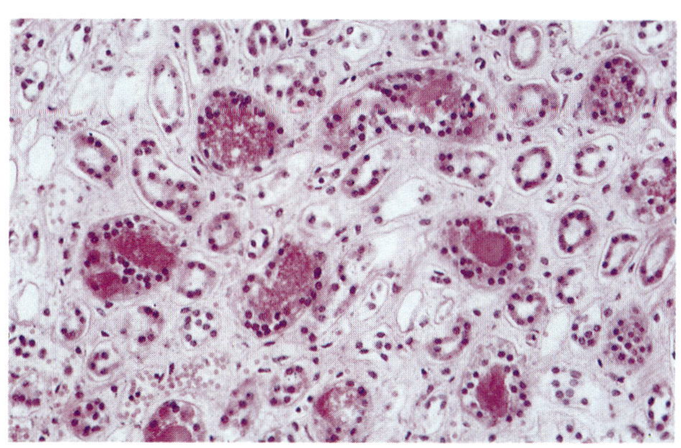

346 **Kidney.** Shock-kidney (haemoglobinuric nephrosis). Protein casts and erythrocytes can be seen in the renal tubules. (*H&E ×100*)

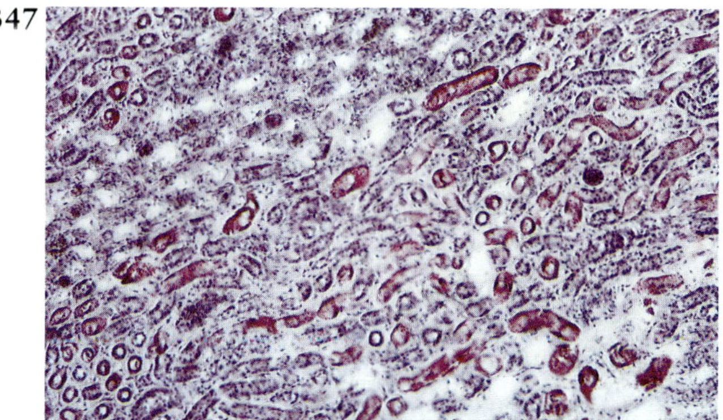

347 **Kidney.** Haemoglobinuric nephrosis caused by septic shock. The epithelial cells of the collecting tubules contain small fat droplets. (*Sudan stain ×100*)

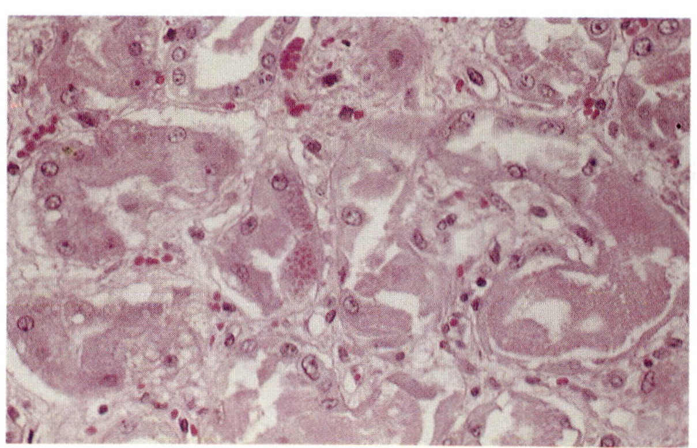

348 **Kidney.** Septic shock. Shwartzman–Sanarelli phenomenon with swelling and necrosis of proximal renal tubular cells. Individual cells contain small eosinophilic droplets. (*H&E ×400*)

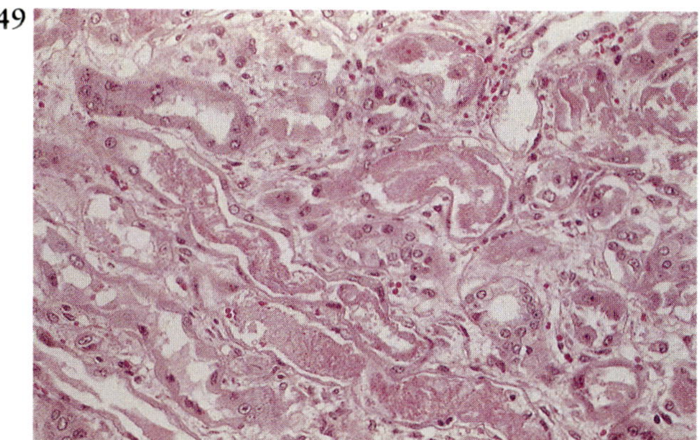

349 **Kidney.** Septic shock. Shwartzman–Sanarelli phenomenon. Numerous protein casts can be seen in the distended collecting tubules. (*H&E ×250*)

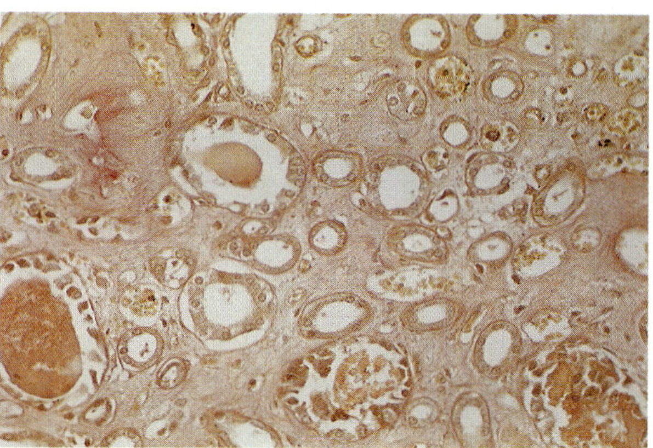

350 **Kidney.** As in **349**. In some tubules, epithelial cell disruption and necrosis (lower middle, lower right) can be seen, as can proteinaceous material in distended tubules. (*van Gieson ×250*)

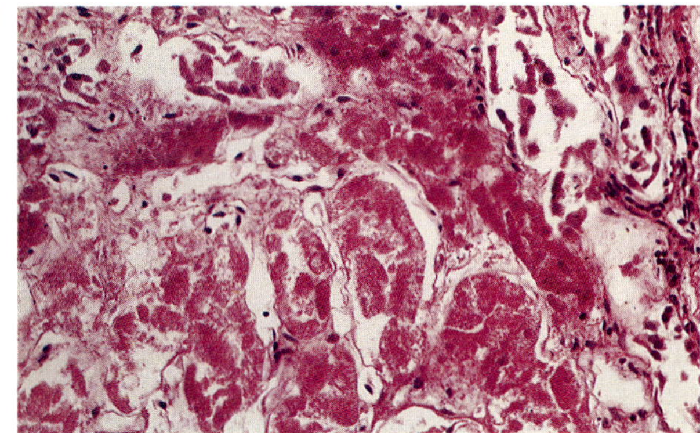

351 Kidney. Crush-kidney (chromoprotein-kidney) in a patient who was injured by falling sand. Extensive necrosis of the proximal convoluted tubules and marked degenerative changes, including necrosis, of the distal convoluted tubules can be seen. (*H&E ×250*)

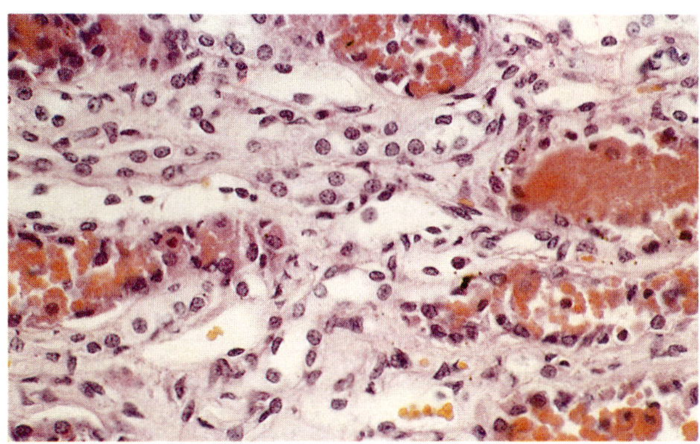

352 Kidney. Crush-kidney, showing the presence of erythrocytes, as well as fine granulated proteinaceous casts (upper right) in the lumen of renal tubules. (*H&E ×400*)

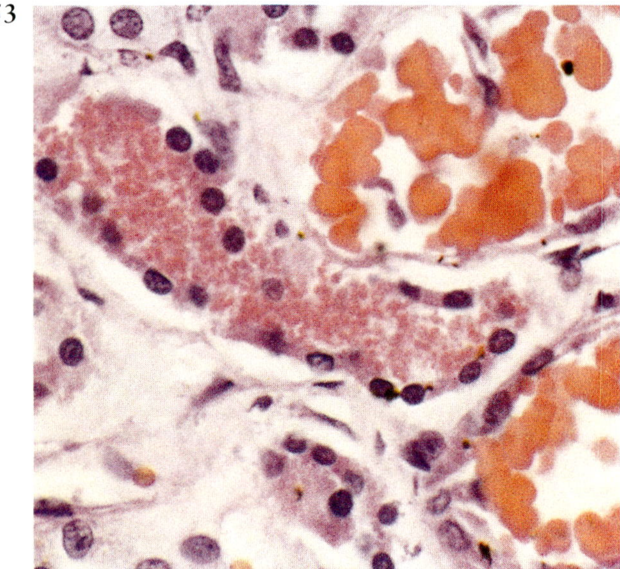

353 Kidney. As in **352**. This underlines the morphological difference between erythrocytes in a tubule (lower right) and a tubular proteinaceous cast. (*H&E ×400*)

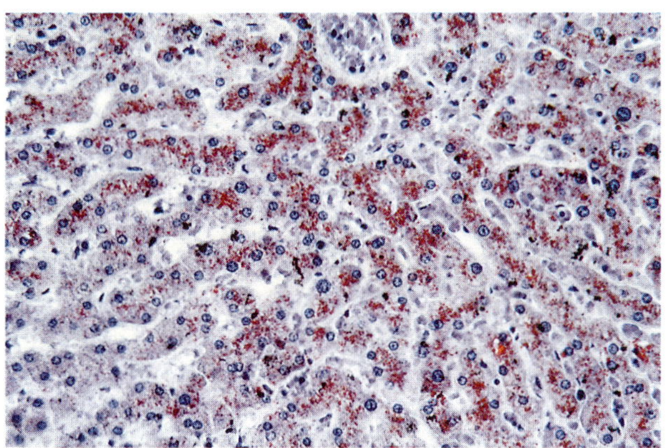

354 Liver. Post-traumatic fat accumulation (red) in hepatocytes following severe head injury in a 25 year-old male. Post-traumatic survival time: 9 days. (*Sudan stain ×250*)

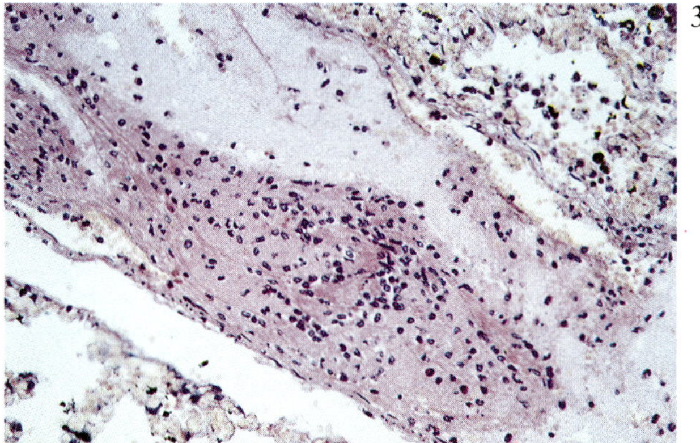

355 Lung. Thrombus in a branch of a pulmonary artery in a patient who died 8 days after severe blunt head injuries. The formation of an endothelial cell layer can be seen at the lower edge of the thrombus. (*H&E ×250*)

9 Morphological changes due to shock

According to Janssen (1977), the following histological alterations indicating the presence of shock can be established:

- Sludge phenomenon (aggregation of erythrocytes and thrombocytes) in dilated arterioles, capillaries and venules of affected organs, in particular, lungs, gastrointestinal tract, kidneys, liver and brain.
- Presence of intravascular hyaline bodies ('globular clots', 'shock bodies') and microthrombi, especially in the terminal circulation of the lung.
- Swelling and necrosis of capillary endothelium and reticuloendothelial cells, particularly the Kupffer cells of the liver sinusoids.
- Necrosis of the intima and media, especially in the coronary arteries.
- Single-cell necrosis and necrosis of groups of cells in liver and kidney. The hepatic lobular necrosis tends to be centroacinar in distribution.
- Bilateral renal cortical necrosis.
- Villous oedema with epithelial cell loss in the small intestine.
- Generalised or circumscribed areas of haemorrhage signifying disseminated intravascular coagulation.
- Acute erosions and ulceration of gastric and small intestinal mucosa.
- Dilatation of the renal tubular system.
- Presence of megakaryocytes in pulmonary capillaries.

The morphological changes in the liver in shock have been described by Remmele and Loeper (1973):

- Acute venous hyperaemia (principally centroacinar).
- Liver cell necrosis, increasing with the duration of the shock state:
    Up to 10 hours – an exceptional finding.
    10–24 hours – minimal necrosis.
    After 24 hours – in approximately 50 per cent of cases.

A whole spectrum of distribution of necrosis can be observed, from disseminated single-cell necrosis through necrotic groups of hepatocytes to extensive centroacinar lobular necrosis.

Microthrombosis in liver blood vessels: the clot may assume the form of thread-like fibrin precipitates or may be globular.

It should be stressed that it is not always possible to distinguish histologically between hepatic changes due to shock and chronic liver congestion. According to Janssen (1977), the pathological changes observed in the liver in shock tend to show:

- Extensive centroacinar lobular necrosis.
- Minimal hyperaemia or complete absence of hyperaemia.
- Microthrombi, principally in the peripheral sinusoids of the lobules and in the intrahepatic branches of the portal vein.

The histopathological changes associated with acute renal failure in shock have been discussed by Bohle (1965), Brun and Munck (1966), Burck (1969), Kanschina (1970), Mohr (1960) and Schubert and Zollinger (1968).

The glomeruli appear anaemic with collapsed capillaries, especially in the peripheral and middle areas of the renal cortex. The basement membrane of the glomeruli is often thicker. From the second to the eighth day, an eosinophilic, granulated or thread-like exudate can be seen in Bowman's space, along with proteinaceous precipitates, exfoliated cells and remains of erythrocytes. A fairly constant finding on the first or second day, but more usually from the sixth to the eighth day, is an enlargement of the cells lining Bowman's space. They assume a cubic form and are reminiscent of cells from the proximal tubules.

The renal tubules undergo vacuolar and hyaline degeneration. Damage to the cells of the proximal convoluted tubules is regarded as characteristic of a nephrotoxic effect. From the third to the fifth day, the lumen of the proximal convoluted tubules becomes distended. As an explanation, it is thought that renal ischaemia leads to a disturbance of the absorptive capacity of the nephron and thus to an effective increase in the amount of glomerular filtrate, which is responsible for a rise in the intratubular pressure in the proximal nephron.

Morphological studies of 140 cases of clinically diagnosed acute renal failure gave the following results (Schubert, 1968):

- Distension of the lumen of the renal tubules (73%).
- Doubly refractile crystals (65%).
- Collecting tubule cylinders: (a) hyaline (63%); (b) pigmented (44.3%); (c) granular (33.6%).
- Collections of immature blood cells in the medullary blood vessels (45%).
- Oedema of the renal interstitial tissue (39.3%).
- So-called osmotic (vacuolar or hydropic) nephrosis (39%).
- Circumscribed interstitial infiltrates (30%).
- Tubular necrosis (20%).
- Glomerular changes: (a) fibrin thrombi (5%); (b) Shwartzman–Sanarelli phenomenon (a special form of endotoxic shock) (2.1%); (c) suspected Shwartzman–Sanarelli phenomenon (2.9%).
- Alterations to blood vessel walls (1.4%).
- Tubulovenous aneurysms (0.7%).

Bilateral renal cortical necrosis is one of the complications. Its occurrence depends on the duration and intensity of the ischaemia and possibly on the presence of a hyperergic state (Shwartzman–Sanarelli phenomenon). Renal cortical necrosis is observed, especially in pathological pregnancies and following ethylene glycol poisoning.

The disease entity seen in shock-induced acute renal failure has been given a variety of names:

- Nephronephrosis (Mueller, 1906; Volhard and Fahr, 1914).
- Interstitial nephritis and anuria (Kimmelstiel, 1938).
- Tubulovascular renal syndrome (Duff and Murray, 1941).
- Crush syndrome (Bywaters, 1944).
- Traumatic anuria (Bywaters *et al.*, 1942).
- Lower nephron nephrosis (Lucké, 1946).
- Haemoglobinuric nephrosis (Mallory, 1947).
- Erythrolytic nephrosis (Letterer and Masshoff, 1949).
- Acute tubular nephrosis (Bull *et al.*, 1950).
- Anuria with chromoproteinuria (Zollinger, 1952).
- Shock-kidney (van Slyke, 1954).
- Tubulo-interstitial nephritis (Brun and Munck, 1957).
- Toxic-infectious kidney (Tarajew, 1958).
- Acute pigment nephrosis (Saskowski, 1967).

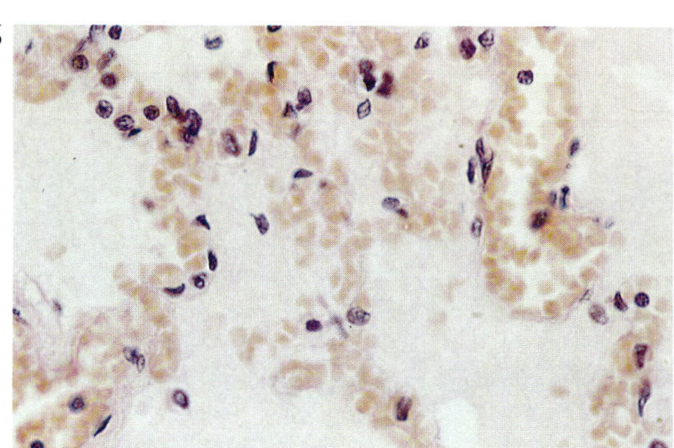

356 Lung. Capillary hyperaemia with formation of intra-alveolar pulmonary oedema. A few erythrocytes can be seen in the alveoli. Material from a 24 year-old male who suffered polytrauma, resulting in hypovolaemic shock. (*H&E* ×640)

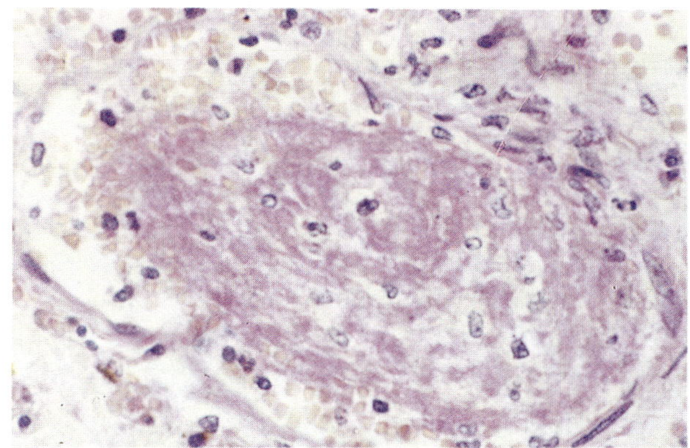

357 Lung. Recent fibrin thrombus in a small branch of the pulmonary arterial tree. This lesion is a result of hypovolaemic shock. Material from a 27 year-old female who died a few hours after a road traffic accident. (*H&E* ×640)

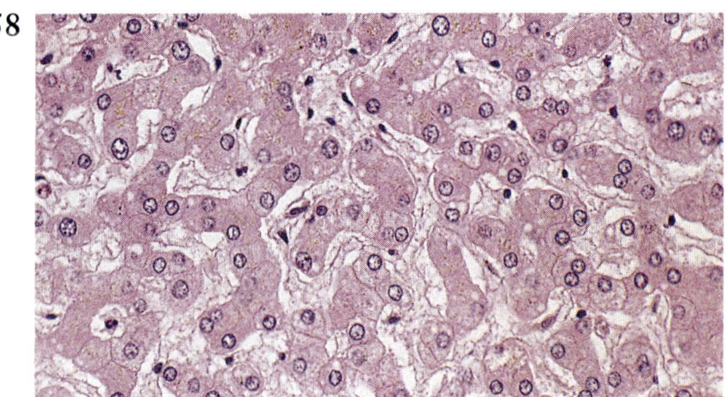

358 Liver. Case of shock due to extensive burns. Serous fluid accumulation in Dissé's space. (*H&E* ×1000)

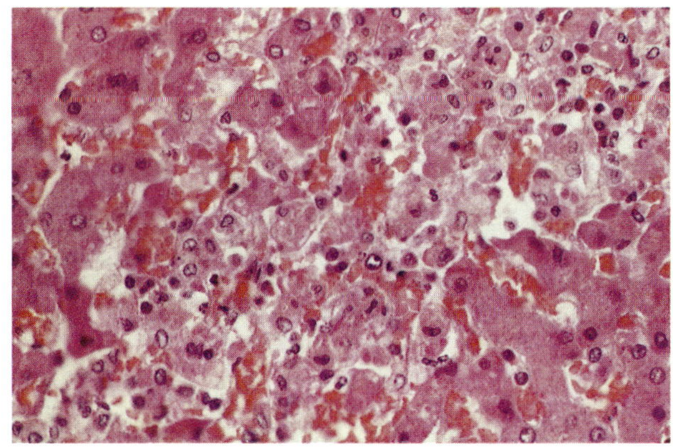

359 Liver. From a case of protracted hypovolaemic shock. Groups of necrotic and dying hepatocytes can be seen (centre) as well as acute congestion of the liver. (*H&E ×1000*)

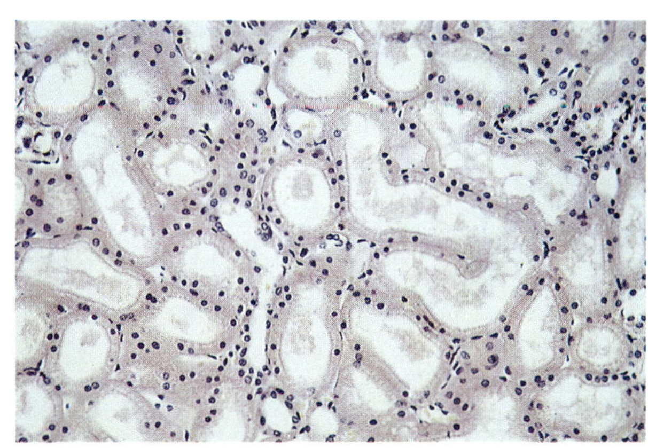

360 Kidney. Tubular dilatation with flattening of the epithelial cells. Material from a patient who died of hypovolaemic shock. (*H&E ×100*)

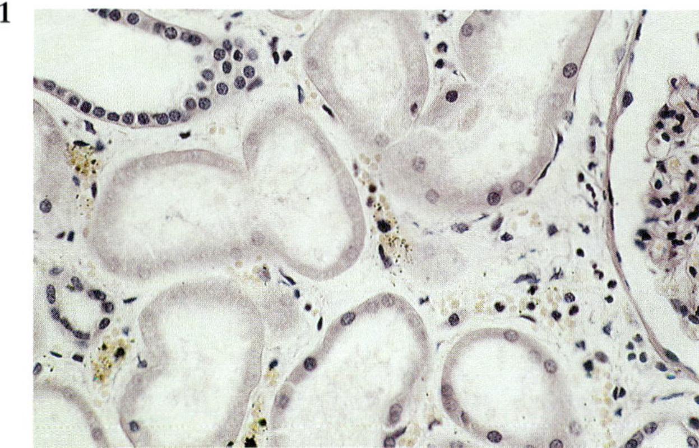

361 Kidney. Same case as 360. Dilatation of proximal renal tubules with flattening and partial necrosis of the tubular epithelial cells. (*H&E ×400*)

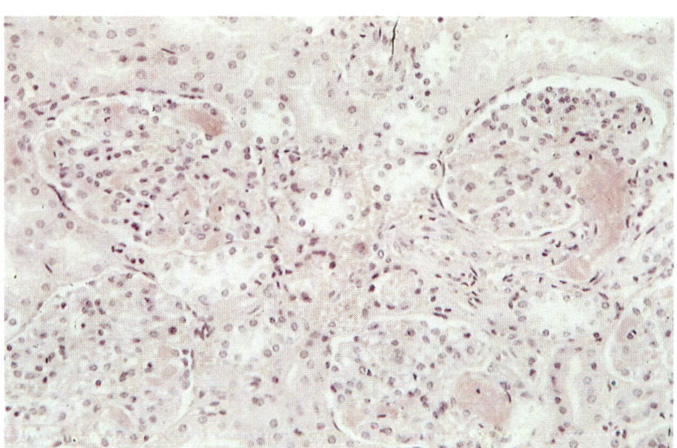

362 Kidney. Fibrin thrombi in the renal glomerula in a patient who died of shock following severe burns. (*H&E ×250*)

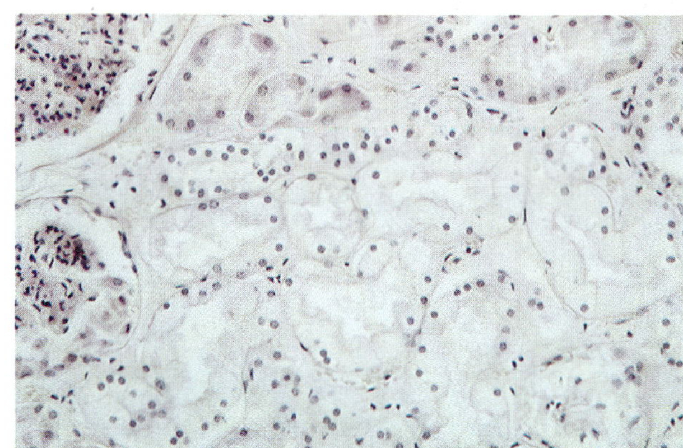

363 Kidney. Osmotic (vacuolar or hydropic) nephrosis following parenteral therapy. The proximal tubular epithelial cells contain fine vacuolation of the cytoplasm. (*H&E ×250*)

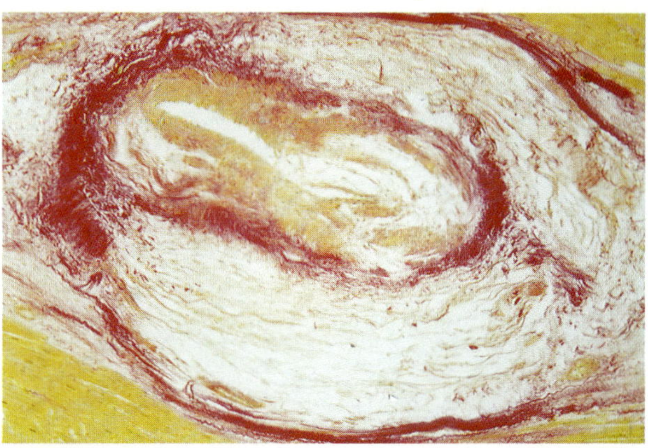

364 Heart. Shock in a 62 year-old female. The adventitia of the depicted arterial branch and the perivascular region show a marked oedema. (*van Gieson ×100*)

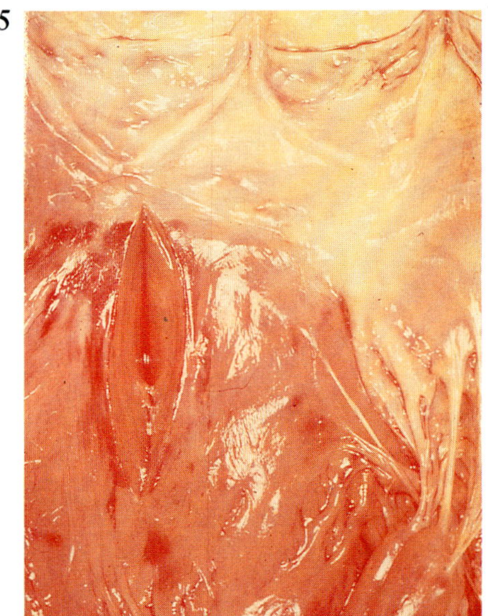

365 Heart. Subendocardial haemorrhage due to shock.

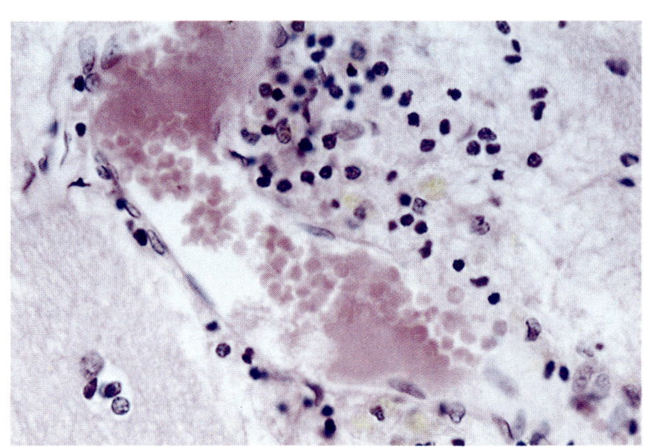

366 Brain. Shock. Venule containing fibrin thrombus (sludge phenomenon). A perivascular cellular reaction is also visible. (*H&E ×250*)

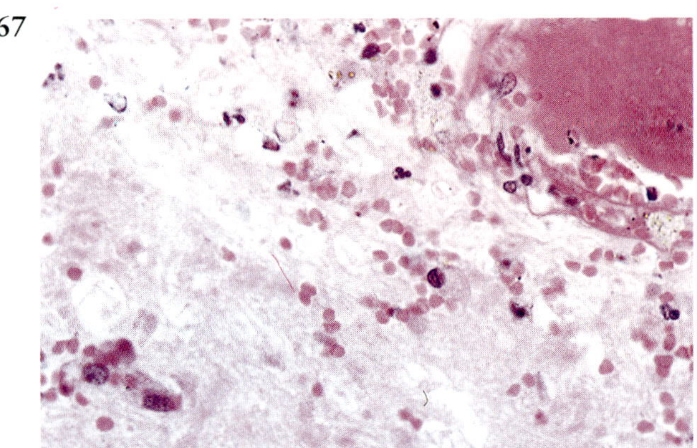

367 Brain. Shock. Fibrin thrombus (upper right), perivascular oedema and haemorrhage (numerous erythrocytes). (*H&E ×640*)

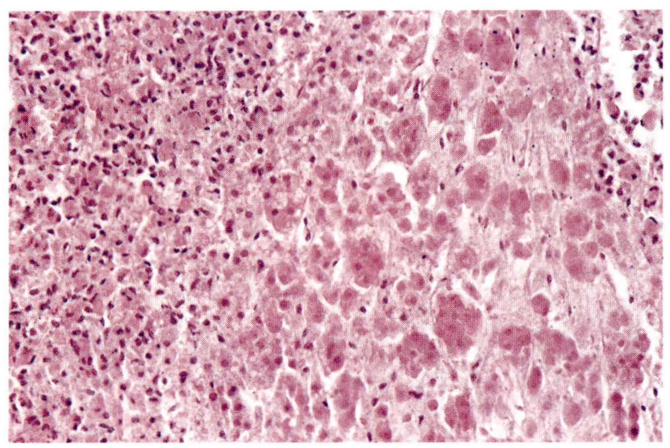

368 Adrenal gland. Area of necrosis in the adrenal cortex. The cells are eosinophilic with poor or absent nuclear staining reaction. A polymorphonuclear cell reaction is also visible. The patient died in shock 4 days after a road traffic accident. (*H&E ×250*)

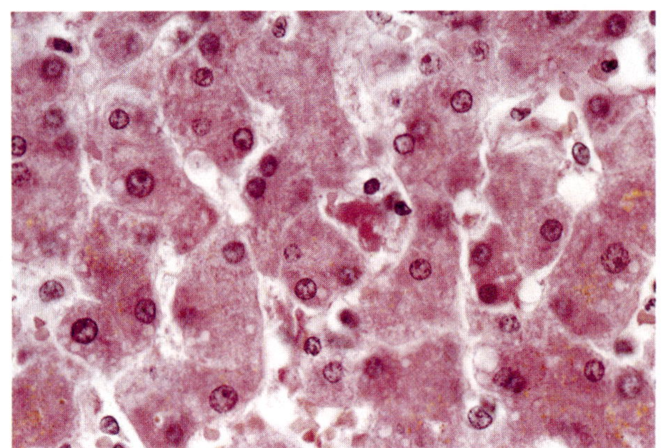

369 Liver. Shock-body in a liver sinusoid. The patient died of septic shock. (*H&E ×640*)

10 Histological age determination

Below is a time scale of wound healing based on work of different authors using various models:

After 4–8 hours	extravasation of fibrin and leucocytes.
After 18 hours	commencement of fibroblast proliferation, appearance of macrophages.
After 26 hours	sprouting of angioblasts.
After 1–5 days	breakdown and removal of necrotic tissue, altered blood and bacteria; leucocytes, histocytes and relatively large amounts of protein can be found in the surrounding oedema fluid.
After 3–5 days	formation of capillaries and fibroblasts (granulation tissue); formation of haemosiderin.
After 4–6 days	increased content of reticulin fibres; increasing amount of collagen fibres; continued formation of granulation tissue; few capillaries, considerable quantities of haemosiderin.
After 7 days	presence of plasma cells.
After 8 days	continued formation of capillaries; argyrophile fibres.
After 8–9 days	reconstruction of epithelial covering.
After 10–14 days	decrease in capillary number and increase in amount of collagen; scar tissue formation.
After 2–3 weeks	maximal formation of collagenous connective tissue; synthesis of elastic fibres.
After 7 months	numerous elastic fibres.
After 6–12 months	modification of collagenous connective tissue with removal of excess collagen fibres.

There are individual variations: for example, according to Berg (1972), collagen fibre formation begins after 4–5 days and reaches a maximum after 12–18 days. Capillary formation starts on day 3.

Janssen (1977) used the results of histological, histochemical and biochemical investigations to compile a synopsis of the most important features used in the age determination of injuries. *Haemosiderin* can be identified after 2–3 days at the earliest;

it is more usual to find it after 4–9 days.

Krauland (1973) discovered haemosiderin in fibroblasts of the meninges no earlier than 5 days after injury. Caution is needed in assessing the significance of the presence of haemosiderin, because it can remain in tissues for years on account of its poor solubility. Haematoidin, which is a bilirubin-like pigment formed from haemoglobin under conditions of reduced oxygen pressure, can be detected after approximately one week.

According to Aufdermaur (1971), meniscus injuries are characterised in the first three weeks by regressive changes, from cellular degeneration to small areas of necrosis and reactive changes (cell proliferation). While degenerative and reparative (eg. removal of cell debris) changes take place in the first few days after injury, reactive changes tend to dominate the later phases.

Healing in bones

In, for example, fractures of the femoral neck, the fractured ends of the cortical bone and cancellous trabeculae show histologically a 1–6 mm band of necrotic tissue. After 4–5 days, a loose tissue rich in blood vessels and cellular components invades the fracture haematoma, for the purpose of resorbing and organising it. The bone fragments and dead cancellous trabeculae are resorbed. After about 9 days the first signs of new bone formation are seen, not in the fracture line, but around and between the destroyed trabeculae of the femoral neck. The fracture is to a large extent obliterated by callous tissue after 6 weeks at the earliest, more often after 8–10 weeks (Fischer & Spann, 1967).

According to Fischer (1968), fractures of the skull are at first filled with blood along the fracture line. Areas can be seen with increased fibrin and blood pigment deposition. Then follows increasing organisation by a granulation tissue rich in blood vessels and a cellular connective tissue originating in the periosteum. There is no ordered structure in the newly formed bone.

Potanina's investigations (1960) of skull trephination have shown that the regeneration process takes place principally from the endosteum of the spongiosa. However, the endosteum cannot be responsible for the formation of compact bone at the bone edges. Potanina (1960) formulated the following regeneration stages:

Up to 2 months appearance of granulation tissue and a border of osteoid along the edges of the trephination.

3–12 months development of bony tissue in the osteoid; further differentiation of the granulation tissue.

After 1 year remodelling of the newly formed bone occurs with fat accumulation in the bone marrow in these areas.

In the *brain*, the healing processes involve three main stages.

Stage 1 (up to day 4)
Poor or absent staining reaction in the damaged tissue; degeneration of the medullary sheaths and the axis cylinders; the neurones appear as ghosts (cloudy swelling); oedema.

Stage 2 (day 4–5)
Proliferation of connective tissue components at the edge of the necrotic areas; increased formation of capillaries; compound granular corpuscles are visible with their foamy cytoplasm in the mesh of connective tissue.

Stage 3 (after about 1 week)
Degeneration of the compound granular corpuscles; formation of cavities with strands of connective tissue; the connective tissue meshwork is seen in the absence of compound granular corpuscles; predominantly glial scar tissue formation is seen in smaller lesions.

Three stages of healing are recognisable after *spinal cord* contusion, also for contusion of the cerebral cortex.

Stage 1 (stage of haemorrhage and necrosis)
- Haemorrhage arising with the application of the force causing the injury.
- Tissue necrosis; this is evident if the patient survives for approximately 24 hours.

Stage 2 (stage of resorption and organisation)
- Proliferation of connective tissue components of blood vessels as early as 2–3 days.
- Appearance of mesodermal phagocytosing cells (compound granular corpuscles).
- Beginning of the degenerative process in the white matter, especially in the anterior roots.

Stage 3 (final stage, scar tissue formation)
- Formation of scar tissue, comprising collagen fibres.
- Formation of glial scar tissue after partial necrosis (pure parenchymal necrosis).
- Formation of cysts.

Histological appearances in *subdural haematoma* (Minckler, 1971):

Up to 24 hours Dilatation of capillaries and venules; appearance of a few polymorphonuclear leucocytes; swelling of endothelial cells and cells of the dura.

2–5 days Invasion of the haematoma by fibroblasts and macrophages.

5–10 days Increase in the number of fibroblasts and phagocytes, which invade the haematoma from the dura; some capillaries can be seen.

10–20 days Further proliferation of fibroblasts and considerable formation of blood vessels (granulation tissue); membrane formation around the haematoma; at this stage the erythrocytes are poorly stained.

20–30 days The granulation tissue becomes more compact; erythrocytes are visible in the newly formed capillaries; the outer membrane becomes thicker.

30 days–3 months Completion of the outer membrane; parallel bands of connective tissue with numerous blood vessels, including arteries; occasionally, recent haemorrhage in the form of thin-walled organised subdural haemorrhages; groups of phagocytes containing iron pigment.

6 months onward After 6 months, an age assessment is no longer possible, as no significant changes occur in, for example, the thickness of the membrane; occasionally, signs of a chronic inflammatory reaction can be seen.

Krauland (1973) described the following stages in the healing process of subdural haemorrhage:

After 5 days Appearance of fibroblasts.
After 9 days Appearance of capillaries.
After 18 days Connective tissue demarcation and formation of giant capillaries.

After many years of survival the appearance of a subdural can vary markedly, from a thin-walled cyst containing clear colourless fluid to a calcified mass similar to bone marrow. Thick-walled cysts containing viscid dark brown material are not uncommon.

Although symptoms may be present they are frequently absent and the presence of the lesion may be detected only by the forensic pathologist following death due to reasons entirely unconnected with the subdural haematoma.

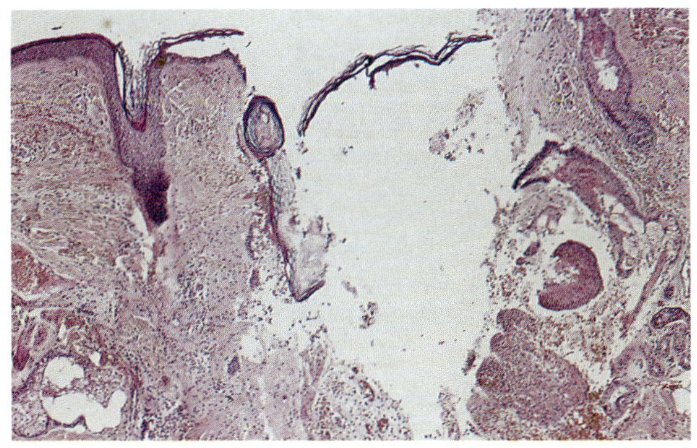

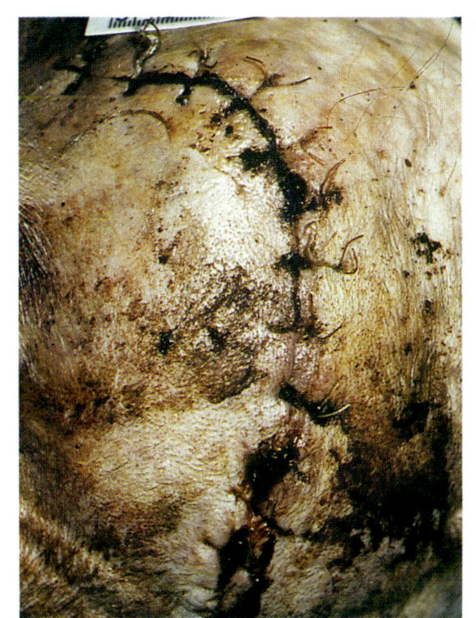

370 Skin (scalp). Recent injury. The victim was struck by a train and death was instantaneous. Haemorrhage is seen at the wound edges, which contain epidermal components (due to trauma). No cellular reaction. (*H&E ×100*)

371 Surgical wound in the scalp following skull trephining; 4 days old.

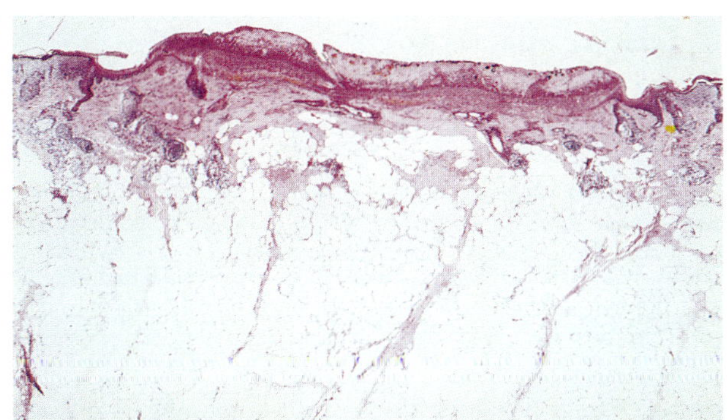

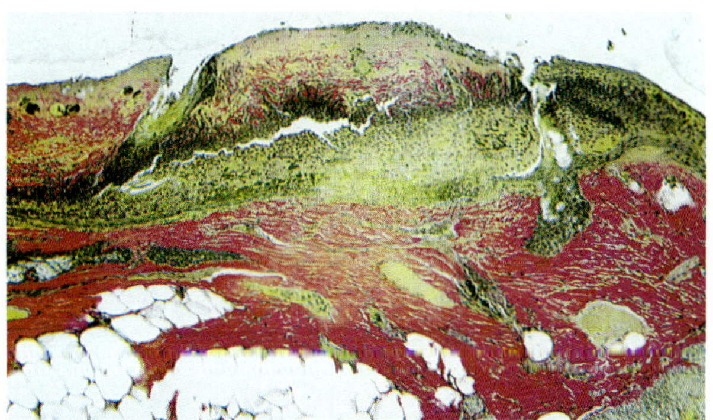

372 Skin (forehead). 10 days after injury, low-power view. (*H&E ×10*)

373 Skin (forehead). 10 days after injury. Formation of new epithelial components with increasing amount of collagenous connective tissue (red). A thicker section was cut in this case, in order to preserve the structure of the friable tissue. (*van Gieson ×100*)

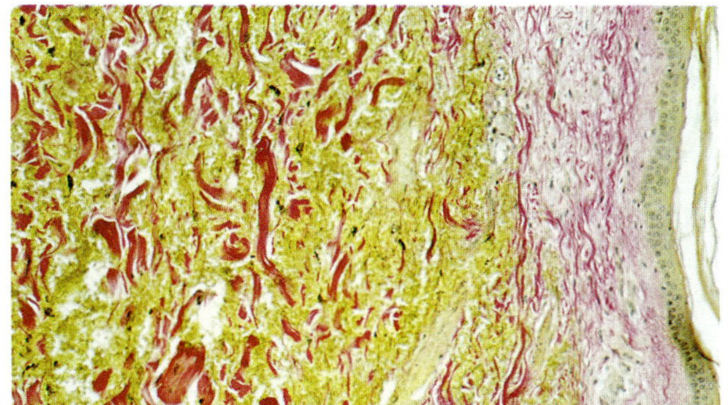

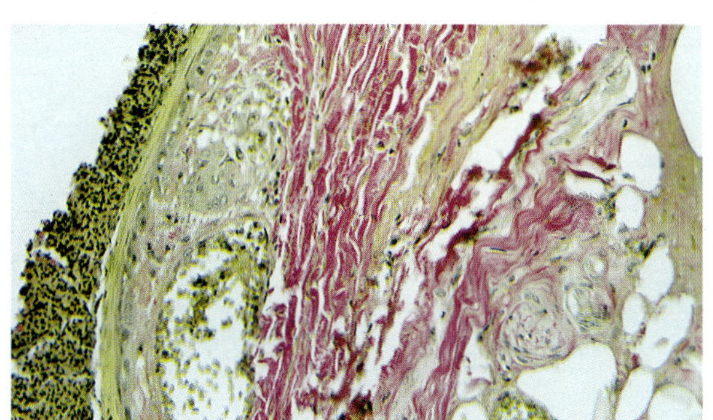

374 Skin (forearm). 14 days after blunt trauma with a fist. Numerous erythrocytes are visible between the disrupted subcutaneous collagen fibres (red, left). (*van Gieson ×160*)

375 Skin (knee). Fall on the knee 11 days previously. Abrasion with pus formation in the scab (left) and the formation of epithelium with epithelial nests. (*van Gieson ×250*)

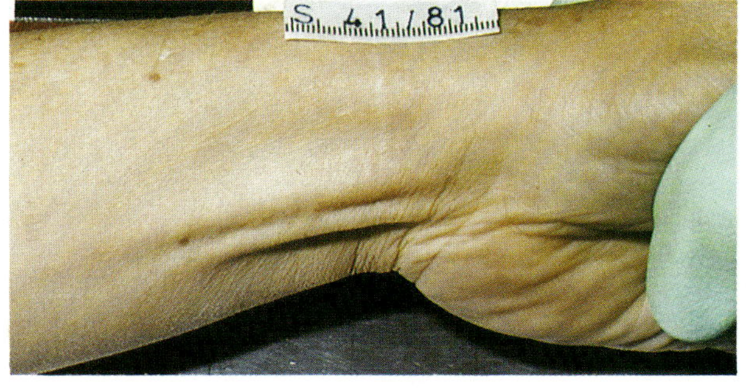

376 **Left wrist.** Fine, almost invisible scar, months, maybe years, old. Healed incision wound in an attempted suicide.

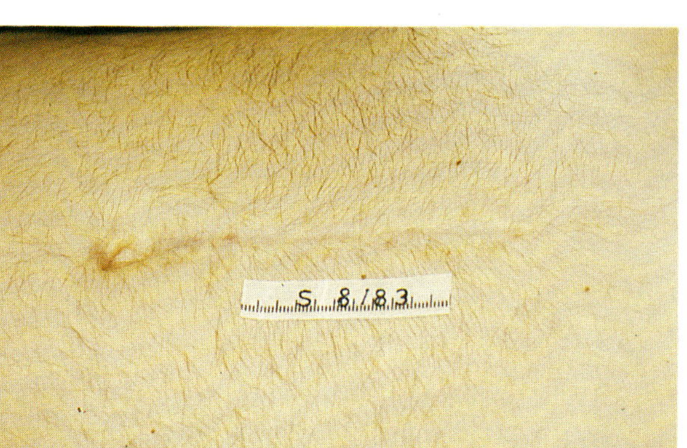

377 **Healed surgical scar,** months, maybe years, old.

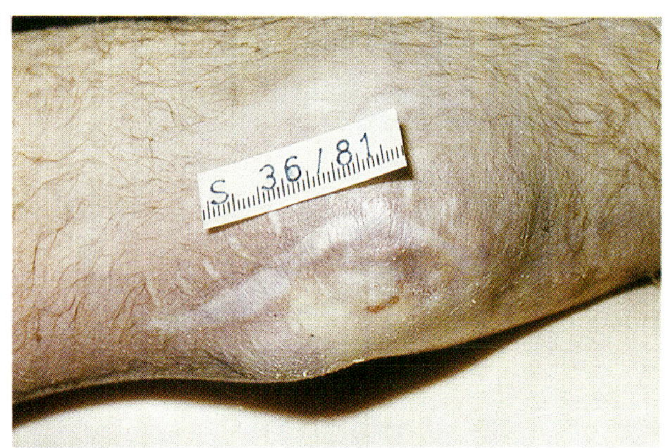

378 **Broad scar,** well healed, following an operation.

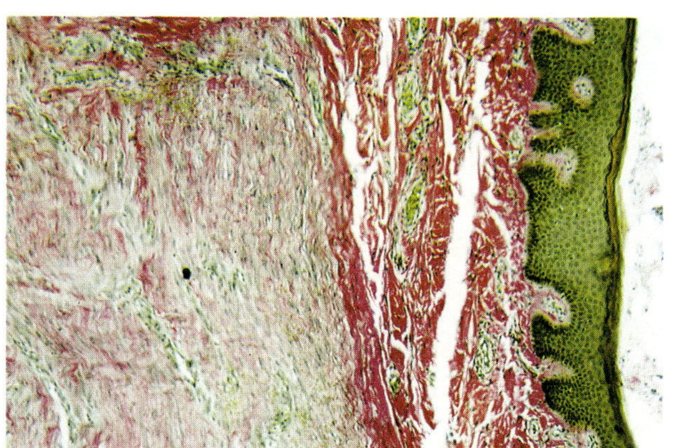

379 **Skin.** Scar tissue formation. In the upper part of the dermis connective tissue components can be seen which contain few cells. In the lower dermis (left) there is much more cellular tissue with some capillary sprouts. Note the absence of skin appendages. (*van Gieson ×100*)

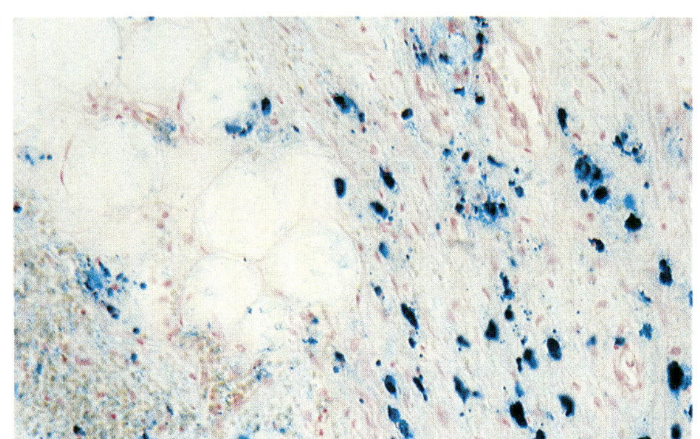

380 **Soft tissue injury (foot).** 17 days after injury. Predominantly connective tissue with few cells and some adipose tissue; large amounts of haemosiderin (blue) can be seen. (*Prussian blue ×250*)

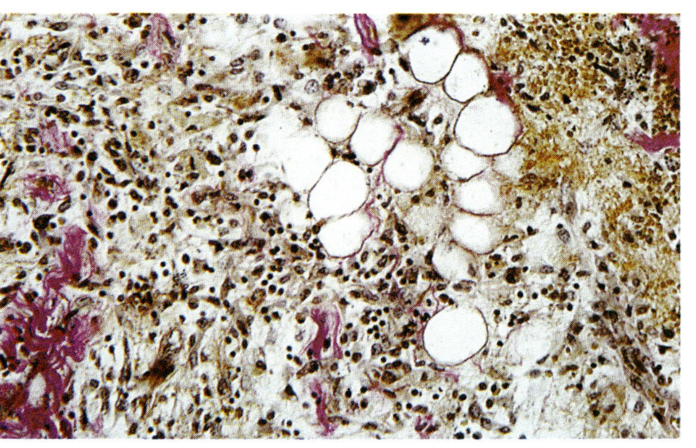

381 **Subcutaneous tissue (neck).** Injury from blows with the fist 8 days before. Haemorrhage, disruption of connective tissue components (red) and a marked inflammatory cell reaction can be seen. (*van Gieson ×250*)

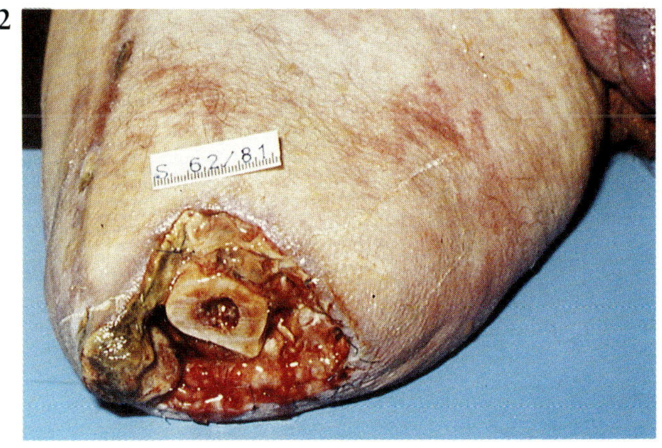

382   Thigh. Stump following amputation a few days previously.

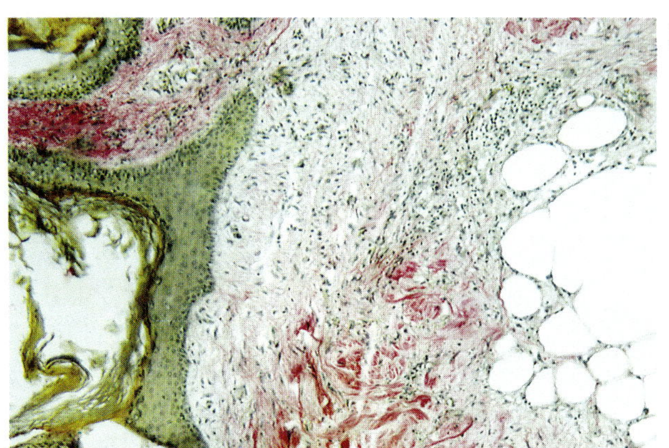

383   Skin (upper arm). Amputation of the arm 14 days previously. Formation of scar tissue with reduction in the number of capillaries in the collagenous connective tissue (right). A new epithelial covering (left) has already been formed with marked synthesis of keratin. The vertical band in the picture is an artefact caused during sectioning. (*van Gieson ×100*)

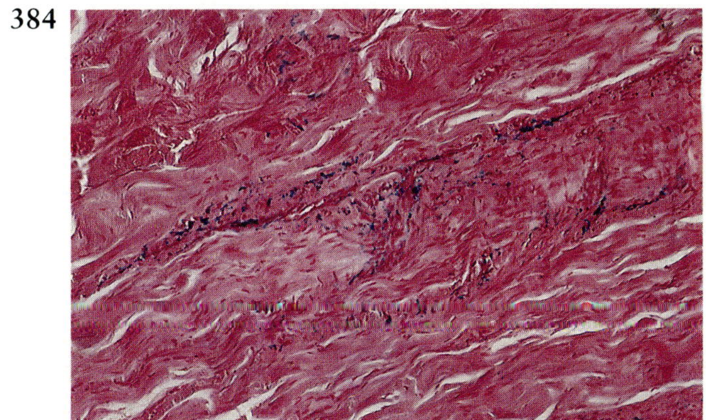

384   Extensor tendon (finger). Tendon rupture some months previously, showing evidence of old haemorrhage (haemosiderin, blue). (*Prussian blue ×250*)

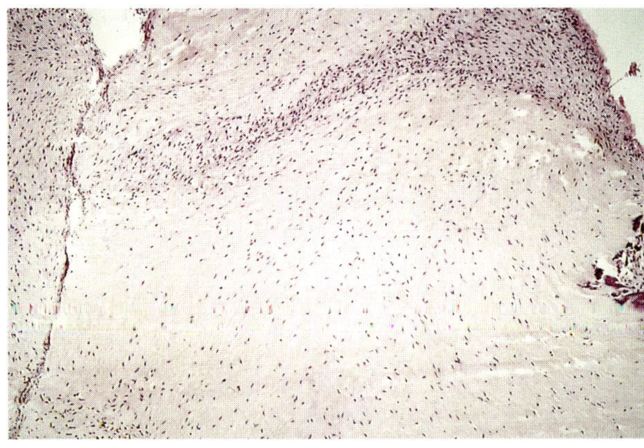

385   Meniscus (knee joint). Meniscus tear 3 weeks previously. Note the cellular reaction to the injury (top) as well as areas of calcium deposition (extreme right), a finding independent of the recent trauma. In the lower right, artefacts can be seen, the result of sectioning the partially calcified tissue. (*H&E ×80*)

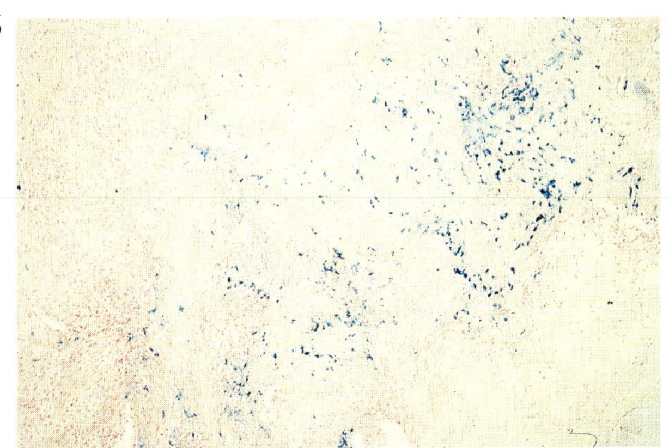

386   Meniscus (knee joint). Same as **385**. Meniscus tear 3 weeks previously. Large amounts of haemosiderin (blue) can be seen at the edge of the area of repair. (*Prussian blue ×80*)

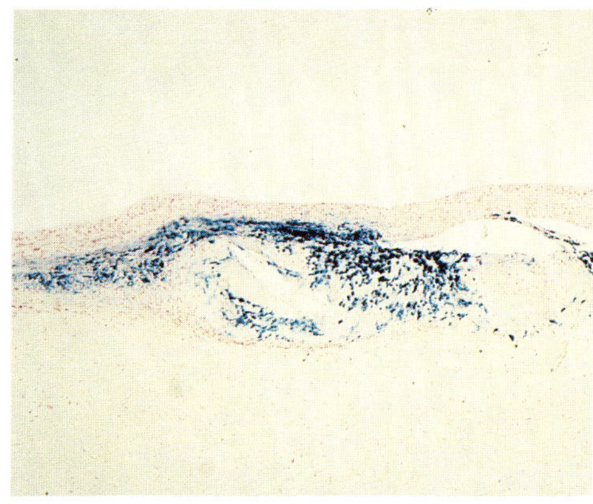

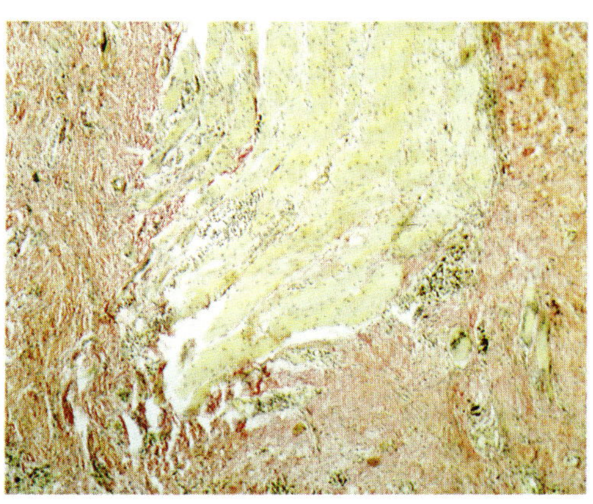

387 Stratum synoviale (knee joint). Remains of subsynovial haemorrhage (haemosiderin, blue) caused by a blunt injury several weeks previously. (*Prussian blue ×80*)

388 Muscle (biceps femoris). Muscle tear 4 months previously. Note the remaining muscle (green-yellow) surrounded by collagenous connective tissue (red) and capillary sprouts. (*van Gieson ×80*)

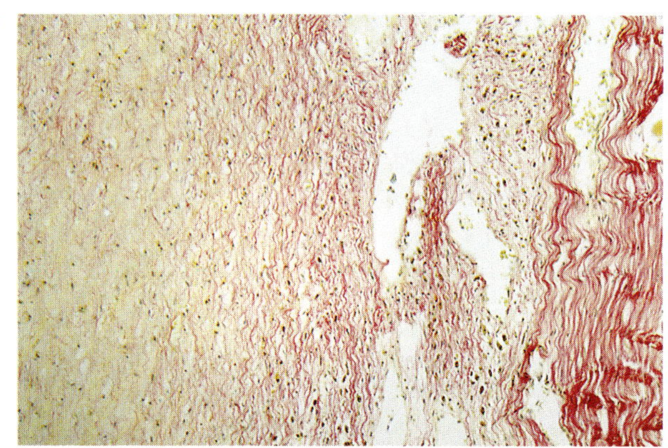

389 Dura mater. Subdural haematoma 7 weeks before death. Note the dura (right) and the organised haematoma with fine collagenous connective tissue components (red, left). (*van Gieson ×100*)

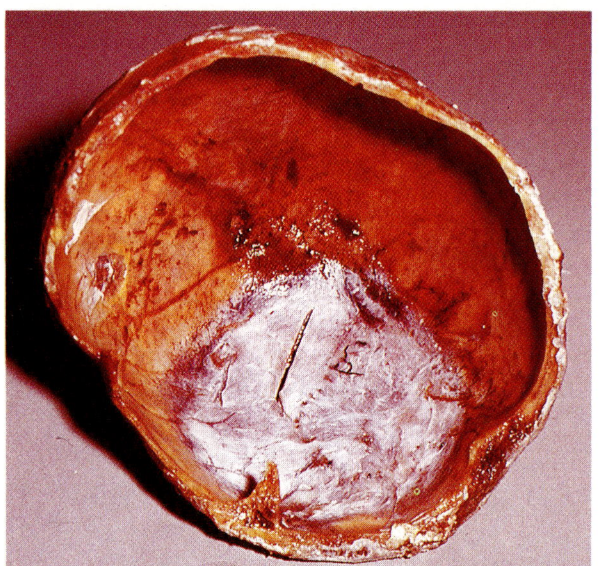

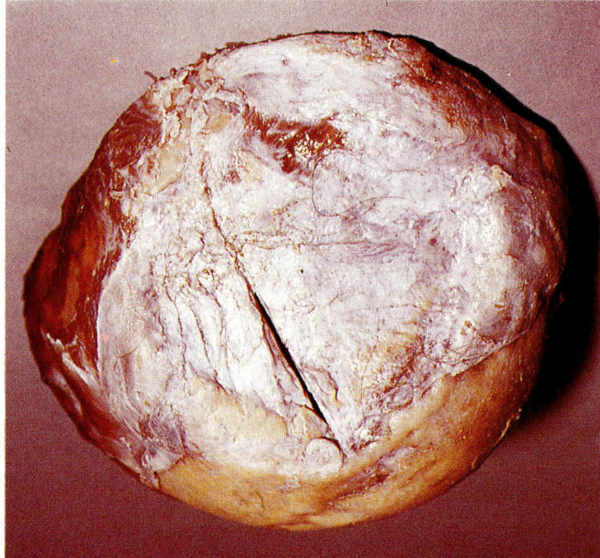

390 Reconstructive surgery (many years before death) of a comminuted fracture of the right squamous temporal and occipital bone in a 40 year-old man. The duraplasty has completely filled the defect (internal aspect).

391 Same case as in **390** (external aspect).

11 Cadaver changes and artefacts

Autolytic processes cause a diffuse red staining of the intima of blood vessels and other tissue as a result of the diffusion of haemoglobin out of erythrocytes. After the autolytic processes have gone on for some time, the colouring becomes brown to dark grey. Hydrogen sulphide produced in the intestine enters adjacent tissue and reacts with haemoglobin to produce sulph-haemoglobin which renders the tissue grey–green. If haemosiderin pigment is present in an organ (for example, in the liver) a further reaction with hydrogen sulphide is possible, namely the formation of ferrous sulphide. The affected organ takes on a brownish-black colouration (pseudo-melanosis).

Furthermore, gastric juice causes breakdown of the gastric mucosa, pancreatic enzymes digest the pancreatic tissue and bilirubin can penetrate the gallbladder wall, giving a yellowish colouration. The warmer the environment, the more rapid the onset of autolysis.

Autolytic changes can also be observed at cellular level. The enzymatic breakdown of nucleic acids leads to a loss of the basophilic staining reaction in the nucleus and later to the loss of normal nuclear structure (pyknosis, karyorhexis, karyolysis). The cytoplasm takes on an opaque appearance caused by water uptake by the mitochondria. Loss of cytoplasmic basophilia results from enzymatic breakdown of ribonucleic acid. Autolytic processes are especially noticeable in the liver, kidneys, heart and skeletal muscle, as well as in ganglion cells.

Lipids rich in phosphatides are released from membrane lipoproteins and are deposited in concentric rings in the cytoplasm — so-called myelin figures.

Heart

Cardiac muscle cell nuclei remain stainable for a relatively long time after death. However, loss of the cytoplasmic cross-striations can be clearly seen as a post-mortem change.

Liver

Dissociation of hepatic trabeculae occurs. Autolytic alterations in hepatocytes develop rapidly in areas already damaged by dystrophic disease processes.

Kidney

The proximal renal tubular epithelium is especially sensitive to autolytic change. Capillary dilatation, particularly in the glomeruli, is also encountered. A differentiation between pathological necrosis of the renal tubuli and autolytic changes is extremely difficult, if not impossible, to make.

Lung

Blood vessel dilatation and distension of alveoli with weakly eosinophilic fluid represents a post-mortem change.

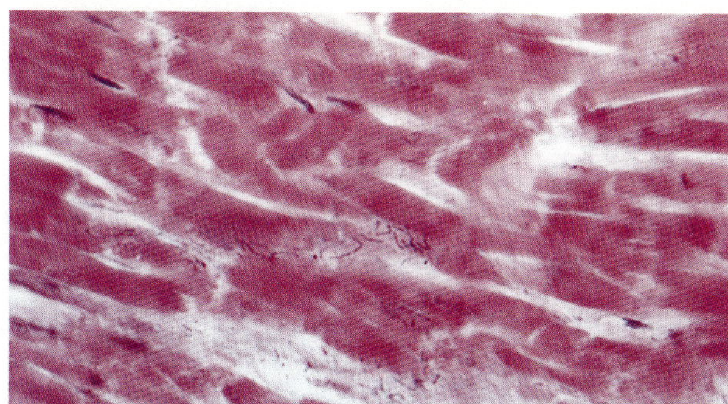

392 Heart. Autolytic alterations of the cardiac muscle cells, with complete absence of nuclear staining reaction. Only individual pyknotic nuclei in the connective tissue surrounding muscle fibres can be seen. Bacterial growth (rods) is also in evidence. (*H&E ×640*)

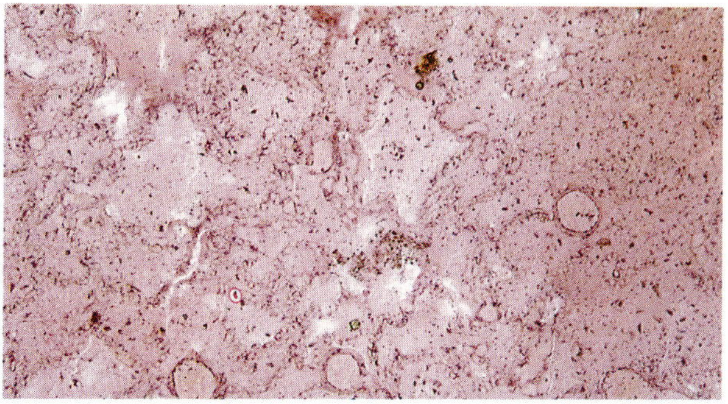

393 Lung. Autolytic change. The features here are the poor or absent staining reaction of the nuclei and the presence of haemolytic fluid in the alveoli, giving a cloudy appearance. A further artefact is the presence of large amounts of formalin pigment (brown–black), which is common in fixed decomposed tissue. (*H&E ×100*)

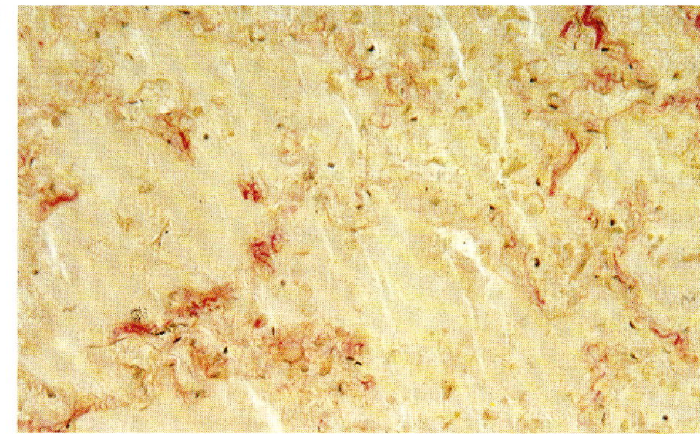

394 Lung. Autopsy material showing advanced decomposition. The picture highlights the value of a connective tissue stain (in this case the van Gieson stain) to demonstrate the structural skeleton of the tissue being investigated. (*van Gieson ×100*)

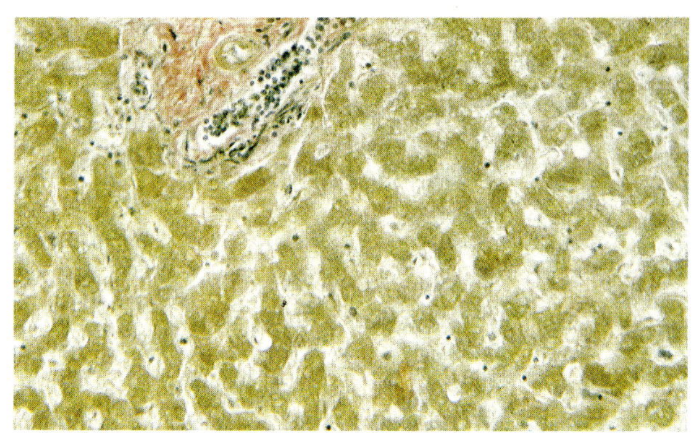

395 Liver. The start of autolytic change with absent staining reaction of the hepatocyte nuclei. (*van Gieson ×250*)

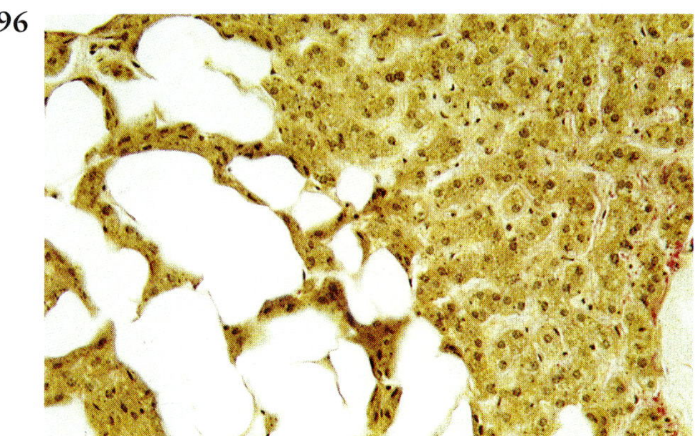

396 Liver. Advanced signs of decomposition with gas formation in the organ. (*van Gieson ×250*)

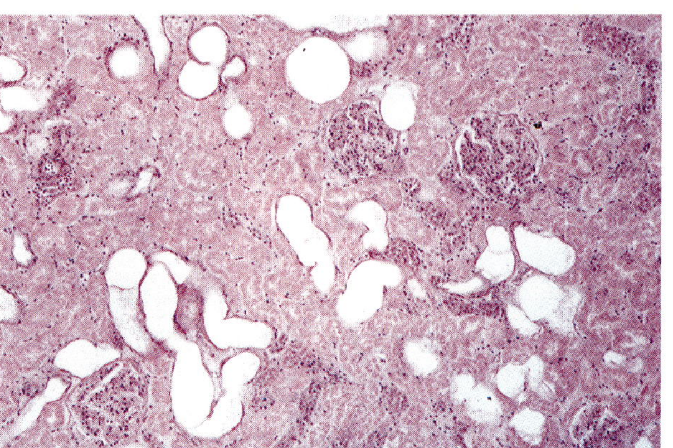

397 Kidney. Autolysis, with poor stainability of the nuclei, particularly of the tubules. Gas formation can also be clearly seen. (*H&E ×100*)

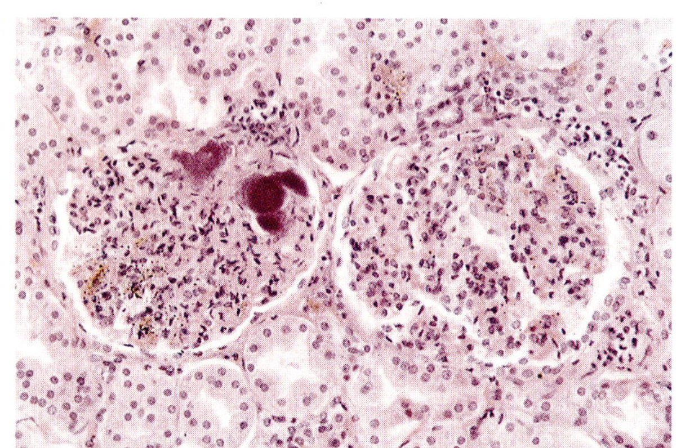

398 Kidney. Decomposition, with bacterial colonies in a glomerulus. (*H&E ×250*)

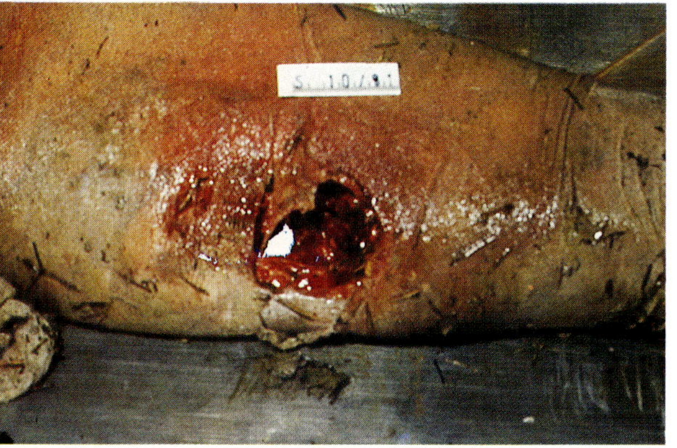

399 Deep laceration on the lateral aspect of the thigh of a corpse which had been in water for 2–3 days.

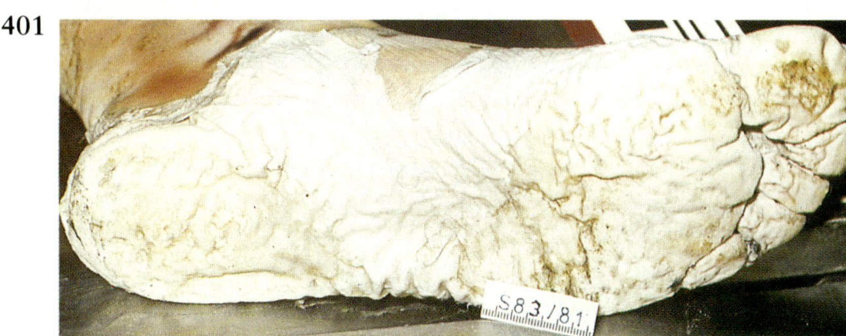

400 **Sole of the foot.** Wrinkled appearance of the skin from a corpse found in the water.

401 **Skin.** Detachment of skin in the ankle region. Corpse removed from water.

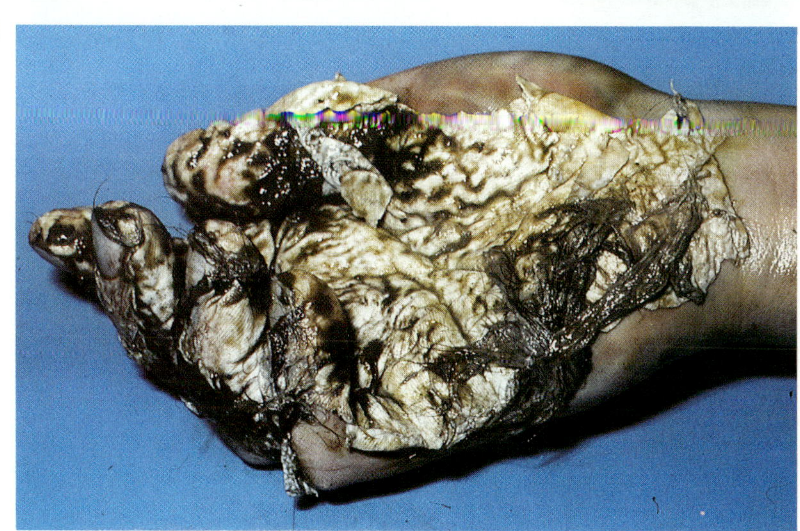

402 **Wrinkled skin** of the right hand with extensive skin detachment.

12 Respiratory interference

The histological findings indicative of damage due to oxygen deficiency or death as a result of suffocation may be summarised in the following way (Janssen, 1977):

- Non-lipid-containing, principally perinuclear vacuoles in hepatocytes and cardiac myocytes, somewhat less marked in the renal tubular cells.
- Swelling of the endothelial cells in the capillaries of the brain and myocardium.
- Mobilisation and proliferation of alveolar cells, occasionally with the formation of multinucleated giant cells (only of significance in healthy lungs).
- Hyaline precipitates in hepatocytes.
- Circumscribed areas of haemorrhage in the lungs and brain.
- Degeneration of ganglion cells with pyknosis and disappearance of the Nissl substance, particularly in the hippocampal region.
- Acute alveolar and interstitial pulmonary emphysema, acute congestion of the internal organs.

The important histological features of the tissues adjacent to a strangulation furrow (hanging, strangulation) in the neck have also been listed:

- Congestion of the blood vessels in the peripheral zones of the furrow.
- Areas of haemorrhage in the region of the furrow.
- Haemorrhage in oblique ridges and in the crests of skin ridges between two strangulation furrows.
- Intraepidermal or subepidermal blister formation with and without content.
- Interruption of tissue continuity with and without haemorrhage.
- Initial signs of an inflammatory reaction with and without cellular infiltration.
- Metachromasia of the cutaneous and subcutaneous connective tissue (revealed by the Mallory stain).
- Destruction of adipose cells and emulsification of cell content.
- Increased uptake of stain by crushed, but not necrotic muscle (revealed by the erythrochromocyanin stain).
- Swelling of nerve endings and axis cylinders.
- Intercolloidal crystals in the thyroid gland.
- Haemorrhage in neck lymph nodes.
- Wax-like degeneration of muscle (resembling Zenker's degeneration).
- Haemorrhage and necrosis in the carotid ganglion or in the surrounding tissue.

Haemorrhage in the absence of tissue destruction is to be viewed with suspicion when a general marked congestion is present.

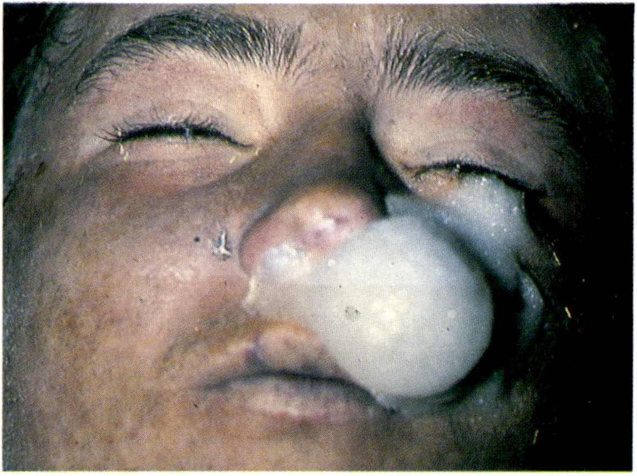

403 **Frothing** at the nose in a case of drowning. Typical macroscopic finding in death by drowning, it can be caused by other phenomena, such as acute drug overdose.

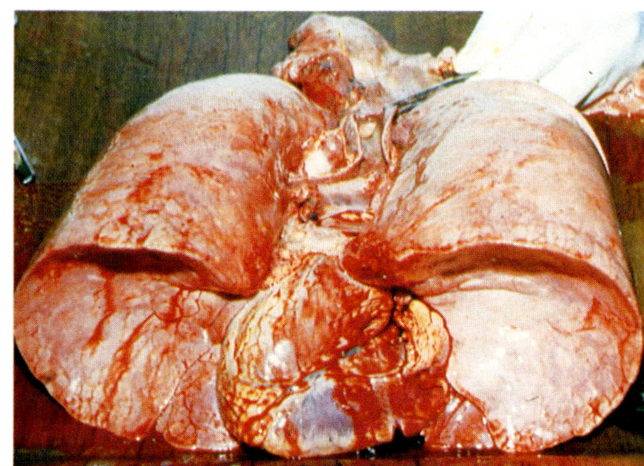

404 **Acute pulmonary emphysema** in a case of drowning.

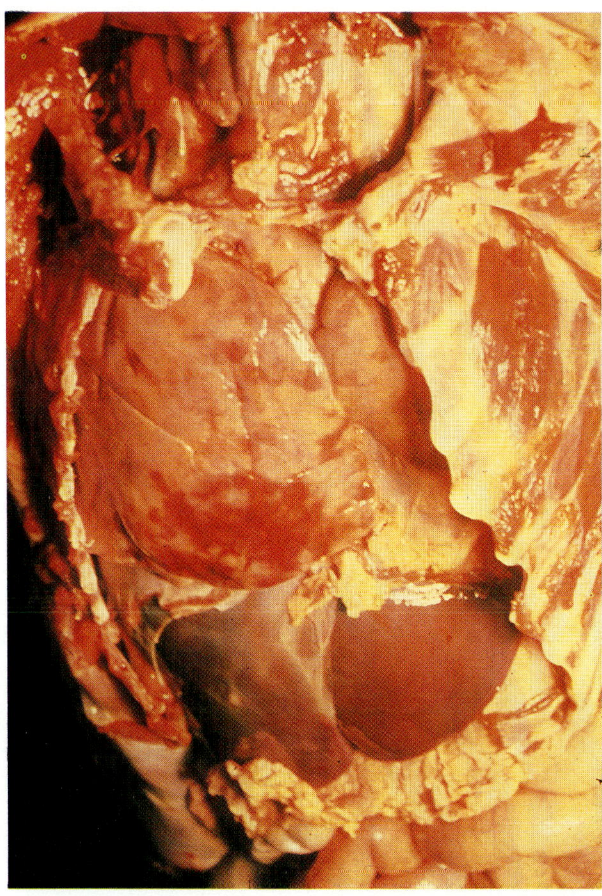

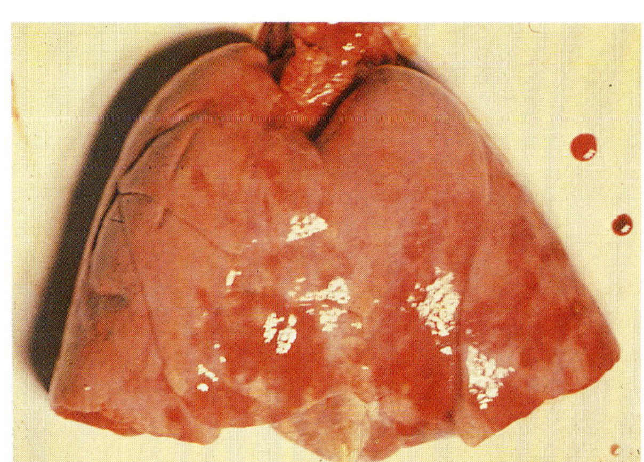

406 Same case as **405**. Close-up view, showing areas of haemorrhage as approximately 1 cm diameter, dark red, indistinct lesions (Paltauf lesions). The apparently white areas are artefacts due to light reflection during photography.

405 **Thorax.** Acute pulmonary emphysema with Paltauf lesions, caused by mixing of water with the products of haemolysis. From a child drowned following abuse.

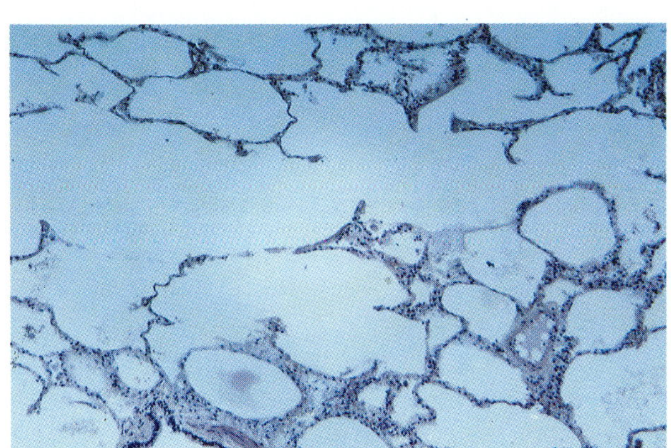

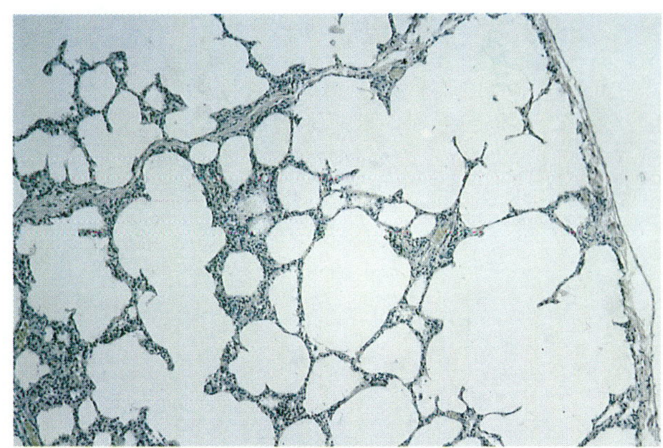

407 **Lung.** Case of drowning. Note the overdistension of the alveoli with tearing of the alveolar septa (emphysema aquosum), and anaemia of the capillaries. From a 25 year-old male. (*H&E ×100*)

408 **Lung.** Case of drowning, showing the marked alveolar hyperdistension in the subpleural regions. (*H&E ×100*)

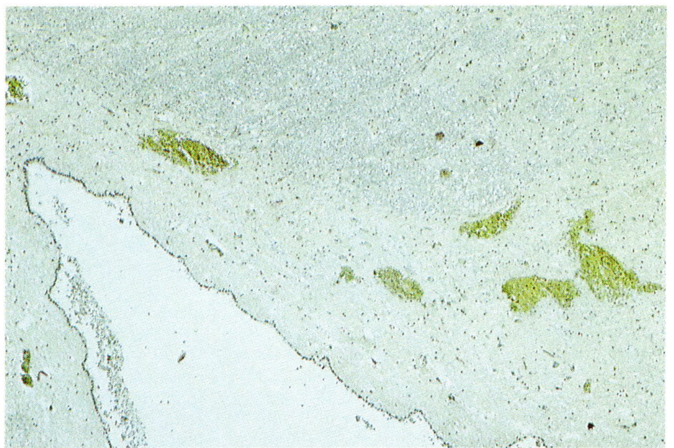

409 Brain. Suffocation caused by massive aspiration of food. Perivascular haemorrhage can be seen in the subependymal regions. Material from a 15 year-old male. (*H&E ×64*)

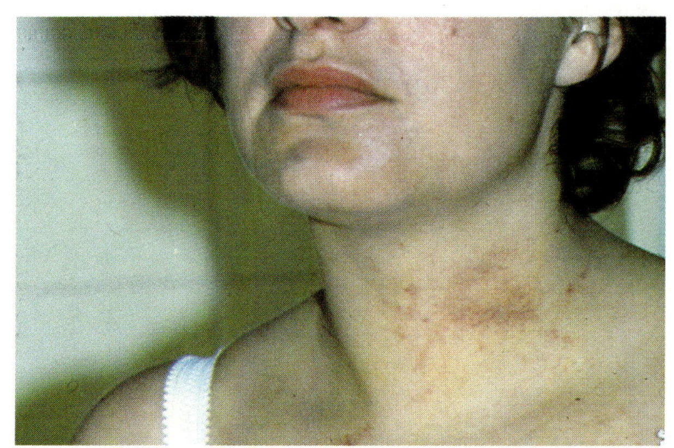

410 Neck. Manual strangulation.

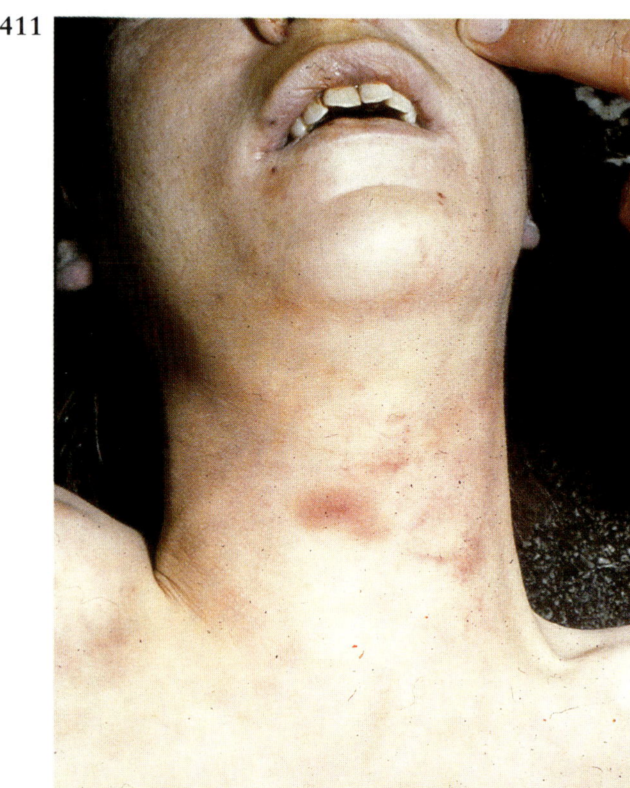

411 Neck. Extensive manual strangulation marks on the neck and over the larynx.

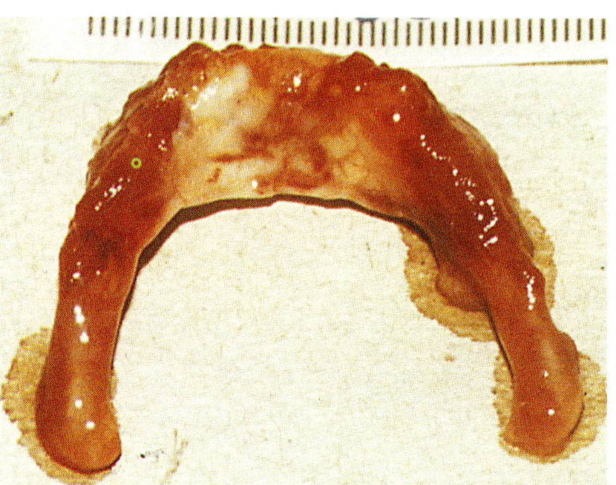

412 Fracture of the cornua of the hyoid bone and marked haemorrhage in a case of manual strangulation. Bleeding and abnormal motion are the clues that lead to the detection of hyoid bone fractures. The hyoid should *always* be removed and carefully examined in every autopsy.

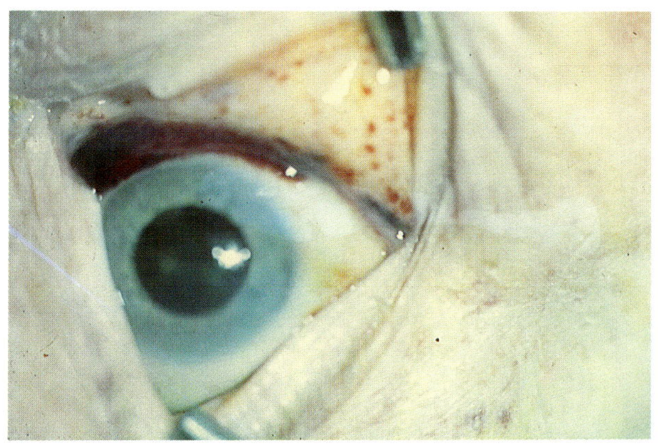

413 Punctate and confluent haemorrhage in the conjunctiva in a case of manual strangulation. Frequently present on bulbar conjunctiva as well, this finding is characteristic of asphyxial deaths, but is also sometimes associated with other causes of death.

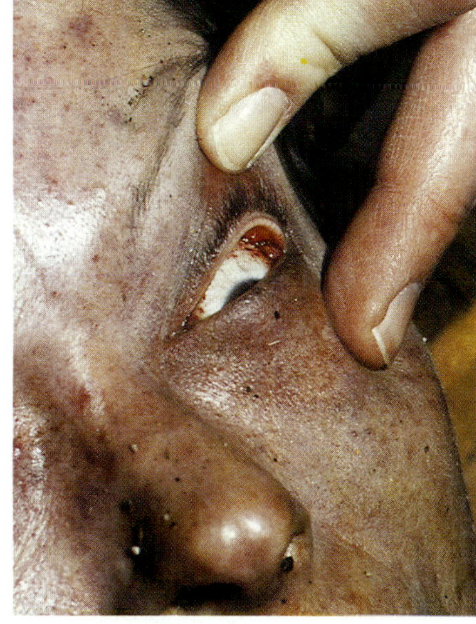

414 Multiple areas of punctate haemorrhage in the facial skin, with more extensive areas of haemorrhage in the conjunctiva in a case of suffocation.

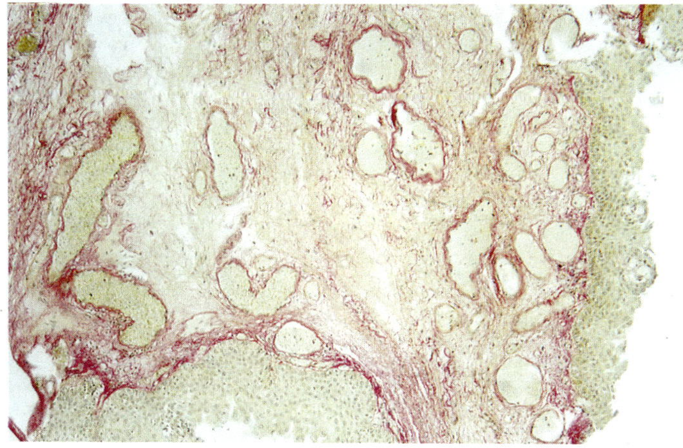

415 Uvula. From a case of manual strangulation. The picture shows marked dilatation and hyperaemia of the blood vessels. (*van Gieson ×100*)

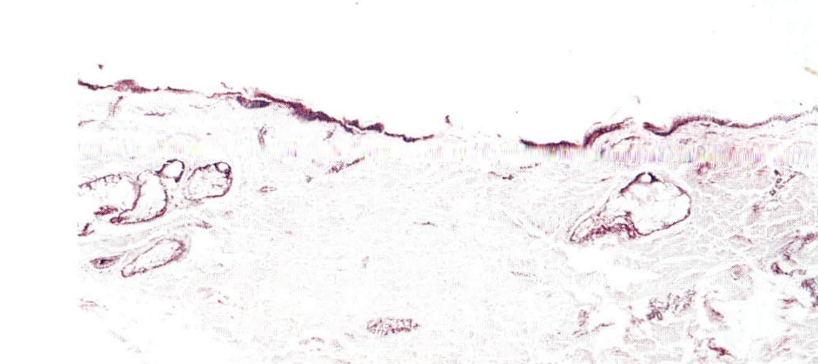

416 Skin (neck). Strangulation. Note the patchy loss of epidermis, in some areas partial thickness, in other areas full thickness. (*H&E ×12*)

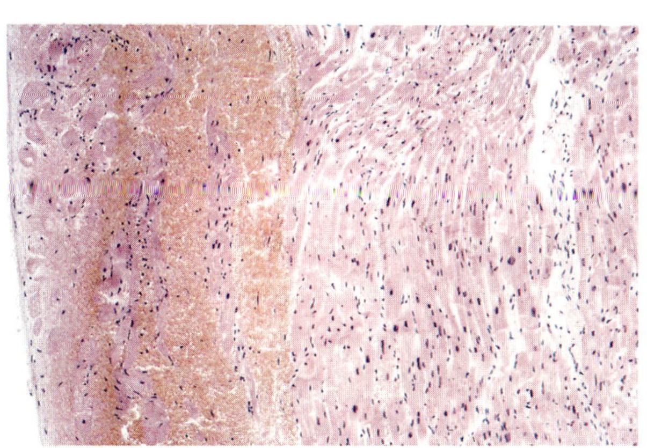

417 Heart. Manual strangulation with extensive sub-endocardial haemorrhage near the conducting system of the heart. (*H&E ×80*)

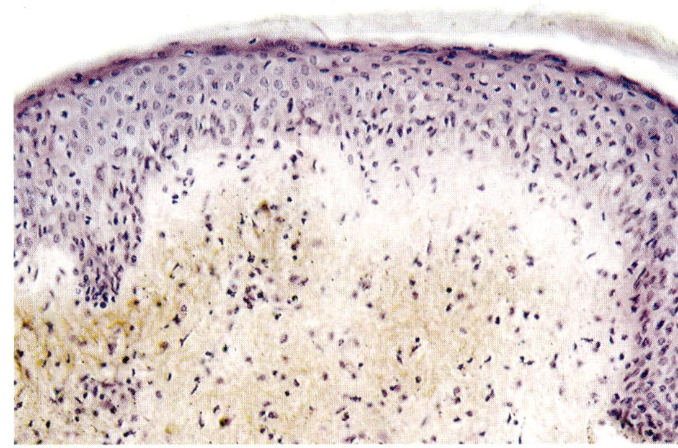

418 Skin (neck). Manual strangulation with massive intradermal haemorrhage. Note that in this case the epidermis is intact. *(H&E ×250)*

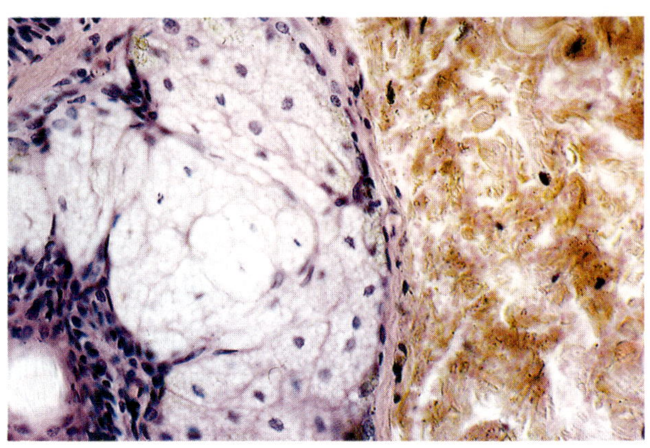

419 Skin (neck). Manual strangulation with haemorrhage (right) around a sebaceous gland. *(H&E ×400)*

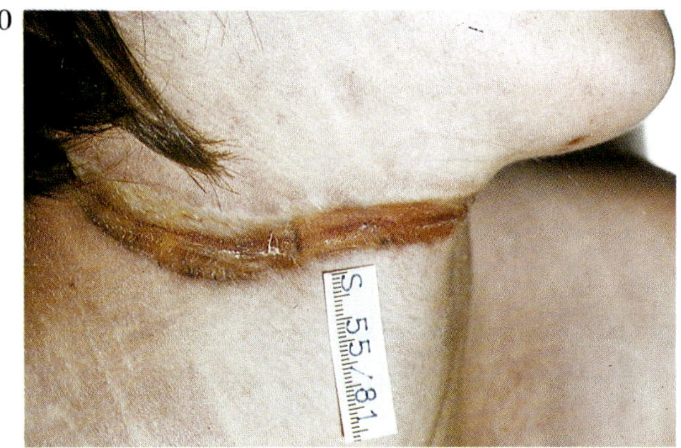

420 Strangulation furrow on the neck with small areas of haemorrhage.

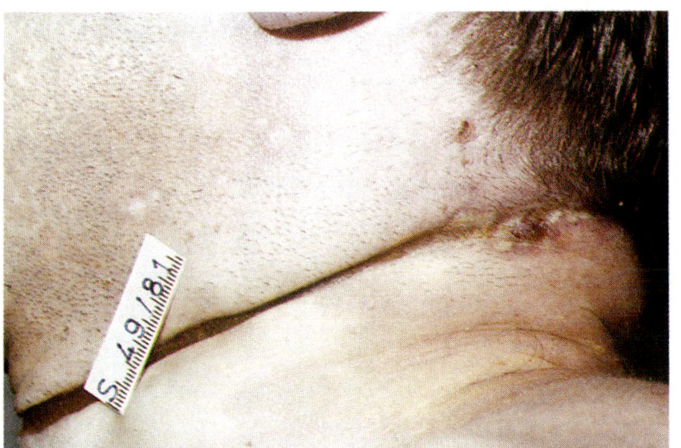

421 Very narrow strangulation furrow with superficial desiccation.

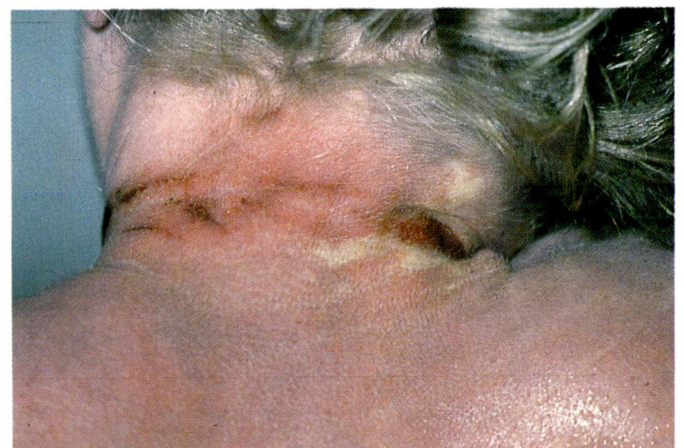

422 Neck. Strangulation mark. Furrows due to strangulation tend to be without the upward angulation found in hanging cases.

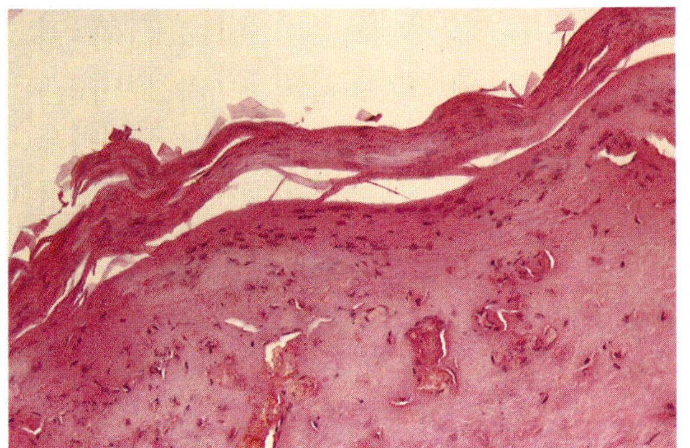

423 Skin (neck). A case of hanging. Epidermal changes resulting from pressure can be seen. The normal layered structure of the epidermis has been disturbed and some epidermal cells show a diminished nuclear staining reaction. *(H&E ×100)*

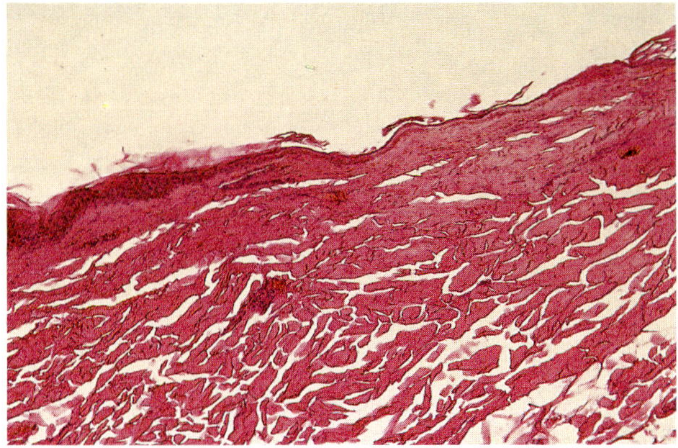
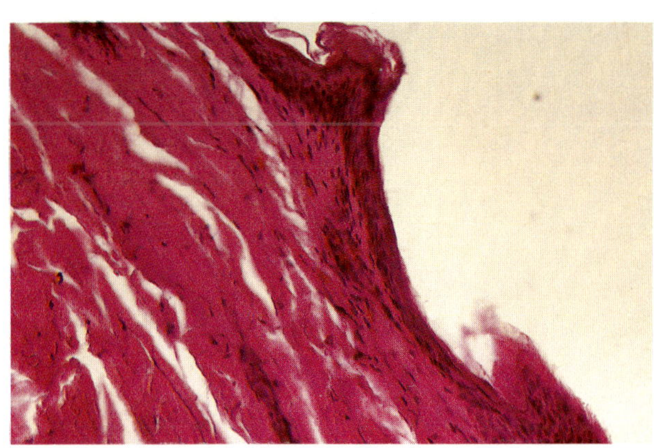

424 **Skin** (**neck**). A case of hanging. Marked loss of epidermis (right) can be seen. The transition zone between the area of denuded skin and normal skin is also depicted (left). (*H&E ×100*)

425 **Skin** (**neck**). As in **424**. This picture depicts the wave-like projections of epidermis which mirror the surface pattern of the rope. (*H&E ×100*)

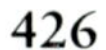
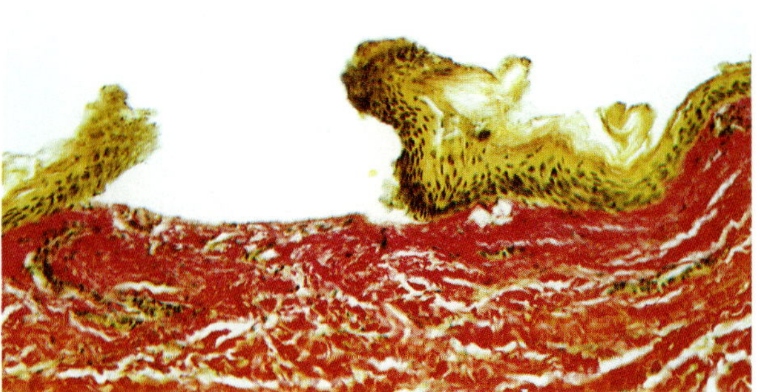
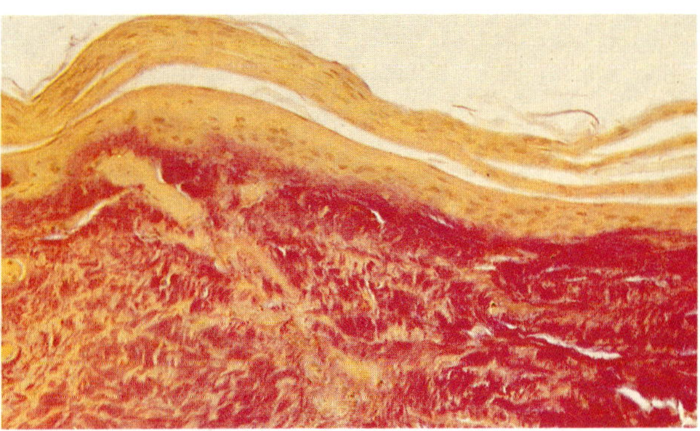

426 **Skin** (**neck**). A case of hanging. The picture shows tearing of the epidermis in the rope furrow. The cellular changes in the epidermis are the result of desiccation. Note the absence of a cellular reaction, as death was instantaneous. (*van Gieson ×250*)

427 **Skin** (**neck**). A case of hanging. A normal staining reaction for collagen (red) can be seen on the right of the picture, whereas on the left, in region of pressure from the rope, the connective tissue stains partly yellow (meta-chromasia). (*van Gieson ×100*)

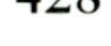
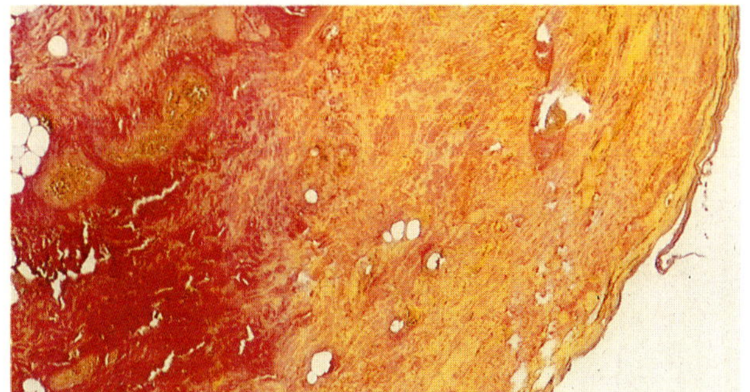
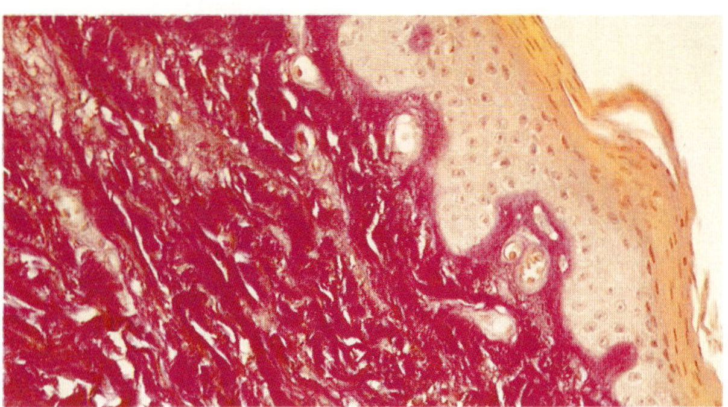

428 **Skin** (**neck**). As in **427**. The altered staining reaction for connective tissue (yellow) can be seen in the immediate subepidermal dermis, which has been subjected to massive pressure. In the deeper regions the normal (red) staining reaction for collagen is evident. (*van Gieson ×100*)

429 **Skin** (**neck**). A case of hanging. *Normal* skin from an area away from the rope furrow is shown. Note the normal structure of the epidermis, as well as the homogenous red staining of the dermal connective tissue (for comparison with **427** and **428**.) (*van Gieson ×250*)

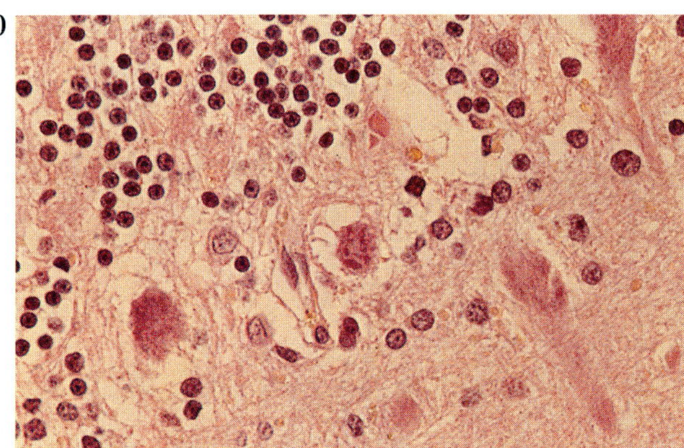

430 Cerebellum. Effects of hypoxia caused by *protracted* respiratory interference. Note the degenerative changes (eosinophilia of the cytoplasm, loss of nuclear structure) in the Purkinje cells (larger cells) and in the smaller cells of the molecular layer. (*H&E ×63*)

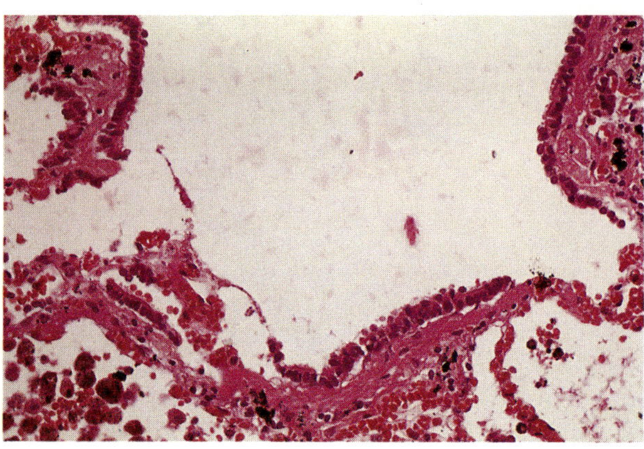

431 Lung. Barotrauma in a diver using a pressurised breathing apparatus. Rupture of a small branch of the bronchial tree with haemorrhage: the cause of death was air embolism. (*H&E ×250*)

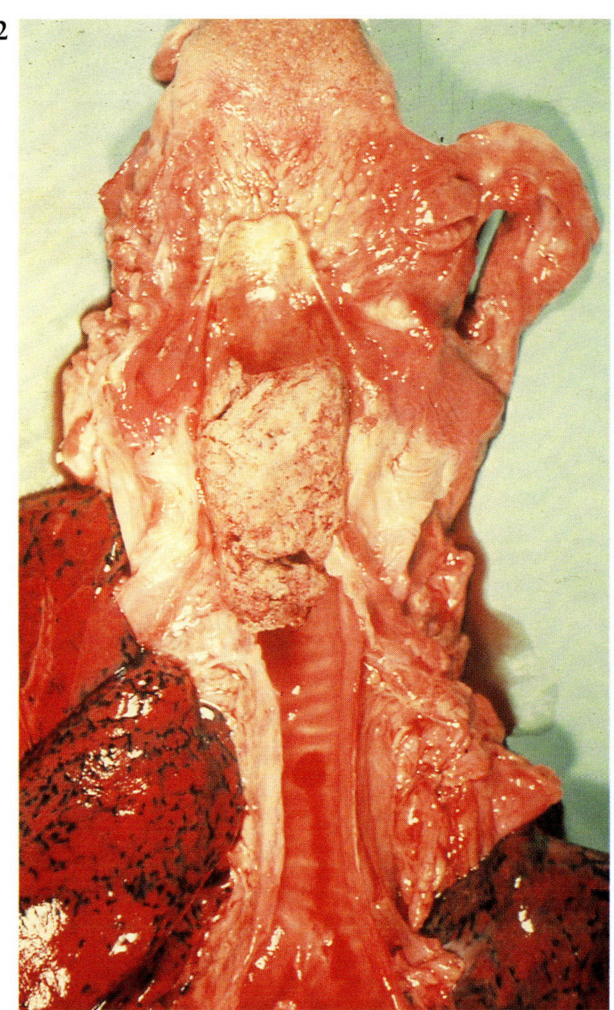

432 Asphyxia caused by an inhaled food bolus ('bolus death'). The bolus is visible just below the epiglottis. This is sometimes called 'cafe coronary'.

13 Trauma in the newborn

The assessment of changes associated with birth trauma requires a good working knowledge of the anatomy and physiology of the newborn, particularly in cases of immaturity.

Viability of the newborn

In *normal respiration* the majority of the alveoli are expanded and the lumen of the bronchial tree is wide. Preterm infants show only a partial expansion of the alveoli. To demonstrate the presence of extended elastic fibres, a longer staining reaction time is necessary than is usually employed. The staining method for elastic fibres is often unreliable and is not always positive in those areas where expanded alveoli are clearly recognisable.

In the absence of respiratory function no expansion of the alveoli can be seen and the lungs will show a characteristic glandular appearance. Individual alveoli may be distended with amniotic fluid.

Pulmonary immaturity, Grade I: occasional tubular structures with cuboidal epithelium. Nevertheless, alveoli dominate the picture. The alveolar wall contains capillaries in the immediate subepithelial region.

Pulmonary immaturity, Grade II: rudimentary alveolar ducts in the form of tubules with a cuboidal epithelium may be found in an abundance of loose connective tissue. The lung tissue contains an incomplete capillary network. Distended vessels with a primitive wall are present in the interstitium and contain blood.

Pulmonary immaturity, grade III: compact parenchyma. Numerous acinar structures with a high cuboidal epithelium. No alveoli are present. The vascularisation of the lung is poor, with occasional capillaries which are not in contact with the tubules (Moragas *et al.*, 1976).

According to MacGregor (1960), differentiation between primary and secondary atelectasis is extremely difficult, if not impossible. In cases of amniotic fluid aspiration the alveoli, bronchioles and bronchi contain solid components, such as vernix scales, skin (squamous epithelia with eosinophilic cytoplasm and pyknotic nuclei), amnion epithelia (flat or cuboidal epithelium) and lanugo hairs. The keratinised epidermis cells stain well with the van Gieson stain, giving them a yellow–brown colour.

In meconium aspiration abundant brownish amorphous material can be found in alveoli and bronchioles. According to Ahvenhainen (1948), amniotic fluid is always present in the lungs of the newborn, albeit in small quantities. It has no damaging effect. Substantial aspiration can lead to suffocation, in which case the lungs are partially aerated.

A few breaths are sufficient to cause a mature lung to expand. The central regions of the alveolar tree are the first to expand, followed by the peripheral regions. Aspiration of amniotic fluid, as well as the presence of hyaline membranes can lead to a delay in expansion. Hyaline membranes are seen as a homogeneous eosinophilic layer (H&E stain) lining the wall of expanded alveoli. Their presence alone should not be regarded as a sufficient explanation of the cause of death (Ahvenhainen, 1948). The quantity and extent of the hyaline membranes, as well as the clinical picture and other disease processes, must be taken into consideration. Further information on the histological appearance of the newborn lung will be found in the publications of Morison (1970) and Potter (1962).

Liver

In the mature newborn, only sparse areas of haemopoiesis are to be found, contrasting with the numerous regions in the immature newborn.

Kidney

In the immature newborn, the nephrogenic region of the kidney contains numerous incompletely developed glomeruli. These are only occasionally found in full-term infants.

Brain

Areas of *anoxia-induced haemorrhage* are found (Morison, 1970):

- In subependymal regions or in the choroid plexus.
- Occasionally with penetration into the ventricles and the subarachnoid space.
- Localised in the pia mater.
- In subependymal areas with terminal rupture into the lateral ventricles.

In *traumatic haemorrhage* the following may be found (Morison, 1970):

- Rupture of the superior cerebral veins.
- Subdural haematoma.
- Rupture of the great cerebral veins with subtentorial haemorrhage at the base of the skull.
- Medial tentorial tears in the straight sinus or lateral sinus into the transverse sinus, with subtentorial or more widespread haemorrhage.
- Rupture at the junction of the falx cerebri and tentorium cerebelli.

Table 1. Cause of death in 1177 newborn infants (1951–1960) (Schnaars, 1965).

	Without artificial respiration	With artificial respiration
Atelectasis[*]	28.9%	21.4%
Cerebral haemorrhage	19.0%	12.8%
Aspiration	14.5%	21.4%
Hyaline membranes	9.0%	12.8%
Bronchopneumonia	6.8%	17.1%
Pulmonary haemorrhage	3.5%	12.8%
Interstitial emphysema	0.5%	30.0%

[*] No clear distinction could be made between primary and secondary atelectasis because of the many intermediate forms.

According to Schnaars (1965), artificial respiration expands the airways instead of expanding the peripheral regions involved in respiration. This leads to insufficient unfolding of the alveoli.

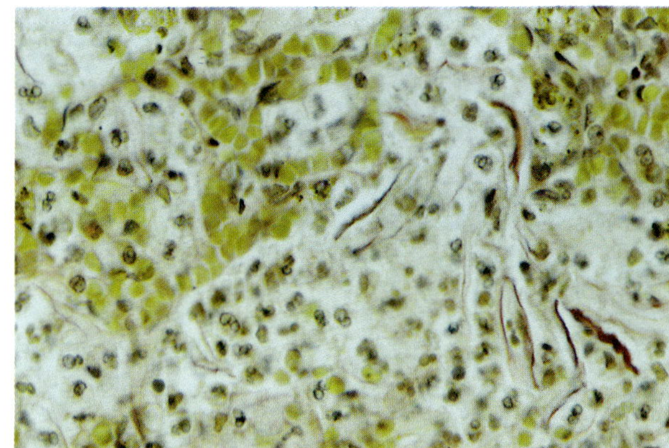

433   **Lung.** Amniotic fluid aspiration. Numerous keratin lamellae can be seen in the alveolar lumen. (*van Gieson ×640*)

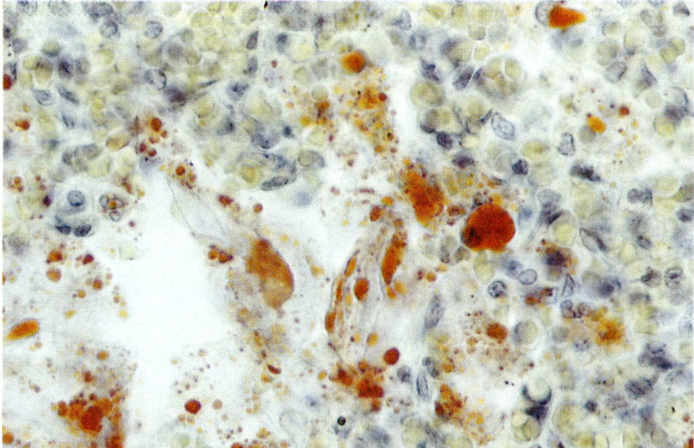

434   Same as **434,** showing the high lipid content of alveolar lining cells present in the lumen. (*Sudan stain ×640*)

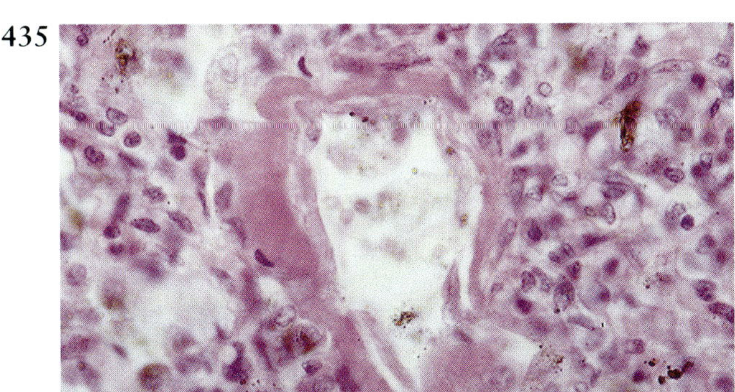

435 Lung. Hyaline membranes: lining of the alveolar wall with homogeneously staining eosinophilic material. The neighbouring lung tissue is atelectatic. (*H&E ×640*)

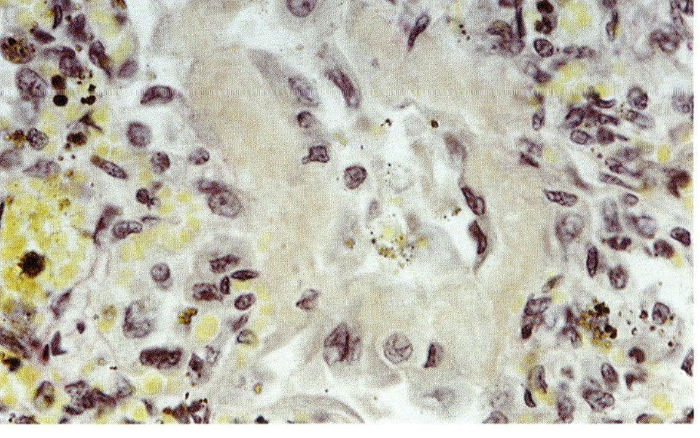

436 Lung. Hyaline membranes in the lung (*van Gieson's stain ×640*).

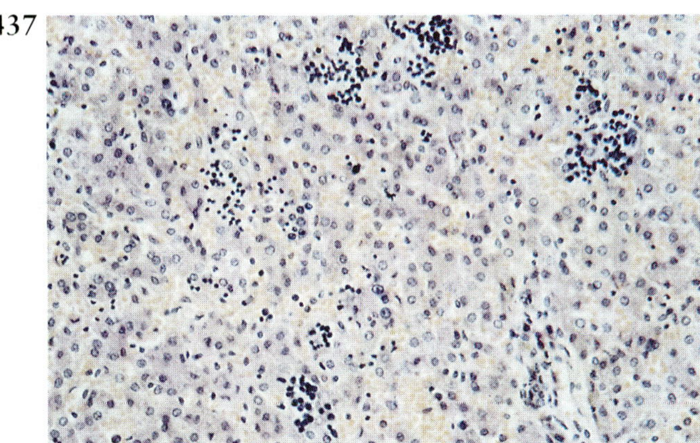

437 Liver. Areas of haemopoiesis in the liver in a mature newborn. Groups of erythroblasts, myeloblasts, myelocytes and megakaryocytes can be seen in the liver sinusoids. (*H&E ×250*)

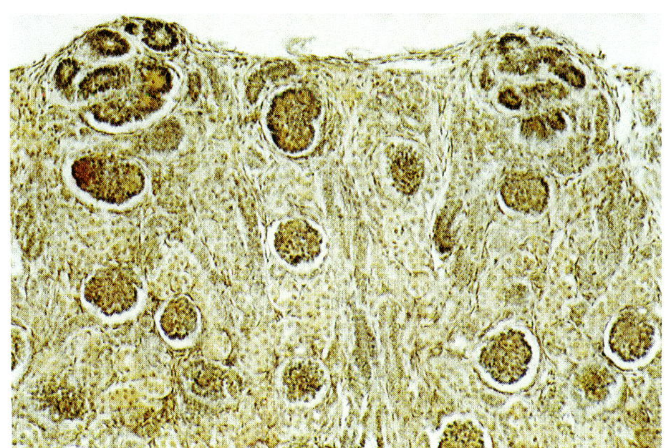

438 Kidney. Nephrogenic zone, showing immature glomeruli in the subcapsular area. Material from a preterm baby. (*van Gieson ×160*)

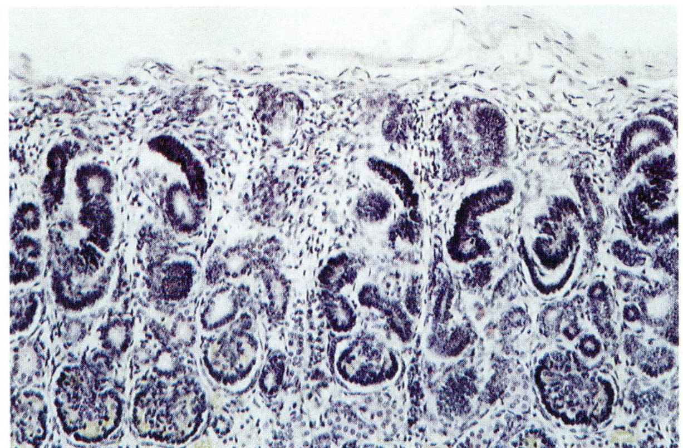

439 Kidney. Nephrogenic zone in a 7 month-old fetus, with numerous immature glomeruli in the subcapsular area. These glomeruli show an even more immature stage than those depicted in **438**. (*H&E ×200*)

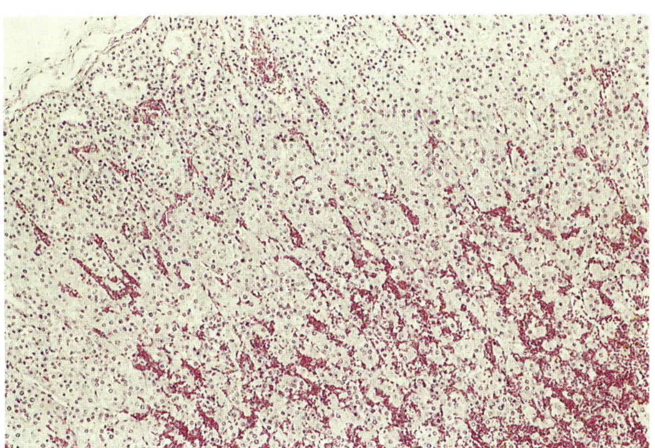

440 Adrenal gland. Haemorrhage in the deeper regions of the adrenal cortex in a 29 week-old fetus. (*H&E ×100*)

14 Ionising radiation injuries

Rather than detail the numerous injuries arising from the therapeutic use of ionising radiation, some examples of typical lesions are given.

The risk of injury from ionising radiation during the course of industrial or scientific use is small, provided that the necessary precautions are taken. Nevertheless, in the case of radiation accidents or catastrophies the dangers to human health are considerable.

In considering the injuries caused by radiation it is important to distinguish between partial body irradiation and whole body irradiation. In the former a dose of 6–120 Gy (600–12000 rem) can cause acute skin damage within a period from seconds up to a few days after exposure. Chronic skin lesions are to be expected above a minimum dose of 30–50 Gy.

Pathological changes may be observed in a variety of organs.

Bone marrow. Reduction or loss of granulopoiesis (agranulocytosis), erythropoiesis (anaemia) and destruction of megakaryocytes (bleeding abnormality).

Gastrointestinal tract. Formation of ulceration and mucosal atrophy.

Lymphatic tissue. Lymphopenia with subsequent impairment of host defence against infection.

Gonadal tissue. Loss of germinal cells; atrophy and fibrosis of gonads. For example, in the *testis* there is atrophy, thickening of the walls of the tubules, tubular necrosis, interstitial fibrosis, hyperplasia of Leydig cells and hyaline changes in blood vessel walls.

Blood vessels. Diffusion of plasma components into the vessel wall with subsequent fibrosis, leading to narrowing of the lumen (radiation vasculopathy). The latter is responsible for ischaemia in the tissue supplied by affected blood vessels.

Skin. Early changes — radiation dermatitis. Late changes — increased pigmentation, epilation, formation of telangiectasia.

Connective tissue. Swelling due to oedema; sclerosis.

Lungs. Radiation fibrosis and vascular changes.

Kidneys. Cell necrosis in glomeruli and tubules.

Eyes. Cataract.

The histopathological changes associated with ionising radiation are well described by Zollinger (1960), Rubin and Casarett (1968), Thurner (1970), Goessner (1972), Janssen (1977) and Casarett (1980).

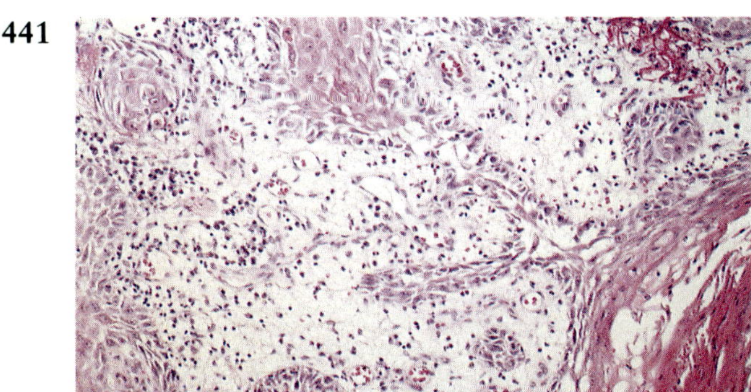

441 Skin. Radiation-induced (X-ray) squamous-cell carcinoma of the skin with oedema of the dermis. (*H&E ×100*)

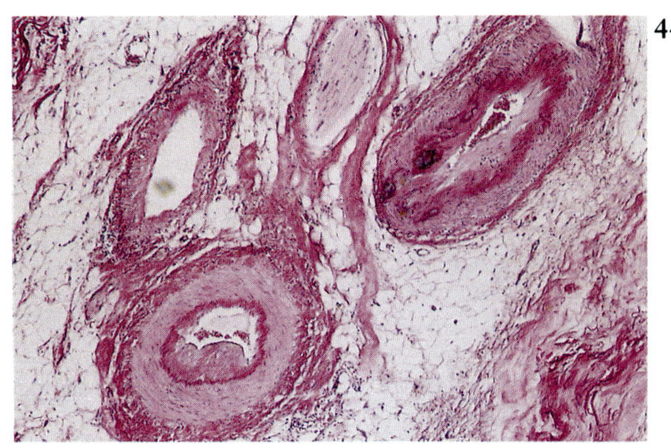

442 Subcutaneous tissue (from the case shown in **441**), showing thickening of the intima and calcification of the media of arteries, a late finding in cases of irradiation. (*H&E ×100*)

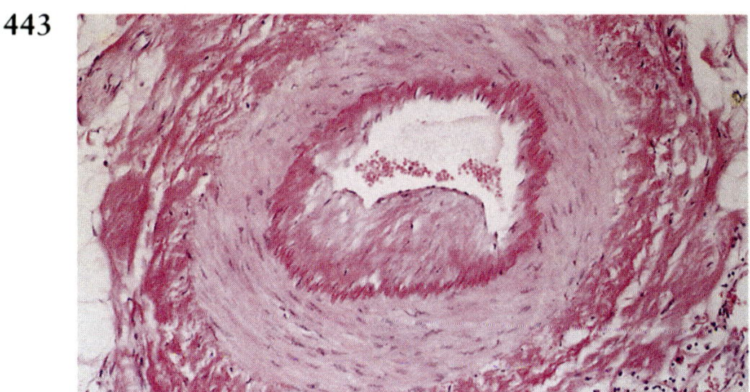

443 Irradiated subcutaneous tissue as in **441**, showing marked intimal proliferation. (*H&E ×400*)

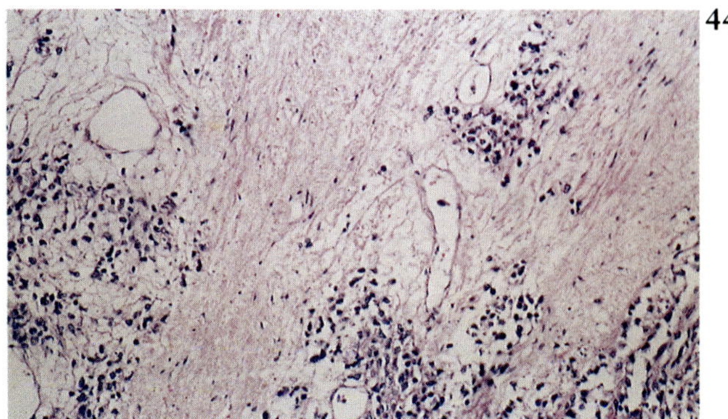

444 Irradiated oat-cell carcinoma of the lung, demonstrating a late change of irradiation — desmoplastic reaction, with production of large amounts of fibrous tissue. (*H&E ×64*)

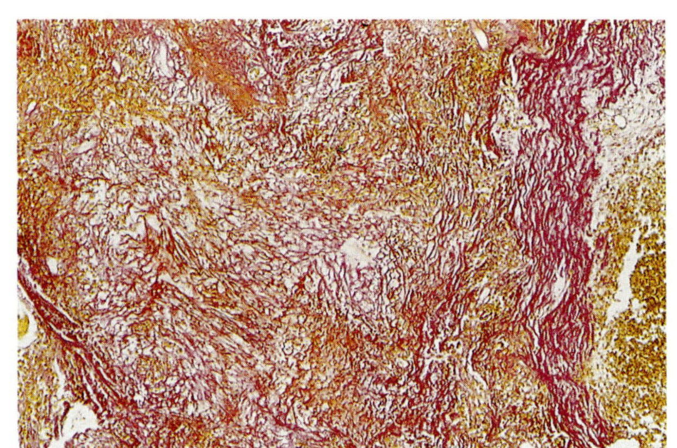

445 As in **444**, showing the presence of collagenous connective tissue. (*van Gieson ×64*)

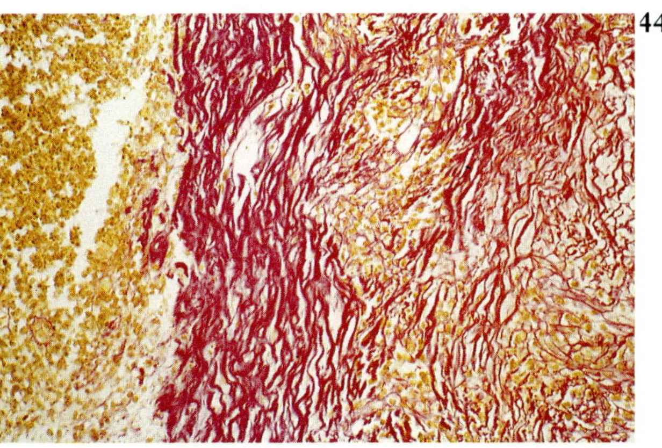

446 Lung. Marked fibrosis in the neighbourhood of an oat-cell carcinoma of the bronchus, treated by radiation. (*van Gieson ×100*)

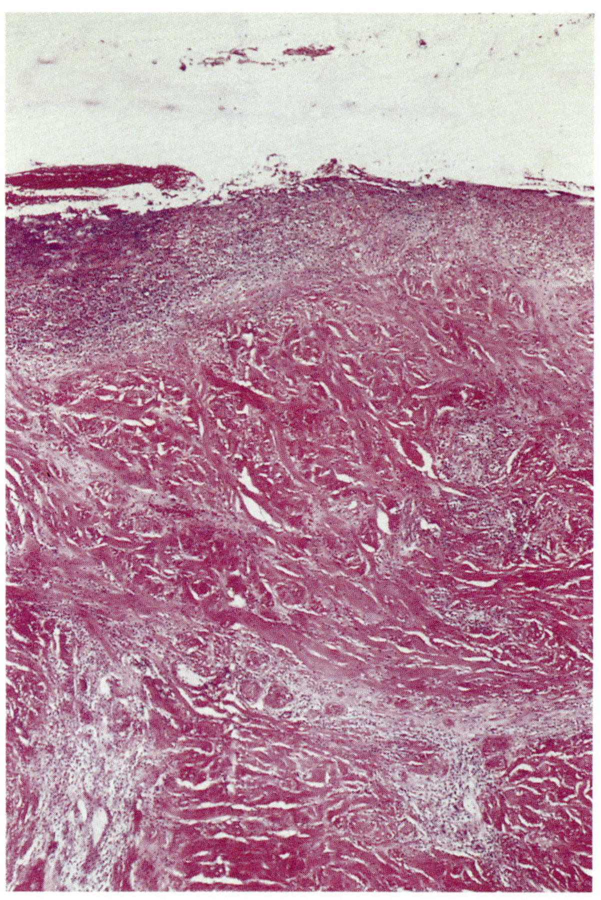

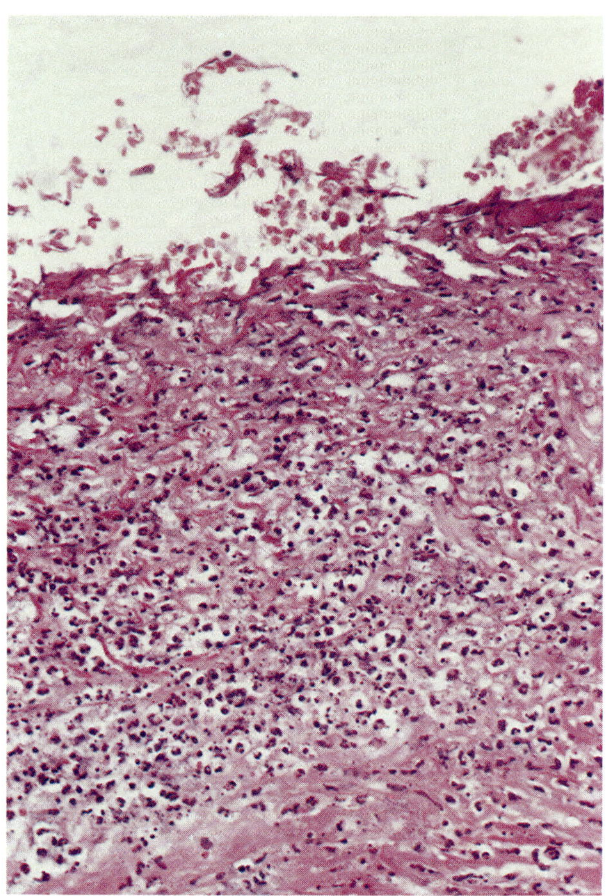

447   Skin. Radiation ulcer (skin from the back) in a 42 year-old male. Replacement of the epidermis (top) by an area of ulceration which is healing. (*H&E ×60*)

448   Same case as in **447**, showing necrosis, infiltration of the skin with numerous polymorphonuclear leucocytes, and fibrous tissue (bottom). There is evidence of healing. (*H&E ×250*)

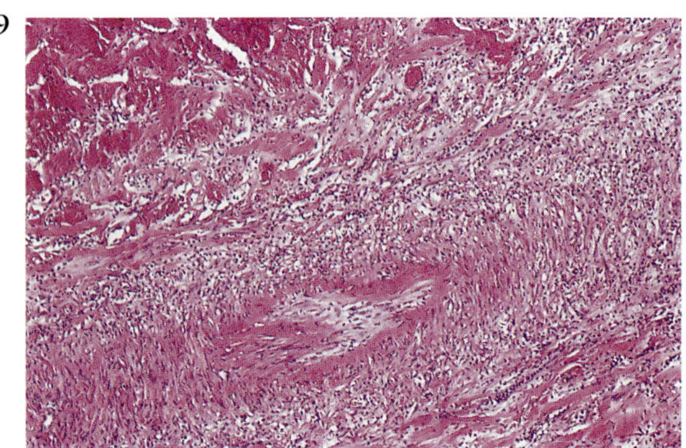

449   Same case as in **447**, showing massive acute inflammatory cell infiltration of the deep layers of the dermis. (*H&E ×150*)

15 Mild trauma and existing disease

This chapter deals with a topic of major importance to the pathologist involved in assessing trauma cases. The interpretation of the sequelae of trauma, and in particular its contribution to the cause of death, is often extremely difficult in victims of trauma who suffer from various existing diseases. Pathological changes in vital organs may severely restrict the capacity of the body to react to stress or shock. Several disease complexes are presented as examples of existing disease which may complicate the assessement of the contribution of trauma to the cause of death.

Coronary atherosclerosis

Even moderate focal atherosclerosis of the major coronary arteries may cause attacks of angina pectoris, especially when coupled with vascular spasm. More severe reduction in the size of the blood vessel lumen (for example, at a site approximately 2 cm distal to the branching of the anterior descending left coronary artery) may lead to acute coronary insufficiency when the body is subjected to physical stress, demanding an increased cardiac output.

Signs of ischaemic heart disease are often seen as disseminated small scars or, after extensive infarction, larger areas of scar tissue. Reduction of the cross-section of a coronary artery by more than 50 per cent caused by atherosclerosis markedly increases the risk of myocardial infarction and thus the possibility of a fatal outcome following even minor trauma.

Nevertheless, a cautionary note needs to be sounded. It is well established that almost complete stenosis of a coronary artery or some of its branches does not make infarction inevitable, especially when sufficient arterial anastomoses are present. Documentation of cardiac pathological findings has also made it clear than even large areas of myocardial infarction may be clinically silent.

Influenza-like infection

Depending on the type of virus involved, various morphological changes, ranging from dilatation and hyperaemia of blood vessels in the tracheal and bronchial walls with detachment of the superficial epithelial cells to extensive haemorrhagic inflammation, may be observed in influenza-like respiratory tract infections. Focal areas of haemorrhagic oedema are usually seen in the alveoli. In certain cases the number of erythrocytes in the alveoli is so large that the term 'haemorrhagic pneumonia' is sometimes used. Often an accompanying cerebral oedema is established at autopsy. Cerebral, cardiac and circulatory failure is usually the final cause of death.

Cystic medionecrosis of the aorta (Gsell and Erdheim)

In this condition there is loss of the elastic lamellae in the tunica media of the aorta, usually without marked reparative changes. Small cavities filled with a mucoid substance arise. This mucoid-cystic degeneration of the media may lead, apparently spontaneously, to the formation of a dissecting aneurysm and rupture of the aorta.

Cerebral arterial aneurysm

This usually takes the form of a saccular or spindle-shaped dilatation of the wall of the cerebral arteries at the base of the skull. The cause is usually a congenital weakness in the blood vessel musculature. Spontaneous rupture, for example during an episode of arterial hypertension, leads to a more-or-less massive subarachnoid haemorrhage.

Myocarditis

This acute or chronic inflammatory disease of the cardiac muscle has many causes, several of which come under the heading of infectious diseases. The extensive inflammation leads to a muscular insufficiency.

Lesions of the cardiac conducting system

Pathological changes in the conducting system of the heart may lead to arrythmias which can be fatal. The pathologist may be confronted with a situation which, at first sight, seems to be death from trauma, but which in fact is really death due to severe arrhythmia. The cardiac conducting system may be involved in, for example, congenital heart disease, in systemic diseases such as lupus erythematosus, or as isolated lesions following infections (viral, bacterial, parasitic), to name but a few.

Diabetes mellitus

In cases of death associated with trauma the pathologist is sometimes faced with the problem that the extent of the injuries is insufficient to adequately account for the fatal outcome. One of the important disease processes in the differential diagnosis is diabetic coma.

Morphological evidence of an underlying diabetes mellitus must be sought. Although not specific for diabetes mellitus, fatty change in the liver and nuclear glycogenation along with increased intra-cytoplasmic glycogen accumulation are important pointers. Among the other important morphological indicators are hyalinisation of the pancreatic islets of Langerhans; Kimmelstiel–Wilson glomerulosclerosis, usually as focal deposition of hyaline material in the glomerular tufts; hyaline thickening of both the afferent and efferent arterioles of the kidney; and, in cases of severe glycosuria, deposition of glycogen in the epithelium of the proximal convoluted tubules and the loop of Henle, seen as vacuolation of the epithelial cells — an appearance known as Armanni–Ebstein change. Chemical studies of blood or urine glucose can also provide clues.

Intoxication

In cases of death associated with trauma the pathologist must also keep in mind the possibility that drugs and/or alcohol may have played a major role in the cause of death. Detailed forensic investigations and careful appraisal of the morphological changes in the various organs are essential.

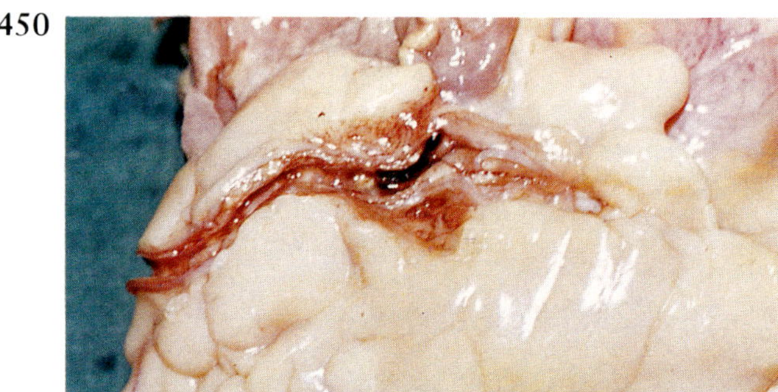

450 Atherosclerosis of a coronary artery with recent coronary thrombosis in a 63 year-old man. Acute coronary death.

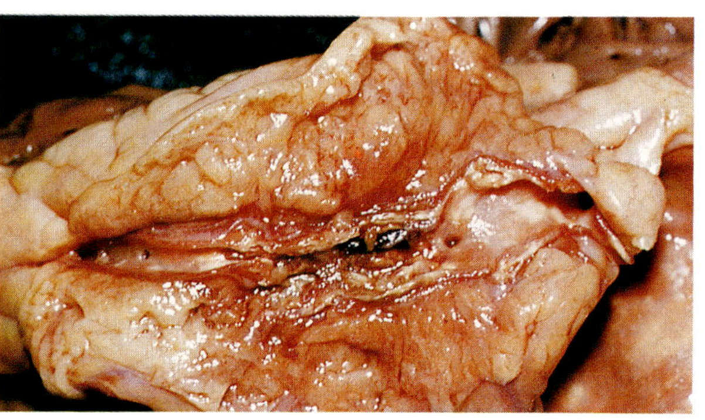

451 Recent thrombosis in a coronary artery affected by severe atherosclerosis (with stenosis and calcification). Sudden death in a 56 year-old man.

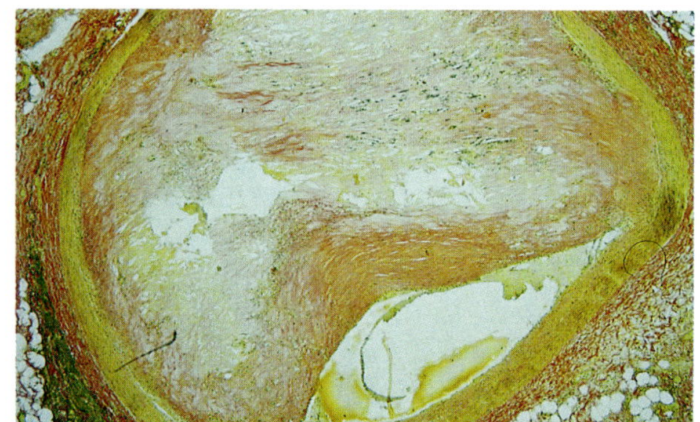

452 Heart. Severe stenosing coronary atherosclerosis with deposition of cholesterol. Fatal acute coronary insufficiency can arise when the lumen is narrowed by 50 per cent or more. (*van Gieson ×15*)

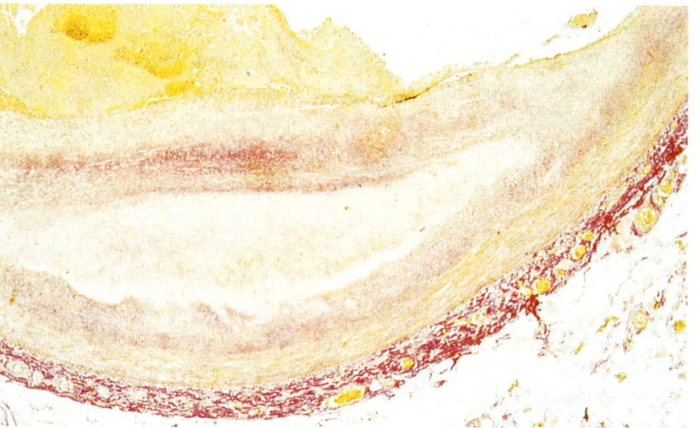

453 Heart. Recent coronary thrombosis (at most a few days) in a coronary arterial branch affected by coronary atherosclerosis. The 28 year-old victim suffered only mild trauma. (*van Gieson ×15*)

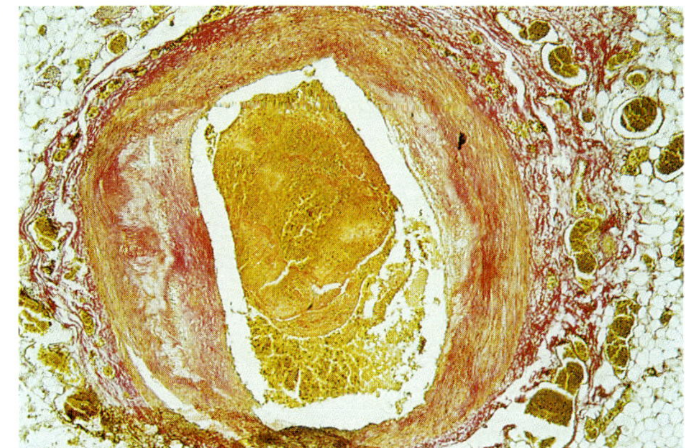

454 Heart. Moderate coronary atherosclerosis with thrombus in the vessel lumen. Material from a 32 year-old male who collapsed suddenly and died: foul play was suspected, hence the autopsy. (*van Gieson ×12*)

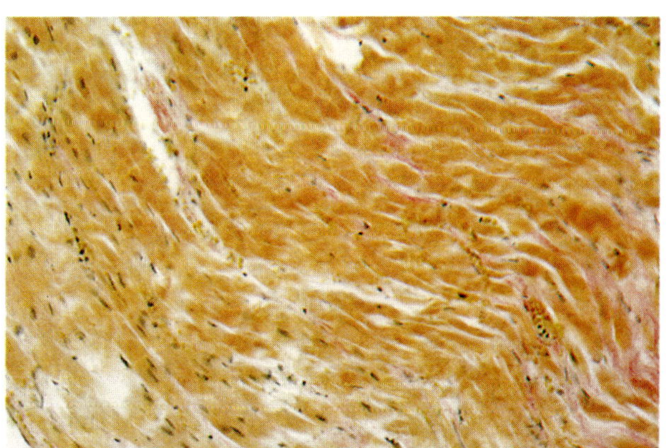

455 Heart. Acute myocardial infarction with necrosis of cardiac myocytes in the absence of a cellular reaction. The staining reaction of the nuclei of the perimysial cells is retained. Material from an 80 year-old male who developed a coronary thrombosis and fell from his bicycle. (*van Gieson ×250*)

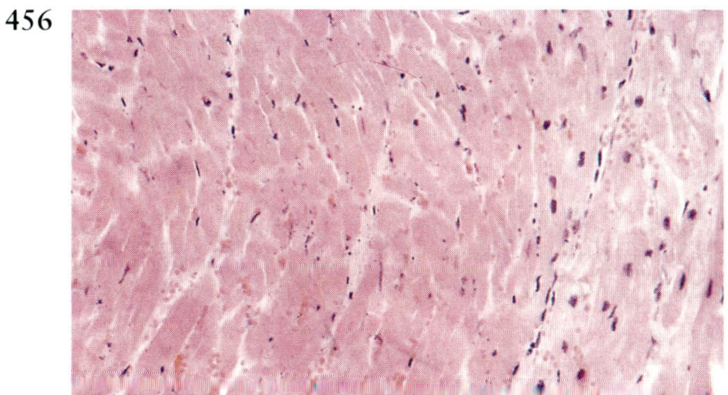

456 Heart. Recent myocardial infarction. Important features are the absence of any nuclear staining reaction in the cardiac myocytes (centre and left), capillary stasis and maintenance of the staining reaction of the perimysial cell nuclei. (*H&E ×100*)

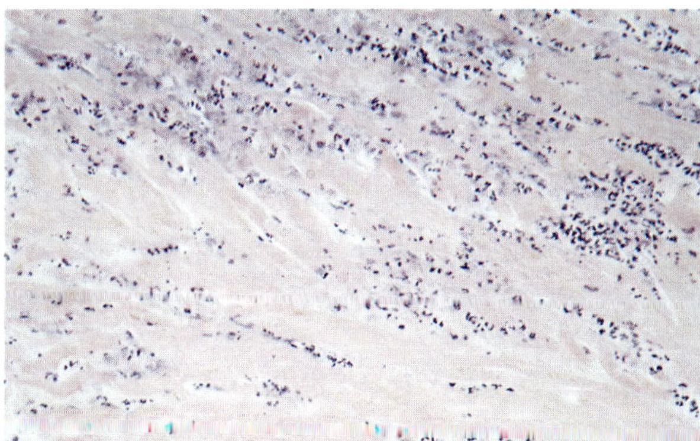

457 Heart. Acute myocardial infarction with myocardial cell necrosis and a marked peripheral cellular reaction. Some of the polymorphonuclear granulocytes show signs of degeneration. The patient died 48 hours after the infarction. (*H&E ×100*)

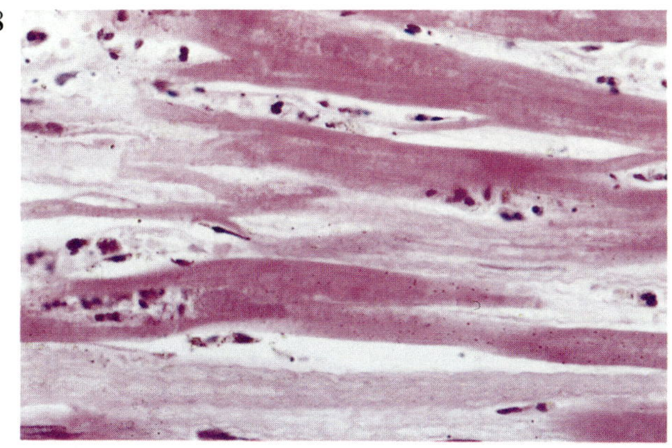

458 Heart. Approximately 8 hours-old infarct showing myocardial cell necrosis with commencement of a cellular infiltration (polymorphonuclear leucocytes). Note the lack of cross-striations and reduced staining reaction of the nuclei. Death following a fall by a 54 year-old female who suffered from stenosing coronary atherosclerosis. (*H&E ×640*)

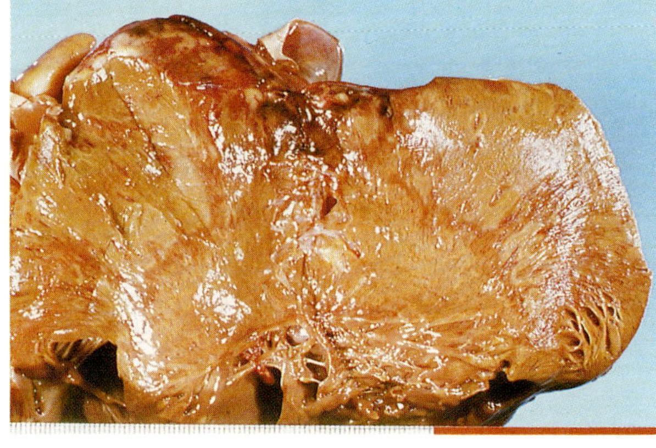

459 Myocardial infarction with extensive areas of necrosis (2–3 days old) in the posterior wall of the left ventricle. Section through septum and posterior wall.

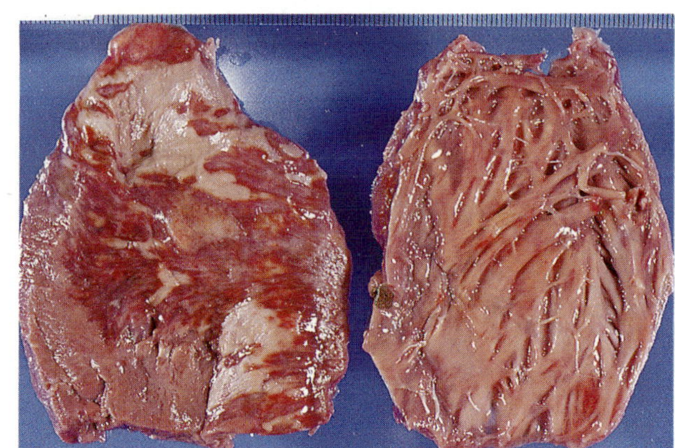

460 Myocardial infarction with geographical map-like areas of necrosis and haemorrhage in the surrounding myocardial tissue.

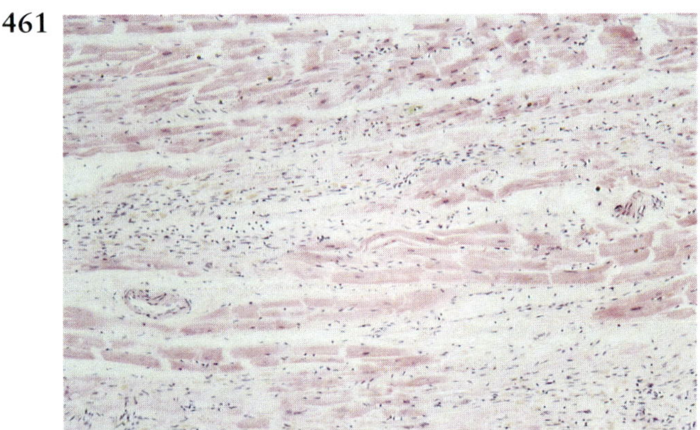

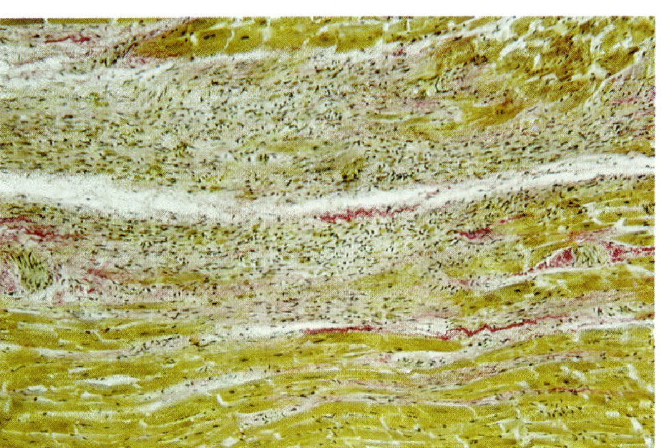

461 and **462 Heart.** A week-old myocardial infarction showing the formation of an immature cellular connective tissue. Note that the collagenous fibres in this tissue are fine and lightly staining in the van Gieson reaction. Some of the remaining myocardial cells show a marked hypertrophy (plump, rectangular nuclei). (*H&E ×100*)

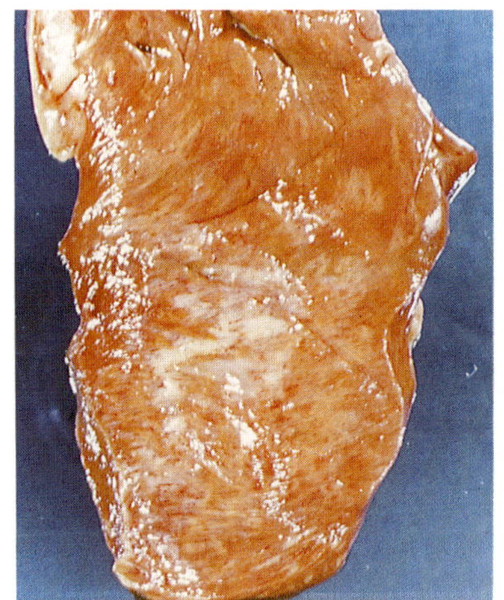

463 Extensive scar tissue in the posterior wall of the left ventricle.

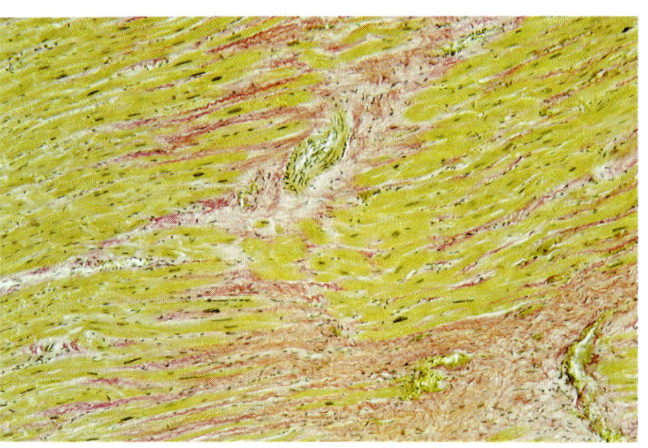

464 Heart. Several weeks old myocardial infarction with formation of a collagen-rich (red-staining fibres) connective tissue containing few cells — formation of scar tissue. Compare with **462**. (*van Gieson ×100*)

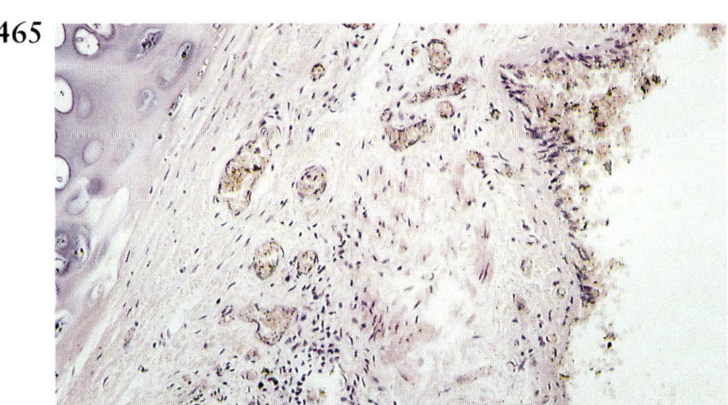

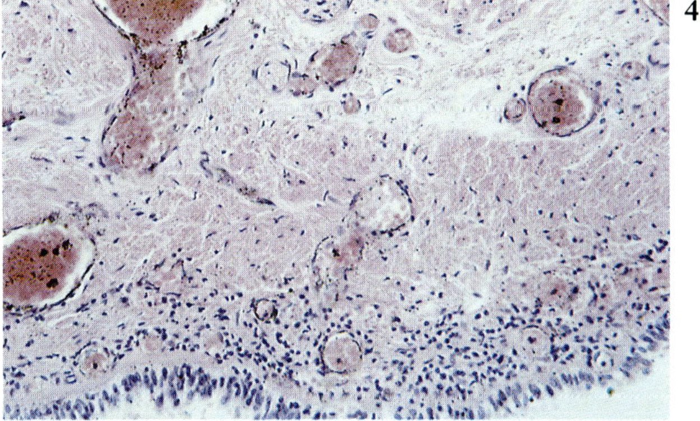

465 Trachea. Influenza-like infection (virus infection), with haemorrhagic deposits on the partially disrupted tracheal mucosa, submucosal oedema, mild cellular infiltration (lymphocytes, occasional plasma cells) and hyperaemia of the submucosa. The black pigment is formalin pigment, an artefact of routine processing. (*H&E ×250*)

466 Trachea. As in **465**. Virus infection with marked dilatation and hyperaemia of the submucosal blood vessels, as well as a minimal chronic inflammatory reaction. (*H&E ×250*)

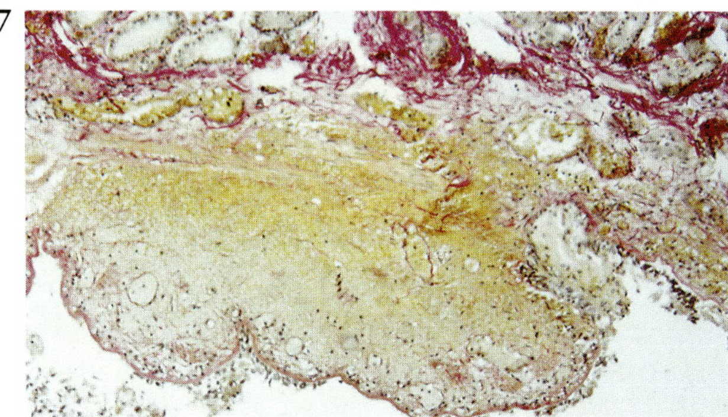

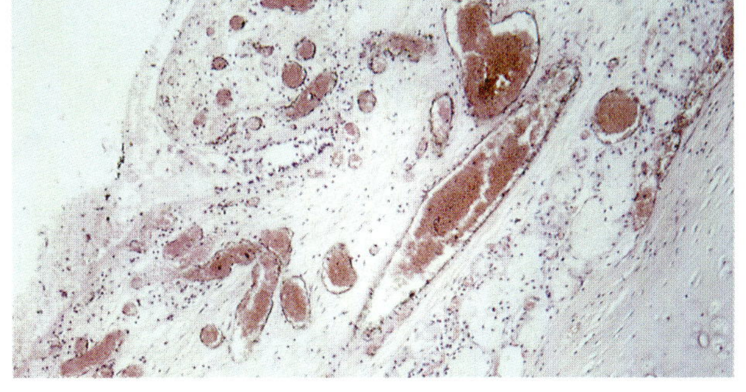

467 Trachea. Haemorrhagic tracheitis as a result of a viral infection. Its features are hyperaemia and dilatation of the blood vessels, oedema and submucosal haemorrhage. (*van Gieson ×100*)

468 Trachea. As in **467**, showing the extent of the submucosal hyperaemia and oedema. (*H&E ×250*)

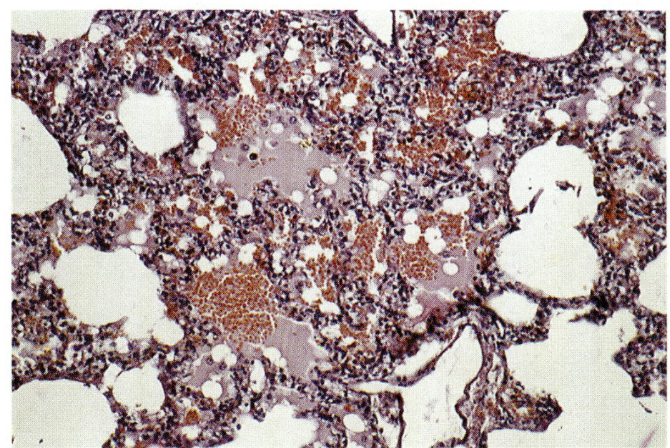

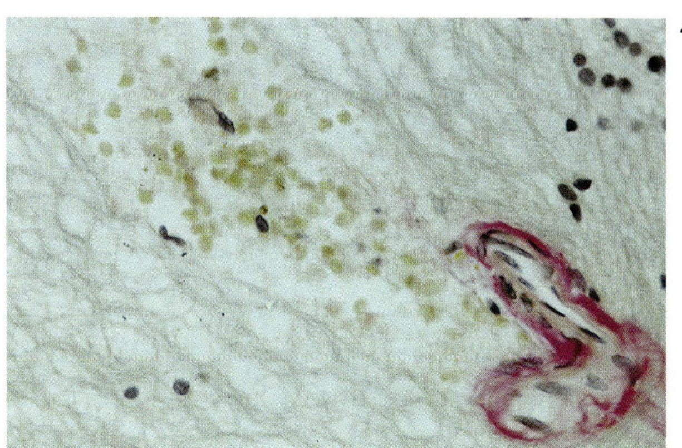

469 Lung. Acute viral infection in a 3 month-old female baby who died suddenly. Note the focal haemorrhagic oedema with over-expansion of neighbouring alveoli. (*H&E ×40*)

470 Brain. Virus infection, showing perivascular oedema and extravasation of erythrocytes. The 35 year-old male victim suffered mild trauma. (*van Gieson ×640*)

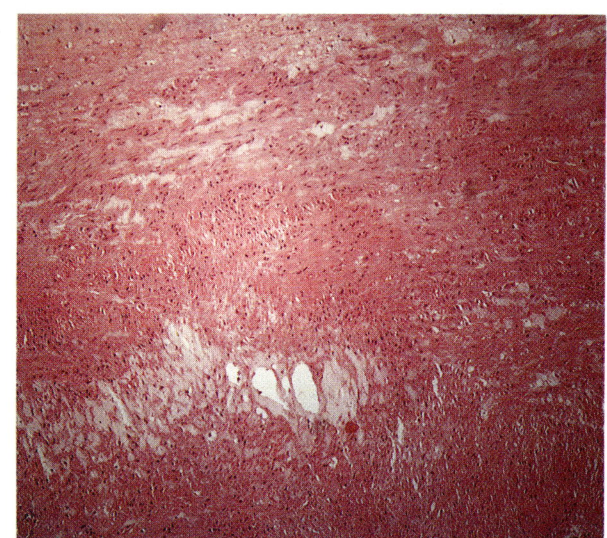

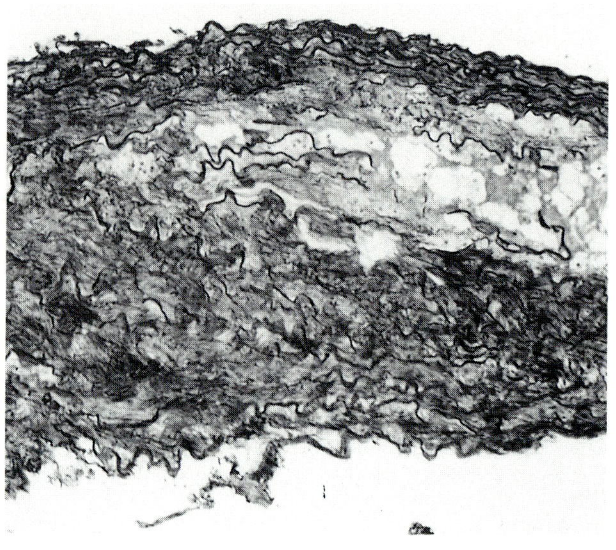

471 Thoracic aorta. Erdheim's cystic medionecrosis, showing oedema of the aortic wall and small areas of cystic change with haemorrhage. Cause of death in the 21 year-old male was haemorrhagic shock following aortic rupture. (*H&E ×250*)

472 Thoracic aorta. Note the areas in the aortic wall with destruction of elastic fibres, mucoid cystic change and oedema. Shows loosening and destruction of elastic fibres. (*Resorcin–fuchsin ×250*)

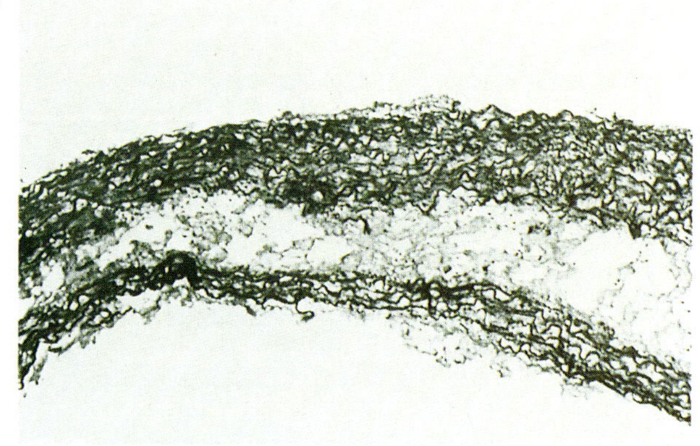

473 Same case as in **472**. Start of aneurysm formation (aortic dissection).

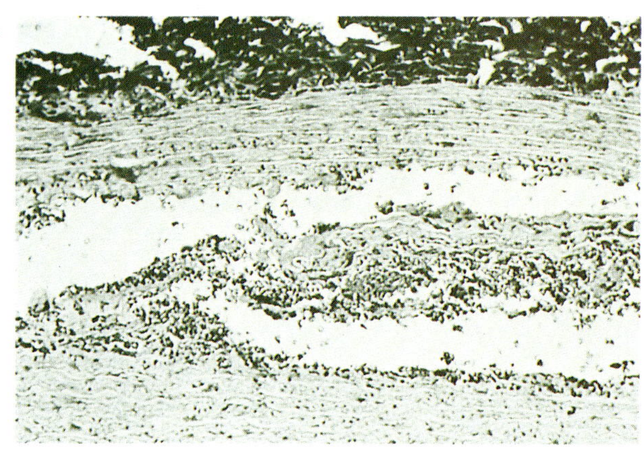

474 Same case as in **472**. Marked aortic dissection.

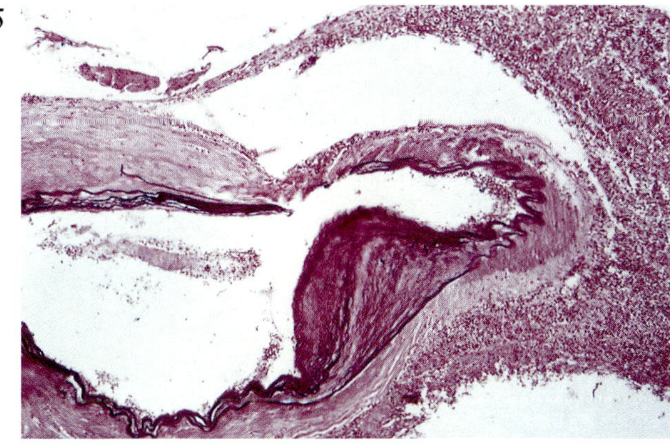

475 Brain. Aneurysm of the anterior cerebral artery in a 41 year-old female. The variation in thickness of the arterial wall is an important feature. (*Elastic stain ×12*)

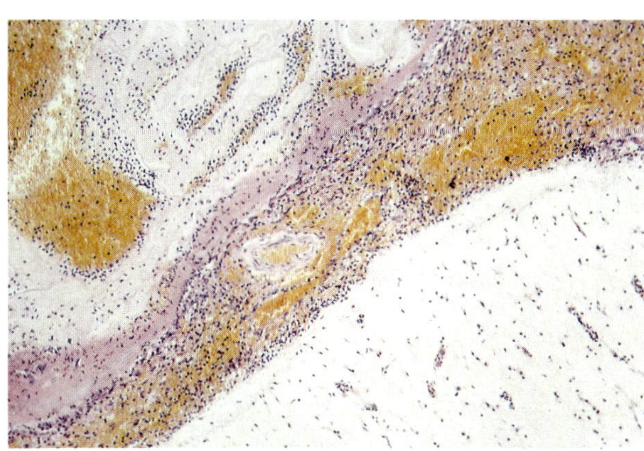

476 Brain. Massive subarachnoid haemorrhage following rupture of a cerebral arterial aneurysm. (*H&E ×100*)

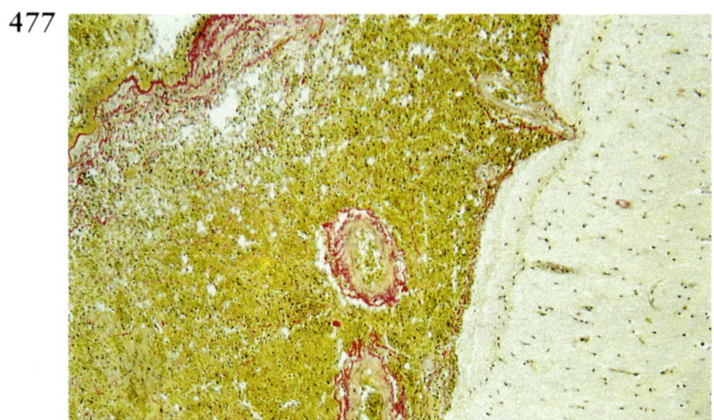

477 Same case as in **476**, showing that the haemorrhage is beneath the arachnoid mater (upper left). (*van Gieson ×100*)

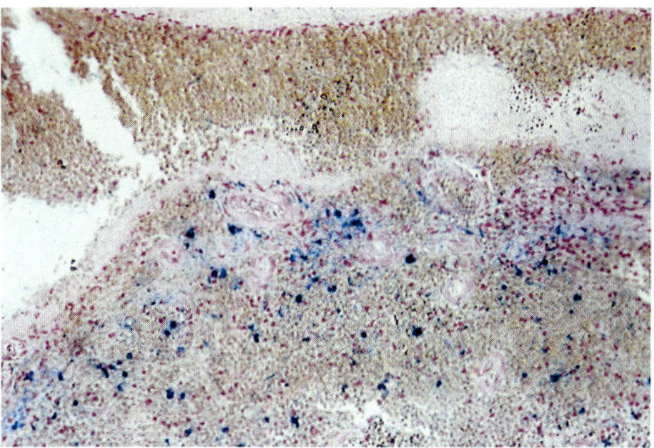

478 Brain. Evidence of previous haemorrhage (blue-staining iron pigment) and recent haemorrhage around the wall of a cerebral arterial aneurysm. The autopsy was necessary to establish that the patient had died from a cerebral areurysm and not from the mild trauma suffered some days prior to death. (*Prussian blue ×200*)

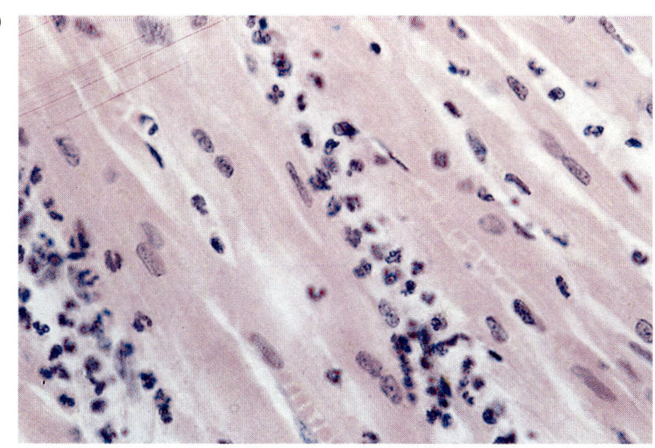

479 Heart. Purulent myocarditis as cause of death in a 10 year-old girl who died suddenly. As foul play was suspected, an autopsy was performed which revealed that death was not caused by trauma. (*H&E ×640*)

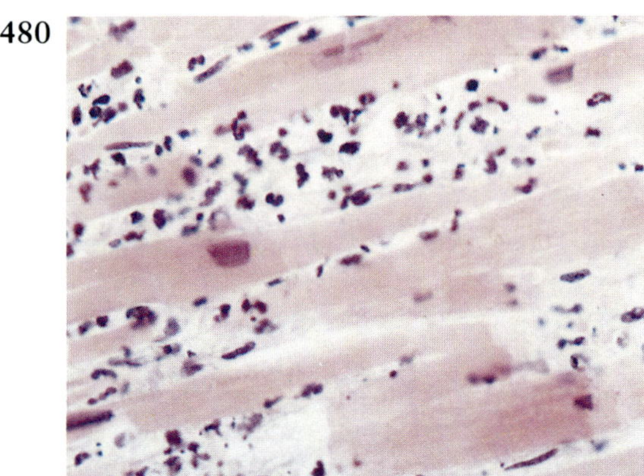

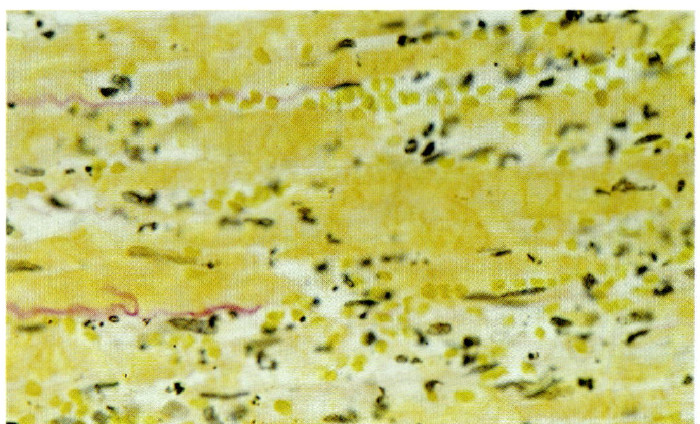

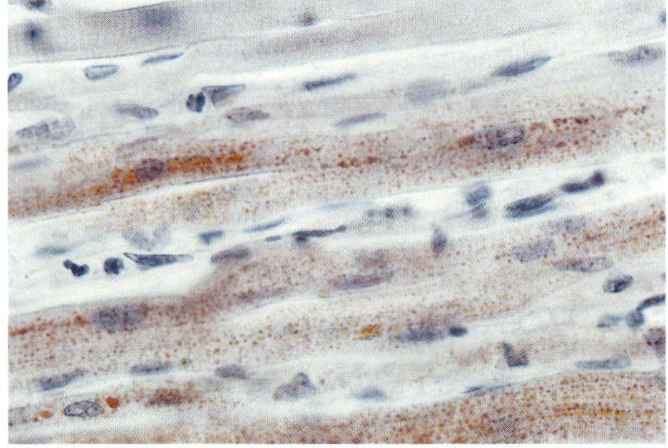

480–482 Heart. Purulent myocarditis in a 27 year-old male who died 3 days after a sudden collapse. The van Gieson stain shows the heterogeneous staining of the myocardiocytes, which is evidence of metabolic changes in these cells. The Sudan stain provides further evidence of metabolic disturbance, with formation of fine droplets of intracellular lipid. (*H&E, van Gieson, Sudan stain ×640*)

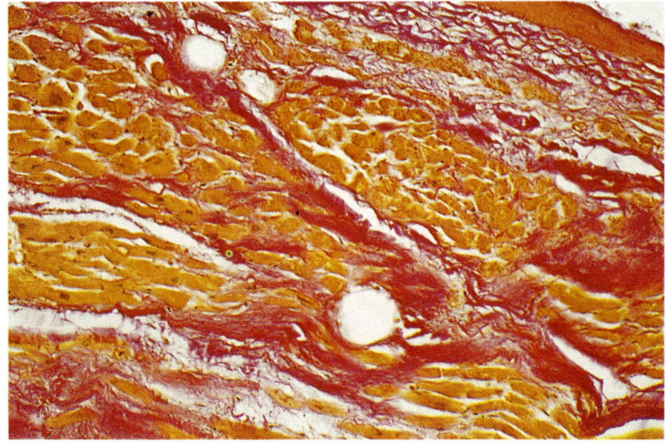

483 Heart. Fine fatty change in myocardiocytes (?toxic or hypoxic origin). The cross-striation pattern is maintained in certain cells. Staining for lipids is an important investigation in cases of sudden death with no apparent cause. (*Sudan stain ×640*)

484 Heart. Fibrotic scars in the region of the cardiac conducting system (Bundle of His) in a 59 year-old man who died suddenly. Arrhythmias and extrasystoles were known from the patient's history. Note the bundles of collagen fibres (red) forming the scar tissue. (*van Gieson ×100*)

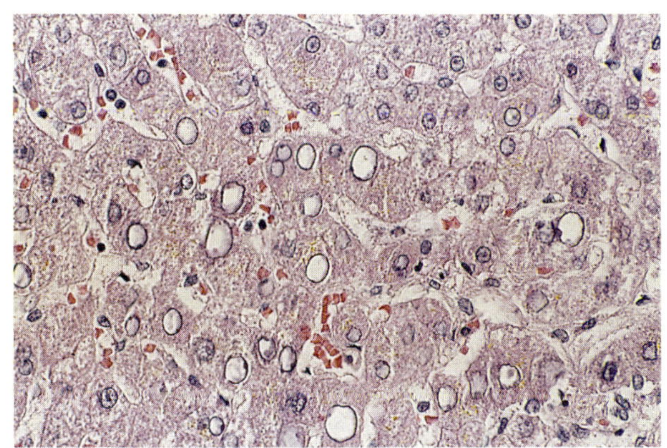 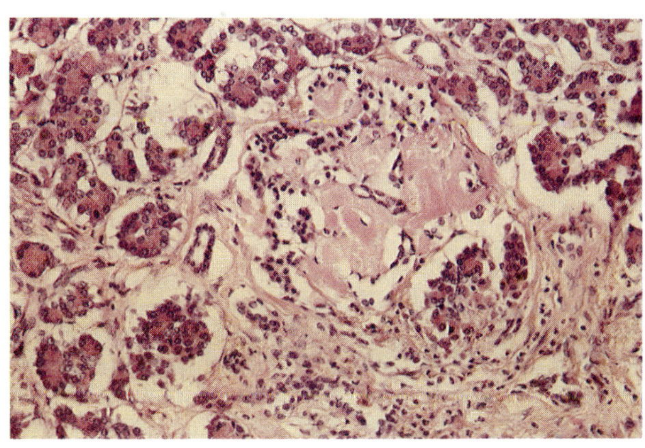

485 **Liver** from a case of diabetes mellitus, showing massive nuclear glycogenation of the hepatocytes, giving the appearance of 'holes' in the nuclei. (*H&E ×40*)

486 **Pancreas** from a case of diabetes mellitus, with extensive sclerosis of the islets of Langerhans. This sclerosis takes the form of a fibrosis of the islets. (*H&E ×100*)

16 Trauma and subsequent manifestations

Trauma may evoke a great variety of tissue changes, which are of major importance in establishing a possible causal link between injury and subsequent disease. Such considerations are vital in the formulation of expert reports. A few examples of such changes will be given.

Following traumatic lesions in muscle the latter may undergo an ossification process – *myositis ossificans*. In some cases this bone formation within the muscle tissue may be so extensive that a tentative diagnosis of osteogenic sarcoma is occasionally made. This metaplastic process involves fibroblasts and osteoblasts which can produce an osteoid, and sometimes a cartilage matrix. Areas of mature bone may also be seen. In differentiating sarcomas and *myositis ossificans*, it should be noted that, in the latter, numerous proliferating cells with visible mitosis are seen in the centre of the lesion, while in the periphery a maturation process occurs with formation of osteoid and bony tissue.

Infection in a wound is often accompanied by a *thrombophlebitis*, in which an acute inflammatory cell infiltration of the vein wall may be seen. The latter is often responsible for thrombosis in the affected vein.

The *suture granuloma* represents a further manifestation of trauma and is caused by a foreign-body reaction to suture material used in the surgical treatment of wounds. This occurs particularly around nonresorbable material. Of differential diagnostic importance is the exclusion of other granulomatous disease processes, in particular sarcoidosis or tuberculosis.

Manifestations of trauma may also be seen in the *adrenal glands*. Under the stimulatory action of ACTH, the lipid-rich spongiocytic cells of the zona fasciculata of the adrenal cortex lose their lipid. This occurs as part of the stress reaction. The adrenal cortex then consists of compact cells typical of the zona reticularis. In severe cases of trauma areas of adrenal cortical necrosis with or without haemorrhage may be encountered.

Serum hepatitis is an 'iatrogenic manifestation' of trauma and usually arises in patients requiring blood transfusion or haemodialysis as a result of severe trauma. The spectrum of pathological changes in the liver is broad, depending on the clinical course and severity of the infection. However, basically, necrosis of hepatocytes and an intense periportal infiltration by histiocytes, lymphocytes and plasma cells are to be seen.

Also within the scope of the stress reaction is the so-called *stress ulcer* of the stomach or duodenum. Erosion of a blood vessel may lead to profuse haemorrhage or alternatively a deeply penetrating ulcer may perforate and cause peritonitis.

487 Marked myositis ossificans around a healed fracture (7 years previously) of the femur. Macerated specimen.

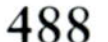

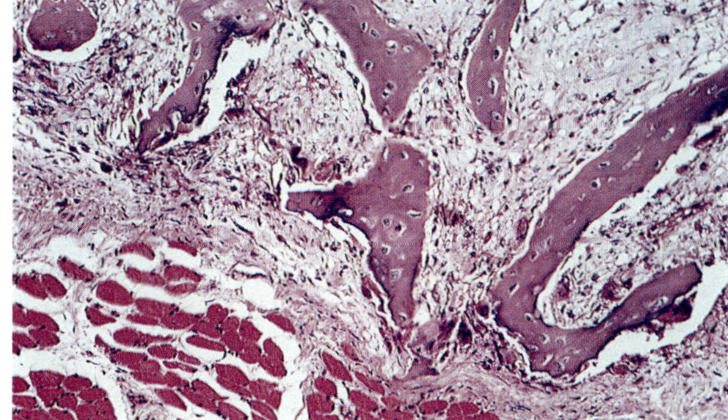

488 Muscle (thigh). Myositis ossificans. The patient suffered a fracture of the femur 18 days previously. A connective tissue with variable cellularity can be seen at the periphery of the muscle, along with newly formed bone lamellae containing osteoblasts. (*H&E ×160*)

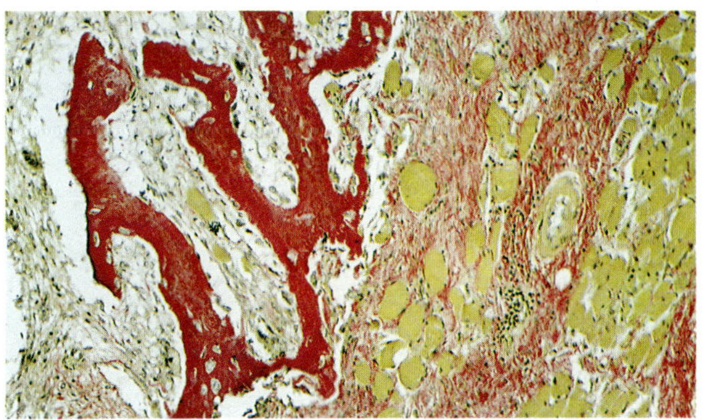

489 As in **488**, showing the typical appearance of bone (dark red) with the van Gieson stain (*×160*)

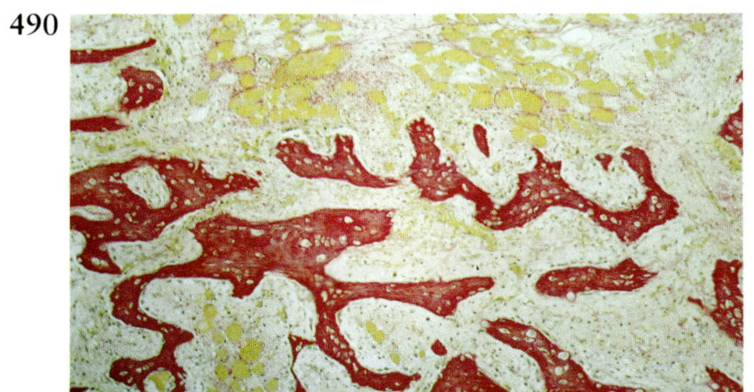

490 Muscle from a further case of myositis ossificans. Muscle fibres (yellow–green) can be seen interspersed between the areas of newly formed bone. (*van Gieson ×160*)

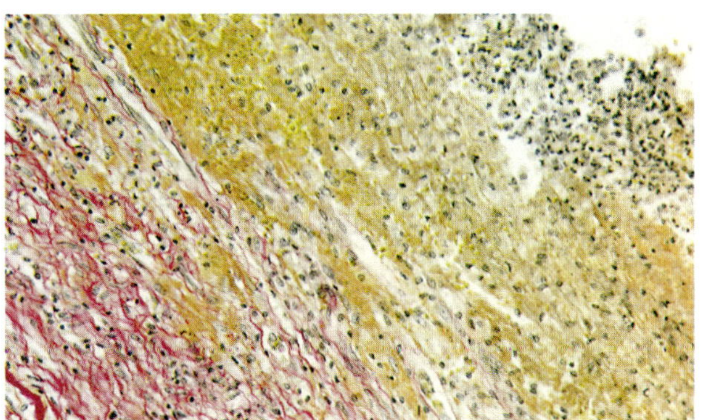

491 Femoral vein. Thrombophlebitis, with inflammatory cell infiltration of the vein wall (left), and deposition of thrombotic material on the intima (yellow–brown) and accumulation of polymorphonuclear granulocytes (upper right). (*van Gieson ×100*)

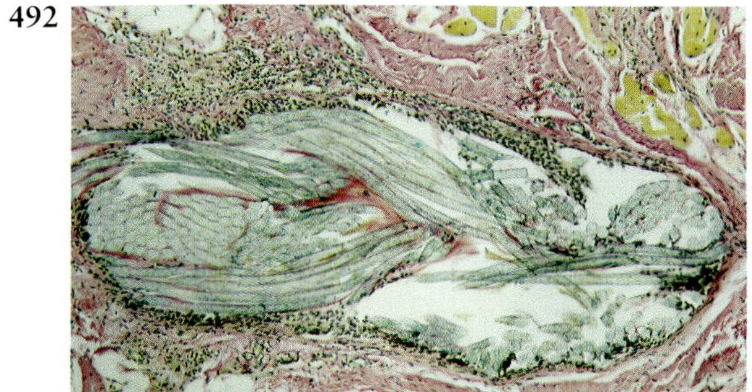

492 Suture granuloma. Suture material is present, surrounded by connective tissue of variable cell density. Material from an old operative scar. (*van Gieson ×100*)

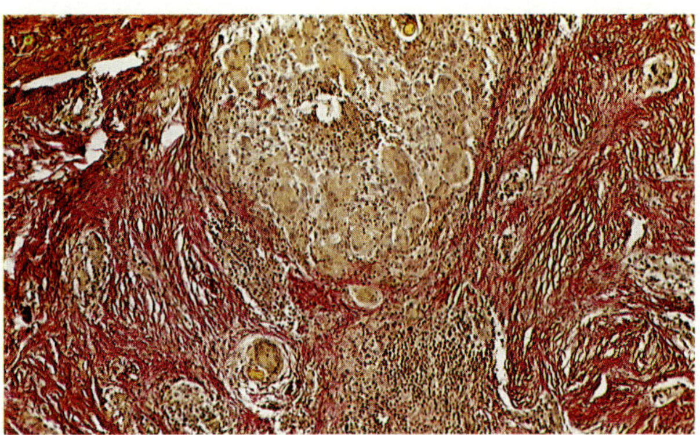

493 Skin (finger). 'Sarcoid-like' foreign-body reaction, with only small amounts of foreign material. Nevertheless, the cellular reaction is marked, with foreign-body giant cells present. In such cases, serial sectioning and polarisation microscopy are recommended in order to demonstrate the presence of the foreign material. (*van Gieson ×100*)

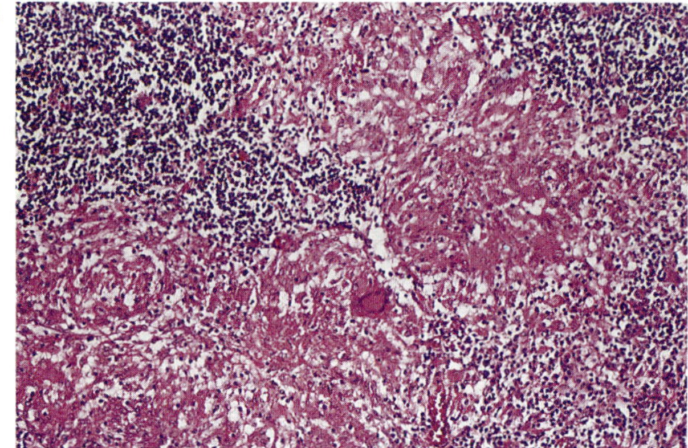

494 Lymph node showing one of the important processes in the differential diagnosis of suture granuloma, namely tuberculosis. The picture shows a small area of caseous necrosis and a cellular infiltration consisting of lymphocytes, epithelioid cells and giant cells. (*H&E ×100*)

495 Same case as in **493**, showing clearly the structure of the epithelioid cells and giant cells. (*van Gieson ×100*)

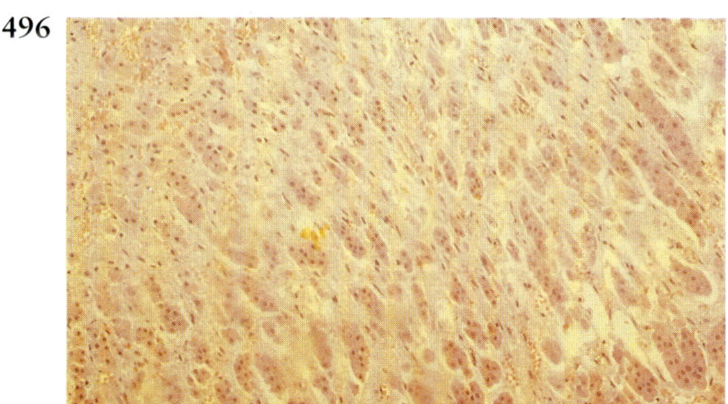

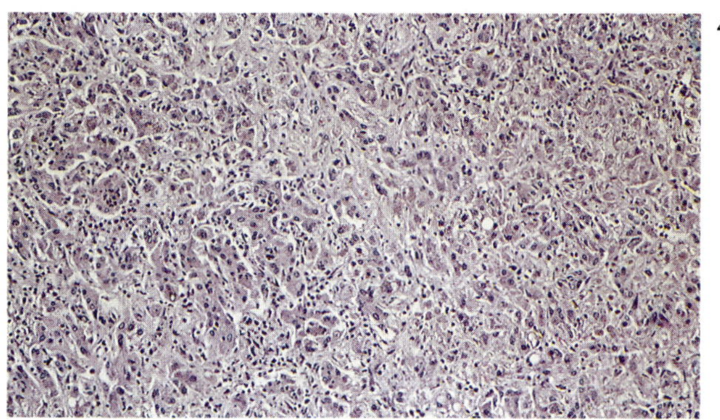

496 Adrenal gland. Material from a 40 year-old male who died 10 days after severe polytrauma. Note the presence of necrotic cortical cells without any cellular infiltration. The cells of the zona fasciculata have been depleted of their lipid content. (*H&E ×60*)

497 Liver. Material from a 67 year-old female who was knocked down in a road traffic accident. Her injuries required treatment by blood tranfusion. Ten weeks later she developed serum hepatitis (hepatitis B), which manifested itself as a severe subacute yellow dystrophy of the liver. The picture shows confluent areas of hepatocyte necrosis. (*H&E ×60*)

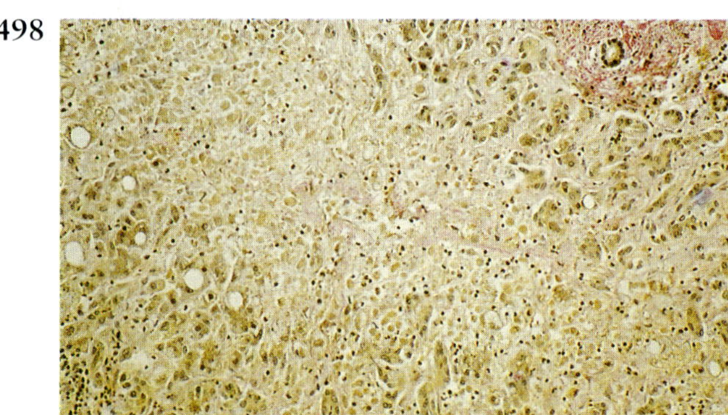

498 Liver. Same case as in **497**, showing the hepatocyte necrosis as well as fine fibres of collagenous tissue (red). (*van Gieson ×60*)

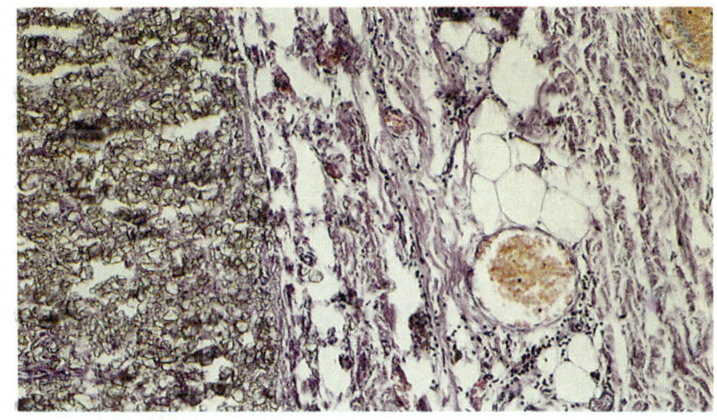

499   Liver capsule/diaphragm. Same case as in **497**. In addition to serum hepatitis, the patient developed a stress ulcer of the duodenum. This became evident during a barium swallow examination. Note the barium sulphate deposits (greyish brown globular material) in granulation tissue from the neighbourhood of the perforated ulcer. (*H&E ×250*)

500   Diaphragm. Same case as **497**, showing the barium sulphate deposits (blackish material, particularly left) on the abdominal aspect of the diaphragm. (*H&E ×250*)

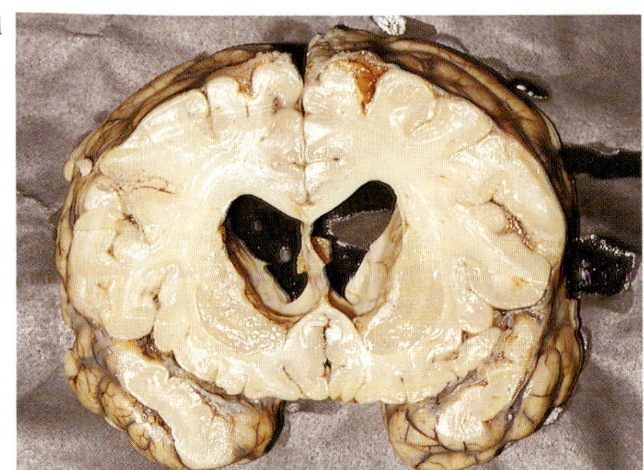

501   Cerebrum from a case of decerebration — decerebrate rigidity. Marked dilatation of the ventricles as a result of widespread damage to the white matter, with oedema, proliferation of microglial cells and small areas of necrosis. Material from a 21 year-old man who suffered blunt head injuries in a motorcycle accident. Survival time: 5 months.

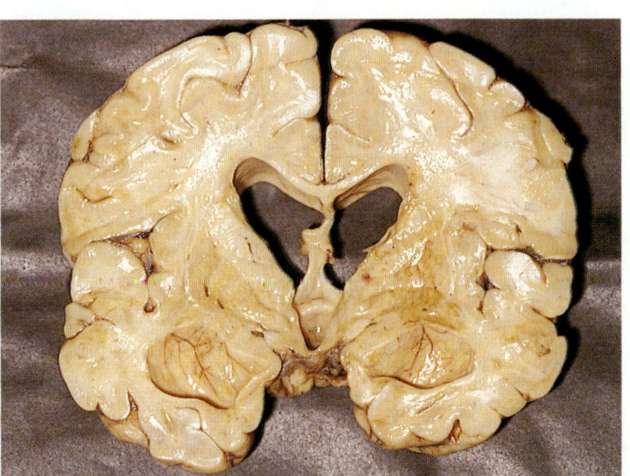

502   Further coronal section of the brain (previous case) showing dilatation of the third ventricle and the lateral horns. Decerebrate rigidity involves severe damage to the brain stem, usually caudal to the red nucleus.

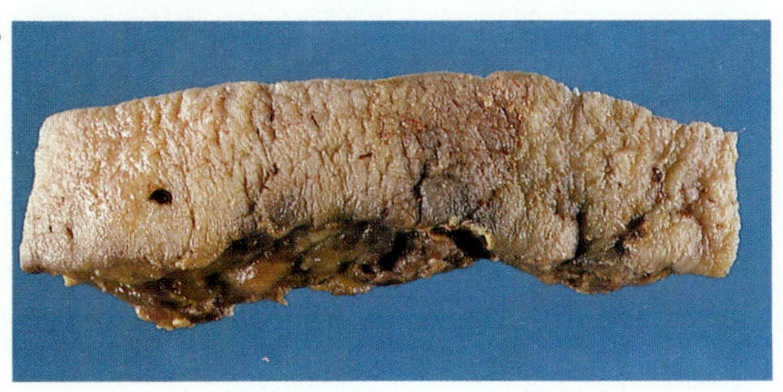

503   Skin and subcutaneous tissue of the thigh from a case of wound infection following amputation. Greyish red discolouration of skin and periphery of the amputation. (*Formalin-fixed tissue*)

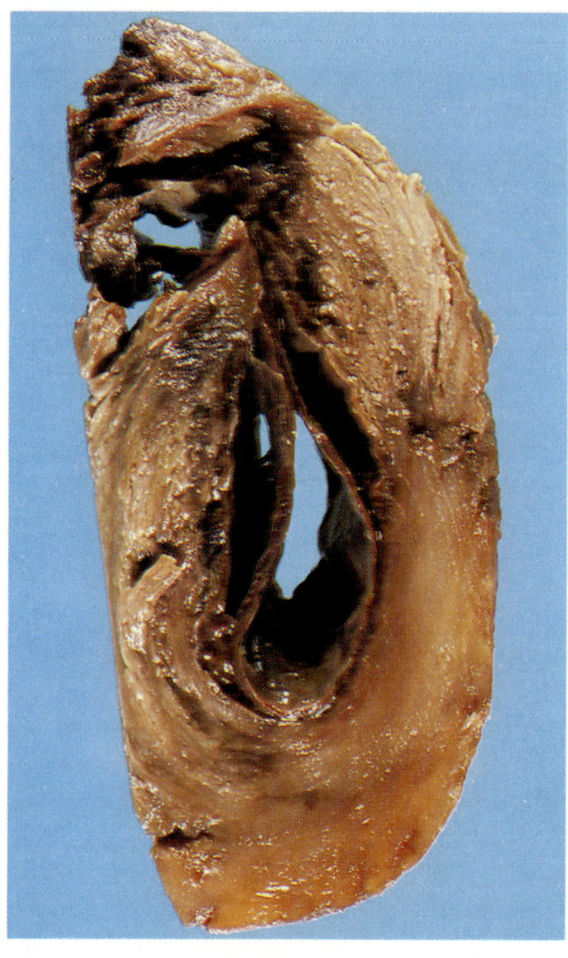

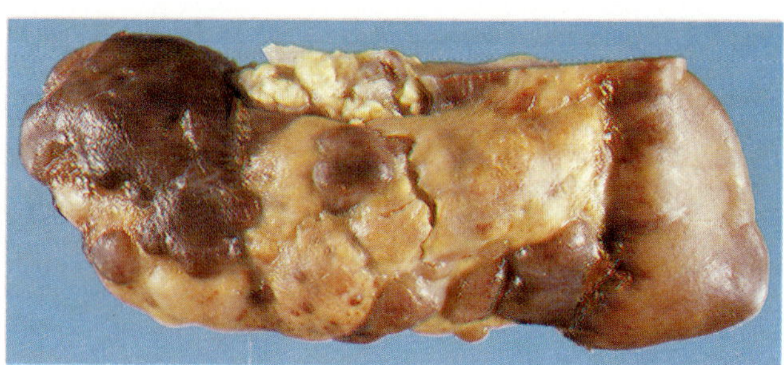

505 Kidney with an extensive healed infarct following severe blunt injury many months before death. The non-functioning kidney was removed at operation. (*Formalin-fixed tissue*)

504 Wound cavity with a partially encapsulated hae-matoma (removed) caused by a penetrating thigh injury some weeks before death. (*Formalin-fixed tissue*)

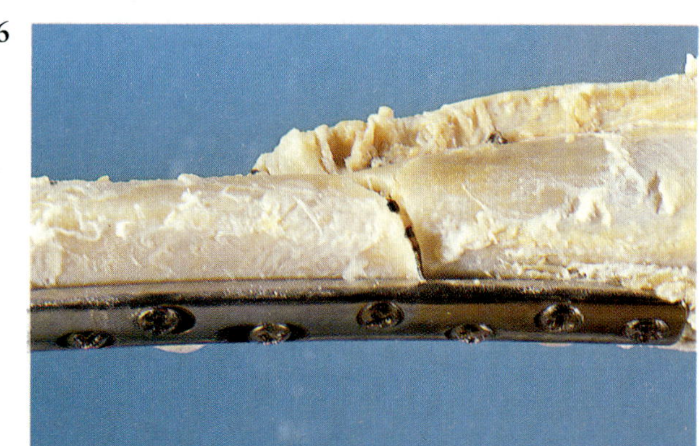

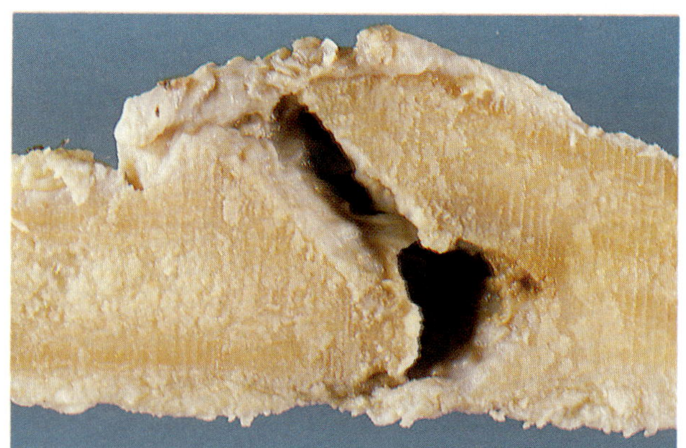

506 Ulnar fracture treated with screws.

507 Pseudoarthrosis of the ulna. This failure of union of the fracture is often associated with movement at the fracture site. (*Formalin-fixed material*)

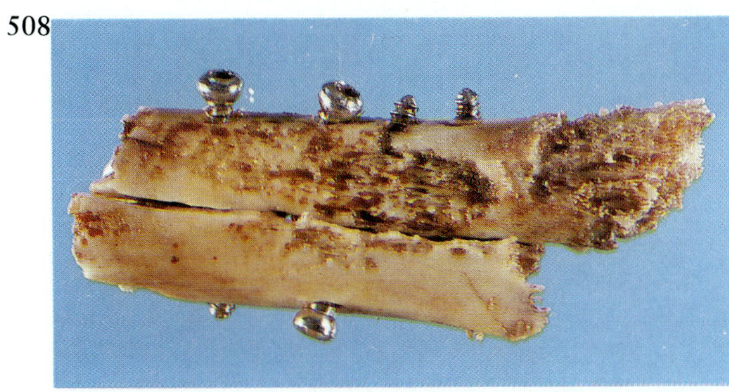

508   **Screw osteosynthesis** of a comminuted fracture of the humerus with subsequent osteomyelitis.

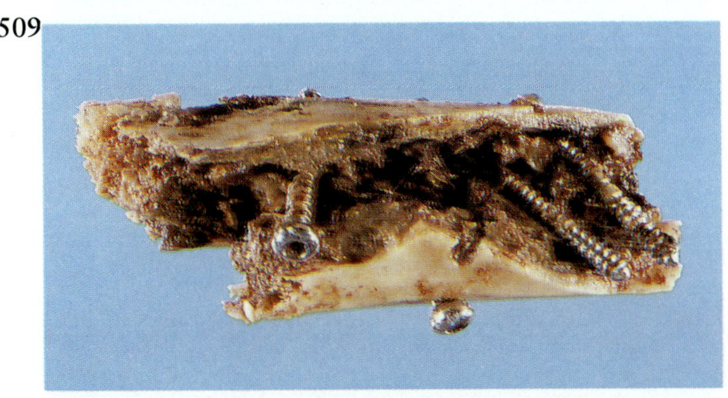

509   Same case as in 508. View of the marrow cavity, showing necrosis of bony tissue with haemorrhage.

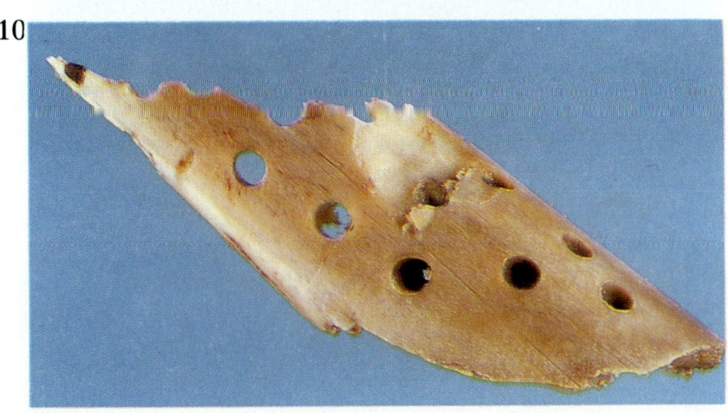

510   Same case as in 508. Bone sequester with numerous drilled holes. Histologically, such sequester shows necrotic bone with loss of osteoblasts, giving empty lacunae.

References

Adelson, L. *The Pathology of Homicide*. Thomas, Springfield, 1974.

Ahvenainen, E.K. On changes in dilatation and signs of aspiration in fetal and neonatal lungs. An experimental and histological study. *Acta Paediatrica*, **35**, Suppl. III, 1948.

Arena, J.M. *Poisoning Toxicology, Symptoms, Treatments*, 4th edn. Thomas, 1979.

Aufdermaur, U. Die Bedeutung der histologischen Untersuchung des Kniegelenkmeniskus. *Schweiz. med. Wschr.*, **101**, 1405–1412, 1441–1445, 1971.

Ballantyne, A. *Forensic Toxicology*. Wright–PSG, 1974.

Beneke, G. Altersbestimmung von Verletzungen innerer Organe. *Z. Rechtsmedizin*, **71**, 1–16, 1972.

Berg, St. Die Altersbestimmung von Hautverletzungen. *Z. Rechtsmedizin*, **70**, 121–135, 1972.

Berg, St. and Ebel, R. Altersbestimmung subkutaner Blutungen. *Münch. med. Wschr.*, **111**, 1185–1190, 1969.

Bohle, A. Pathologische Anatomie des akuten Nierenversagens. *Verh. dtsch. Ges. Path.*, **49**, 54–67, 1965.

Boltz, W. Histologische Untersuchungen an Injektionsstichspuren. *Dtsch. Z. ges. ger. Med.*, **40**, 181–191, 1951.

Brinkhous, K.M. *Accident Pathology. Proceedings of an International Conference*. Sheraton–Park Hotel, Washington, D.C. June 6–8, U.S. Government Printing Office, Washington, D.C., 1968.

Brown, D.L. Wetli, C.V. and Davis, J.H. Sudden unexpected death from primary pulmonary hypertension. *J. Forensic Sciences*, **26**, 381–386, 1981.

Brun, Cl. and Munck, O. Acute renal failure. In Mostofi, F.K. and Smith C.E., *The Kidney*. International Academy of Pathology Monographs Nr. 6, p 82–94. Williams and Wilkins, Baltimore, 1966.

Burck, H.Ch. Häufigkeit und Bedeutung der klinischen und patho-anatomischen Diagnose eines akuten Nierenversagens bei 1000 verstorbenen und obduzierten Kranken. *Med. Klinik*, **64**, 21–30, 1969.

Burck, H. Ch. Das akute Nierenversagen. II. Morphologie; diagnostik 3, Heft 12, 1970.

Casarett, G.W. *Radiation Histopathology*, 2 Vols, CRC Press, Boca Raton, Florida, 1980.

Chapman, A.J. and White, C. Death resulting from lacrimatory agents. Case report. *J. Forensic Sciences*, **23**, 527–530, 1978.

Clarke, R.A. and Henson, P.M. (Eds) *The Molecular and Cellular Biology of Wound Repair*. Plenum Press, 1988.

Cottone, J.A. and Standish, S.M. *Outline of Forensic Dentistry*. Year Book Medical Publishers, Chicago, 1982.

Courville, C.B. Contrecoup injuries of the brain in infancy. *Arch. Surg.*, **90**, 157–165, 1965.

Durigon, M., Campana, J.P., Eliakis, E. and Dérobert, L. Lésions pulmonaires observées chez les victimes d'une catastrophe aerienne. *J. Forensic Sciences*, **6**, 153–163, 1975.

Fatteh, A. *Medicolegal Investigation of Gunshot Wounds*. Lippincott, 1976.

Ferris, J.A. and Friesen, J.M. Definitions of ischaemia, infarction and necrosis. *Forensic Sciences International*, **13**, 253–259, 1979.

Fischer, H. Über das morphologische Bild der Abheilung von Kalottenfraktion des Schädels. *Acta Neurochirurgica*, **19**, 171–182, 1968.

Fischer, H. Das Stress-Ulcus, eine Gefahr für den Unfallverletzten. *Mschr. Unfallheilk.*, **75**, 124–130, 1972.

Fischer, H. Zur pathologischen Anatomie des akuten Nierenversagens, (Literaturübersicht). *Akt. Traumatologie*, **2**, 141–144, 1972.

Fischer, H. Verletzungen des Schädelskelets und ihre Ausheilung. In Burkhardt, L. and Fischer, Pathologische Anatomie des Schädels in seiner Beziehung zum Inhalt; Spezielle Pathologie des Schädelskelets. *Handbuch der speziellen pathologischen Anatomie und Histologie*, 9 Band, 7 Teil, Springer, Berlin, 1970.

Fischer, H. and Spann, W. *Pathologie des Trauma*. Bergmann, München, 1967.

Förster, A. and Goldbach, H.J. Der heutige Stand der histologischen Lungenprobe unter besonderer Berücksichtigung der elastischen Faserfärbung. *Dtsch. Z. ges. ger. Med.*, **45**, 386–393, 1956.

Froede, R.G., Lindsey, D. and Steinbronn, K. Sudden unexpected death from cardiac concussion (commotio cordis) with unusual legal complications. *J. Forensic Sciences*, **24**, 752–756, 1979.

Gerlach, D. Post-mortem investigations of fatal cases of narcotic addiction. *Forensic Science International*, **15**, 31–39, 1980.

Gössner, W. Grundlagen und allgemeine pathologische Anatomie der Strahlenschäden. *Verhandl. d. Dtsch. Ges. Path.*, **56**, 168, 1972.

Grant, W.M. *Toxicology of the Eye*, 2nd edn, Thomas, Springfield, 1974.

Gresham, G.A. *Colour Atlas of Wounds and Wounding*. Kluwer Academic, 1986.

Gresham, G.A. *Color Atlas of Forensic Pathology*. Year Book Medical Publishers, Chicago, 1975.

Gresham, G.A. and Turner, A.F. *Post-Mortem Procedures*. Year Book Medical Publishers, 1979.

Gromov, A.P. and Naumenko, W.G. *Gerichtsmedizinische Traumatologie* (Taschenbuch) (Russian). Meditsina, Moskva, 1977.

Gruber, R.T. *et al. The Pathophysiology of Combined Injury and Trauma*. Academic Press, 1987.

Gurdjian, E.S., Lange, W.A., Patrick, L.M. and Thomas, L.M. *Impact Injury and Crash Protection*. Thomas, Springfield, 1970.

Hackett, C.J. Microscopical focal destruction (tunnels) in exhumed human bones. *Med. Sci. Law*, **21**, 243–265, 1981.

Hadenque, A., Durigon, M., Haertig, A. and Boudène, C. Aspects histologiques des voies respiratoires au cours d'incendies. *Méd. lég. Toxicol.*, **23**, 327–333, 1980.

Harris, R. *Outline of Death Investigation.* Thomas, Springfield, 1973.

Hunt, A.C. Traumatic uraemia. In *Pathology of Injury.* The Report of a Working Party of the Royal College of Pathologists. Harvey Miller and Med Calf Ltd, London, 1972.

Jackson, R.H. The epidemiology of accidents in Europe and the role of health services in prevention, 4 November 1981.

Janssen, W. *Forensische Histologie.* Schmidt–Römhild, Lübeck, 1977.

Janssen, W., Jaecker, O. and Erbach, A. Zur Unterscheidung von Druck und Stauungsblutungen in den Halsweichteilen. *Dtsch. Z. ges. ger. Med.*, **64**, 147–157.

Kanschina, N.F. Pathologische Anatomie der akuten Niereninsuffizienz (Russian). *Arch. Path.*, **32**, 3–15, 1970.

Klein, H. Mikroskopische Beobachtungen an Würgemalen. *Dtsch. Z. ges. ger. Med.*, **45**, 17–20, 1956.

Klein, H. Die gerichtsmedizinische Diagnose des Stromtodes. *Dtsch. Z. ges. ger. Med.*, **47**, 29–54, 1958.

Könn, G. and Meiser, S. Zur morphologischen Pathologie traumatischer Nierenverletzungen und ihrer Spätfolgen. *Beit. path. Anat.*, **137**, 350–372, 1968.

Krauland, W. Über die Zeitbestimmung von Schädelhin verletzungen. *Beitr. Gerichtl. Med.*, **30**, 226–251, 1973.

Krogman, W.M. *Human Skeleton in Forensic Medicine.* Thomas, Springfield, 1978.

Labowitz, D.I., Menzies, R.C. and Scroggie, R.J. Characteristics and wounding effects of a black powder handgun. *J. Forensic Sciences*, **26**, 288–301, 1981.

Lesoine, W. Schwere Oesophagusverätzungen mit Todesfolge. *Med. Klinik*, **60**, 2139–2141, 1965.

Macgregor, A.R. *Pathology of Infancy and Childhood.* Longstone Ltd., Edinburgh, 1960.

Malamud, N., Haymaker, W. and Custer, R.P. Heat stroke: a clinico-pathologic study of 125 fatal cases. *Milit. Surg.*, **99**, 397–449, 1946.

Mason, J.K. *The Pathology of Violent Injury.* Arnold, London, 1978.

McLaughlin, H.L. *Trauma.* W.B. Saunders and Co., Philadelphia, 1959.

Menzies, R.C., Scroggie, R.J. and Labowitz, D.I. Characteristics of silenced firearms and their wounding effects. *J. Forensic Sciences*, **26**, 239–262, 1981.

Minckler, J. *Pathology of the Nervous System, Volume Two.* McGraw-Hill, New York, 1971.

Mohr, H.J. Leitsymptom: Das akute Nierenversagen. Pathologische Anatomie. *Dtsch. med. J.*, **11**, 261–266, 1960.

Moragas, A., Ballabriga, A. and Vidal, M.T. *Atlas der Histopathologie des Neugeborenen*, Thieme, Stuttgart, 1976.

Morison, J.E. *Foetal and Neonatal Pathology.* Butterworths, London, 1970.

Moritz, A.R. *The Pathology of Trauma.* Lea-Febiger, Philadelphia, 1954.

Noren, G.R., Stanley, N.A., Bandt, C.M. and Kaplan, E.L. Occurrence of myocarditis in sudden death in children. *J. Forensic Sciences*, **22**, 188–196, 1977.

Oksala, A. and Salminen, L. Eye injuries caused by tear gas handweapons. *Acta Ophthal.*, **53**, 908, 1975.

Orsós, F. Die vitalen Reaktionen und ihre gerichtsmedizinische Bedeutung. *Beitr. path. Anat. allg. Path.*, **95**, 163, 1935.

Owen-Smith, M.S. *High Velocity Missile Wounds.* Arnold, London, 1981.

Paparo, G.P. and Siegel, H. Histologic diagnosis of sodomy. *J. Forensic Sciences*, **24**, 772–774, 1979.

Parmley, L.F., Manion, W.C. and Mattingly, T.W. Nonpenetrating traumatic injury of the heart. *Circulation*, **18**, 371, 1958.

Peacock, E.E. *Wound Repair*, 3rd edn. Saunders, 1984.

Perper, J.A. and Wecht, C.H. *Microscopic Diagnosis in Forensic Pathology.* Thomas, Springfield, 1980.

Peters, G: Klinische Neuropathologie, 2. Aufl. Thieme, Stuttgart, 1970.

Pierson, K.K. *Principles of Prosecution. A Guide for the Anatomic Pathologist.* Wiley Medical, 1974.

Pisano, R.V., Taylor, M.B. and Sopher, I.M. Dissecting coronary artery aneurysm: a report of two cases. *J. Forensic Sciences*, **24**, 18–25, 1979.

Potanina, M.N. Einige Besonderheiten der Regeneration von Schädelknochen. 1. Mitteilung: Die Knochen des Schädeldaches. *Ref. Die Medizin der Sowjetunion*, 7, 1375, 1960.

Potter, E.L. *Pathology of the Fetus and Infant.* Year Book Second Edition, Chicago, 1962.

Proudfoot, A.T. *Diagnosis and Management of Acute Poisoning.* Mosby, Chicago, 1982.

Raasch, F.O. Hirvonen, J.I. and Stahl, C.J. Timing of injuries in human thermal burns. *J. Forensic Sciences*, **19**, 723–729, 1974.

Rajs, J. Left ventricular subendocardial haemorrhages. A study of their morphology, pathogenesis and prognosis. *Forensic Science International*, **10**, 87–103, 1977.

Rajs, J. and Jakobsson, S. Severe trauma and subsequent cardiac lesions causing heart failure and death. *Forensic Science International*, **8**, 13–21 (1976).

Remmele, W. Zur pathologischen Anatomie des Kreislaufschocks beim Menschen. III. Ansammlung von Blut- und Knochenmarkszellen in den Markgcfäßcn der Niere. *Klin. Wschr*, **46**, 803–809, 1968.

Remmele, W. and Gille, J. Zur pathologischen Anatomie des Kreislaufschocks beim Menschen. II. Renale Tubulusdilatation. *Klin. Wschr.*, **46**, 636–642, 1968.

Remmele, W., Gille, J. and Harms, D. Vergleichende Untersuchungen zur histologischen Schockdiagnostik beim Menschen. *Verh. dtsch. Ges. Pathologie*, **52**, 281–287 IC, 1968.

Remmele, W and Harms, D. Zur pathologischen Anatomie des Kreislaufschocks beim Menschen. I. Mikrothrombose der peripheren Blutgefäß. *Klin. Wschr.*, **46**, 352–357, 1968.

Remmele, W. and Loeper, H. Zur pathologischen Anatomie des Kreislaufschocks beim Menschen. IV. Pathomorphologie der Schockleber. *Klin. Wschr.*, **51**,

10–24, 1973.

Rubin, P. and Casarett, G.W. *Clinical Radiation pathology*, 2 Vols, Saunders, Philadelphia, 1968.

Sandritter, W. Pathologische Anatomie des Schocks. Inreversible Organschädigung durch Thromben. *Dtsch. Ärzteblatt*, **64**, 2061–2062, 1967.

Schnaars, P. Anatomische Lungenbefunde bei Neugeborenen nach Beatmung. *Helvetica Paediatrica Acta*, **20**, 197–215, 1965.

Schubert, G.E. Die pathologische Anatomie des akuten Nierenversagens. *Erg. allg. Path. path. Anat.*, **49**, 1–112, 1968.

Stein, A.A. and Kirwan, W.E. 'Chloracetophenone (tear gas) poisoning': a clinico-pathologic report. *J. Forensic Sciences*, **9**, 374–382, 1964.

Suzuki, T., Kashimura, S. and Umetsu, K. Sudden infant death syndrome: histological studies on adrenal gland and kidney. *Forensic Science International*, **15**, 41–46, 1980.

Teare, R.D. Poisoning by paraquat. *Med. Sci. Law*, **16**, 9–12, 1976.

Tedeschi, C.G. *Forensic Medicine*. Saunders, Philadelphia, 1977.

Thompson, A. and Luna, A.A. *An Atlas of Artefacts*. Thomas, Springfield, 1978.

Thurner, J. *Iatrogene Pathologie*. Urban u. Schwarzenberg, München, 1970.

Tillmann, B. and Engel, H. Klinische und pathologisch-anatomische Spätbefunde nach Wurzelausrissen des Armplexus. *Fortschr. Neurol.*, **42**, 28–37, 1974.

Unterharnscheidt, F.J. Die traumatischen Hirnschäden. Mechanogenese, Pathomorphologie und Klinik. *Z. Rechtsmedizin*, **71**, 153–221, 1972.

Vale, J.A. and Meredith, T.J. *Poisoning: Diagnosis & Treatment*. Kluver, Boston, 1980.

Walker, R.I. *et al. The Pathophysiology of Combined Injury and Trauma*. Aspen Pub. 1985.

Warren, S. Pathologic criteria of radiation injury. *J. Forensic Sciences*, **19**, 709–714, 1974.

Warren, S. Risk of cancer subsequent to low-dose radiation. *J. Forensic Sciences*, **25**, 721–776, 1980.

Watanabe, T., Imamura, T, Nakagaki, K. and Tanaka, K. Disseminated intravascular coagulation in autopsy cases. Its incidence and clinicopathologic significance. *Path. Res. Pract.*, **165**, 311–322, 1979.

Weber, D.L. *Autopsy Pathology, Procedure and Protocol*. Thomas, Springfield, 1973.

Wilson, E.F. Sperm's morphological survival after 16 days in the vagina of a dead body. *J. Forensic Sciences*, **19**, 561–564, 1974.

Winter, H. *Post Mortem Examination of Ruminants*. University of Queensland, Australia, 1978.

Winthrop, S.R., Clearly, P.E. and Minckler, D.S.; Penetrating eye injuries: a histopathological review. *Brit. J. Ophthal.*, **64**, 809–817, 1980.

Zollinger, H.V. *Radio-Histologie und Radio-Histopathologie. Handb. d. Allgem. Path.*, **10**, (1), 127, Springer, Berlin, 1960.

Zollinger, H.V. Die pathologische Anatomie der Niereninsuffizienz, *Wien klin. Wsch.*, **71**, 31, 1959.